Genetic and Epigenetic Regulations of Tumor Progression and Metastasis

Genetic and Epigenetic Regulations of Tumor Progression and Metastasis

Editors

Bozena Smolkova
Julie Earl
Agapi Kataki

MDPI • Basel • Beijing • Wuhan • Barcelona • Belgrade • Manchester • Tokyo • Cluj • Tianjin

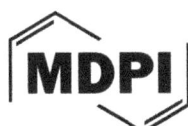

Editors

Bozena Smolkova
Department of Molecular
Oncology
Biomedical Research Center
of the Slovak Academy
of Sciences
Bratislava
Slovakia

Julie Earl
Molecular Epidemiology and
Predictive Markers in
Cancer Group
Ramón y Cajal Health
Research Institute (IRYCIS)
Madrid
Spain

Agapi Kataki
1st Department of
Propaedeutic Surgery
Hippocratio General Hospital
of Athens
Athens
Greece

Editorial Office
MDPI
St. Alban-Anlage 66
4052 Basel, Switzerland

This is a reprint of articles from the Special Issue published online in the open access journal *International Journal of Molecular Sciences* (ISSN 1422-0067) (available at: www.mdpi.com/journal/ijms/special_issues/Tumor_Genetics).

For citation purposes, cite each article independently as indicated on the article page online and as indicated below:

LastName, A.A.; LastName, B.B.; LastName, C.C. Article Title. *Journal Name* **Year**, *Volume Number*, Page Range.

ISBN 978-3-0365-7185-0 (Hbk)
ISBN 978-3-0365-7184-3 (PDF)

© 2023 by the authors. Articles in this book are Open Access and distributed under the Creative Commons Attribution (CC BY) license, which allows users to download, copy and build upon published articles, as long as the author and publisher are properly credited, which ensures maximum dissemination and a wider impact of our publications.

The book as a whole is distributed by MDPI under the terms and conditions of the Creative Commons license CC BY-NC-ND.

Contents

About the Editors vii

Preface to "Genetic and Epigenetic Regulations of Tumor Progression and Metastasis" ix

Bozena Smolkova, Julie Earl and Agapi Kataki
The Metastatic Process through the Eyes of Epigenetic Regulation: A Promising Horizon for Cancer Therapy
Reprinted from: *Int. J. Mol. Sci.* **2022**, 23, 15446, doi:10.3390/ijms232415446 1

Souvik Ghatak, Shakti Ranjan Satapathy and Anita Sjölander
DNA Methylation and Gene Expression of the Cysteinyl Leukotriene Receptors as a Prognostic and Metastatic Factor for Colorectal Cancer Patients
Reprinted from: *Int. J. Mol. Sci.* **2023**, 24, 3409, doi:10.3390/ijms24043409 5

Rania Faouzi Zaarour, Mohak Sharda, Bilal Azakir, Goutham Hassan Venkatesh, Raefa Abou Khouzam and Ayesha Rifath et al.
Genomic Analysis of Waterpipe Smoke-Induced Lung Tumor Autophagy and Plasticity
Reprinted from: *Int. J. Mol. Sci.* **2022**, 23, 6848, doi:10.3390/ijms23126848 27

Federica Ruscitto, Niccolò Roda, Chiara Priami, Enrica Migliaccio and Pier Giuseppe Pelicci
Beyond Genetics: Metastasis as an Adaptive Response in Breast Cancer
Reprinted from: *Int. J. Mol. Sci.* **2022**, 23, 6271, doi:10.3390/ijms23116271 49

Ekta Manocha, Alessandra Consonni, Fulvio Baggi, Emilio Ciusani, Valentina Cocce and Francesca Paino et al.
CD146[+] Pericytes Subset Isolated from Human Micro-Fragmented Fat Tissue Display a Strong Interaction with Endothelial Cells: A Potential Cell Target for Therapeutic Angiogenesis
Reprinted from: *Int. J. Mol. Sci.* **2022**, 23, 5806, doi:10.3390/ijms23105806 71

Sangeetha Hareendran, Bassam Albraidy, Xuyu Yang, Aiyi Liu, Anne Breggia and Clark C. Chen et al.
Exosomal Carboxypeptidase E (CPE) and CPE-shRNA-Loaded Exosomes Regulate Metastatic Phenotype of Tumor Cells
Reprinted from: *Int. J. Mol. Sci.* **2022**, 23, 3113, doi:10.3390/ijms23063113 89

Maria Urbanova, Verona Buocikova, Lenka Trnkova, Sabina Strapcova, Viera Horvathova Kajabova and Emma Barreto Melian et al.
DNA Methylation Mediates EMT Gene Expression in Human Pancreatic Ductal Adenocarcinoma Cell Lines
Reprinted from: *Int. J. Mol. Sci.* **2022**, 23, 2117, doi:10.3390/ijms23042117 107

Manel Benhassine, Gaëtan Le-Bel and Sylvain L. Guérin
Contribution of the STAT Family of Transcription Factors to the Expression of the Serotonin 2B (HTR2B) Receptor in Human Uveal Melanoma
Reprinted from: *Int. J. Mol. Sci.* **2022**, 23, 1564, doi:10.3390/ijms23031564 129

Lenka Kalinkova, Nataliia Nikolaieva, Bozena Smolkova, Sona Ciernikova, Karol Kajo and Vladimir Bella et al.
miR-205-5p Downregulation and *ZEB1* Upregulation Characterize the Disseminated Tumor Cells in Patients with Invasive Ductal Breast Cancer
Reprinted from: *Int. J. Mol. Sci.* **2021**, 23, 103, doi:10.3390/ijms23010103 147

Yen-Yu Lin, Yu-Chao Wang, Da-Wei Yeh, Chen-Yu Hung, Yi-Chen Yeh and Hsiang-Ling Ho et al.
Gene Expression Profile in Primary Tumor Is Associated with Brain-Tropism of Metastasis from Lung Adenocarcinoma
Reprinted from: *Int. J. Mol. Sci.* **2021**, *22*, 13374, doi:10.3390/ijms222413374 . . . . **165**

Jenna Kitz, Cory Lefebvre, Joselia Carlos, Lori E. Lowes and Alison L. Allan
Reduced *Zeb1* Expression in Prostate Cancer Cells Leads to an Aggressive Partial-EMT Phenotype Associated with Altered Global Methylation Patterns
Reprinted from: *Int. J. Mol. Sci.* **2021**, *22*, 12840, doi:10.3390/ijms222312840 . . . . **181**

About the Editors

Bozena Smolkova

Bozena Smolkova earned her undergraduate degree and completed PhD in Genetics from Comenius University Bratislava. She was employed as a research scientist in the Institute of Preventive and Clinical Medicine, Bratislava and currently, she is employed as a senior scientist at the Cancer Research Institute, Biomedical Research Center of the Slovak Academy of Sciences, Bratislava. She focuses on human molecular genetics and epigenetics, particularly on DNA methylation changes in tumor tissues and peripheral blood, including circulating cell-free DNA and circulating tumor cells. She published 73 original research publications in prestigious international journals. She is also a reviewer for national and international journals such as Mutation Research, Food and Chemical toxicology. In addition, she is an active participant in Oncology lectures, supported by the Cancer Research Foundation, where she shares her knowledge and expertise to promote the importance of cancer research in the prevention, detection, and treatment of cancer.

Julie Earl

Julie Earl completed her PhD at the University of Liverpool, UK, in 2002 and her postdoctoral studies at the University of Liverpool from 2002–2008 and the Spanish Cancer Research Center (CNIO) in Madrid, Spain, from 2008–2011. She is a senior researcher in the Medical Oncology department of the university hospital Ramón y Cajal, Madrid, Spain, since 2011 and specializes in cancer genetics and tumor biomarkers, particularly in digestive cancers. She is the coordinator of the Spanish familial pancreatic cancer registry and her lines of research include the genetics of familial pancreatic cancer and the use of the liquid biopsy for the identification and validation of tumor biomarkers. Currently, the group are performing whole exome sequencing to identify novel genes associated with familial cancer and also developing and validating liquid biopsy based tumor markers as prognostic and diagnostic tools. This includes Circulating Tumor Cells (CTC) detection and circulating free tumor DNA detection (cftDNA) in plasma. She is a member of the board of the liquid biopsy group of the Biomedical Research Network in Cancer (CIBERONC) and the coordinator of the in vitro tumor models platform of her institute. She has published more than 40 articles and currently actively participates in several national and international projects related with pancreatic oncology research.

Agapi Kataki

Agapi Kataki is a biologist who completed her MSc and PhD studies in the field of Medical Genetics at the University of Glasgow, UK in 1992. Her postdoctoral experience was gained during her four-year stay in France in Faculté des Sciences—Université de Montpelier, in Centre Hospitalier Régional Universitaire de Nancy and in Institut de Cancérologie de Lorraine—Alexis Vautrin. She is currently a Senior Researcher, but also a Teaching Assistant in Athens Medical School both in undergraduate and postgraduate level. Her interest is focused on Translational Clinical Oncology, Cancer Genetics and Genetic Counselling. She is currently involved in the development of a pancreatic cancer registry, the analysis of pancreatic tumor profile and the application of liquid biopsy as a prognostic and diagnostic tool. Results from her long-term engagement in cancer research have been presented at various National and International Conferences and published in 35 articles. Currently, she is actively participating in several European projects related to pancreatic cancer research.

Preface to "Genetic and Epigenetic Regulations of Tumor Progression and Metastasis"

Cancer is a complex and heterogeneous disease that arises from the accumulation of genetic and epigenetic alterations in cells. Tumor progression and metastasis are the major contributors to cancer-related deaths worldwide. Understanding their underlying genetic and epigenetic mechanisms is essential for the development of effective diagnostic and therapeutic approaches.

The aim of this reprint is to provide a wide range of topics, including the cellular and molecular mechanisms underlying tumor progression and metastasis, involvement of cell signaling pathways, cellular plasticity, and interactions with the tumor microenvironment. This reprint also discusses the role of oncogenes and tumor suppressor genes, chromosomal rearrangements, copy number variations, and epigenetic modifications. Furthermore, it provides the current state of the art in several aspects of cancer diagnosis, prevention, and treatment and highlights emerging therapeutic strategies based on genetic and epigenetic alterations.

The contributing authors are renowned experts in the field of cancer research and treatment. They provide valuable insights into the latest discoveries and advances in cancer research and offer a unique perspective on the challenges and opportunities in the fight against cancer.

We hope this reprint will serve as a valuable resource for researchers, clinicians, and students working in the field of cancer biology and oncology. We believe that the knowledge and insights presented here will inspire further research and innovation in the field of cancer research.

Bozena Smolkova, Julie Earl, and Agapi Kataki
Editors

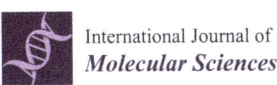

Editorial

The Metastatic Process through the Eyes of Epigenetic Regulation: A Promising Horizon for Cancer Therapy

Bozena Smolkova [1,*], Julie Earl [2] and Agapi Kataki [3]

1. Department of Molecular Oncology, Cancer Research Institute, Biomedical Research Center of the Slovak Academy of Sciences, Dubravska Cesta 9, 845-05 Bratislava, Slovakia
2. Molecular Epidemiology and Predictive Tumor Markers Group, Medical Oncology Research Laboratory, Ramón y Cajal Health Research Institute (IRYCIS), Carretera Colmenar Km 9100, CIBERONC, 28034 Madrid, Spain
3. 1st Department of Propaedutic Surgery, National and Kapodistrian University of Athens, Vasilissis Sofias 114, 11527 Athens, Greece
* Correspondence: bozena.smolkova@savba.sk

Genetic aberrations, including chromosomal rearrangements, loss or amplification of DNA, and point mutations, are major elements of cancer development. However, since epigenetic dysregulation was shown to be strongly related to human disease, especially cancer, the epigenetic component seems equally important. The term epigenetics was first introduced by Conrad Waddington in 1942 [1] in his effort to link the genotype with phenotype. It is currently used to describe the ensemble of several mechanisms that can reversibly modify gene expression profiles without altering the DNA sequence [2]. Epigenetic mechanisms are meant to cooperate with various other regulatory factors to secure time and tissue-specific regulation of gene expression in relation to developmental or environmental cues.

It was long assumed that tumors exhibit cell-to-cell variability, and recent technological advances have provided considerable evidence supporting gene expression and functional phenotypes heterogeneity within malignant tumors. Phenotypic plasticity seems to assist malignant cells in adapting to their environment in order to survive, grow and spread. Although most cancer cells leaving the primary tumor die in circulation, a small population, known as metastasis-initiating cells, survive and retain the ability to seed metastasis. These stem-like malignant progenitors adopt diverse phenotypic stages in response to intrinsic and external stromal signals driving their resistance to therapy and relapse [3]. Consequently, the vast majority of patients with recurrence or de novo metastases die within five years [4]. Acquired epigenetic and subsequent transcriptional changes have been shown as critical events in metastasis [5]. Excessive levels of enzymes that act as epigenetic modifiers have been reported as markers of aggressive cancers and associated with metastatic progression. Analysis of the mutation patterns and overall mutation burden in primary and metastatic cancers has been shown to be largely concordant [6,7]. Still, several recurrent metastasis-associated mutations were identified to be responsible for resistance to specific therapies. Recent studies have found that distinct subgroups of poor-prognosis tumors lack genetic alterations but are epigenetically regulated, confirming the critical role of epigenetic modifications and/or their modifiers to cancer progression [8].

Thus, this Special Issue, with one review and eight original research papers, has focused on deciphering genetic and epigenetic regulation of tumor progression and metastasis, providing novel insights into the mechanisms underlying processes associated with cancer cell plasticity and the development of metastatic disease.

The review of Ruscitto et al. focused on breast cancer, addressing genetic and phenotypic heterogeneity. Whole-genome sequencing of primary tumors and metastases revealed that breast cancer metastasis is a non-genetically selected trait resulting from transcriptional and metabolic adaptation to unfavorable microenvironmental conditions such as hypoxia, low nutrients, endoplasmic reticulum stress, or chemotherapy. However, the nature of the key players in the adaptive responses remains largely unknown [9]. Benhassine et al. analyzed the aberrant expression of serotonin receptor 2B (HTR2B), the most discriminant gene from the 12-gene expression signature, which can efficiently predict metastatic progression in uveal melanoma. The authors confirmed the presence of a STAT putative target site in the HTR2B promoter and showed the impact of IL-4 and IL-6 on HTR2B expression, thus providing evidence that HTR2B expression is modulated by STAT proteins [10].

One of the phenotypic plasticity processes relevant to the development of metastasis is the epithelial-to-mesenchymal transition (EMT), during which epithelial cells lose their polarity and cell–cell adhesion and invade the tumor stroma. Cells with EMT features are present at the invasion fronts of carcinomas [11]. Besides EMT, mesenchymal-to-epithelial transition (MET) endows the metastatic cells with traits needed to spread to distant organs. The dynamic shift between these two phenotypes indicates that the plasticity of EMT could be attributed to epigenetic regulation rather than to permanent genetic mutations [12]. Cancer cells with the mesenchymal state develop increased motility and invasive stem cell-like phenotype, including resistance to treatment [13]. The role of partial EMT phenotypes in prostate cancer progression was investigated by Kitz et al. Knockdown of Zeb1 resulted in partial EMT, inducing co-expression of EMT markers, a mixed epithelial/mesenchymal morphology, and increased invasion and migration. Treatment of knockdown cells with 5-azacytidine mitigated this aggressive phenotype. DNA methylation analysis using Illumina Methylation EPIC BeadChip revealed ten potential EMT targets, which can serve to identify patients who might benefit from 5-aza therapy [14]. Urbanova et al. used DNA methyltransferase inhibitor decitabine, which efficiently decreased DNA methylation by up to 53% and reactivated several silenced EMT-associated genes in four pancreatic ductal adenocarcinoma cell lines. These results confirmed the regulation of these genes by DNA methylation and uncovered possible new targets for epigenetic therapy. EMT plasticity suggests that epigenetic landscapes are implicated in the dynamic events underlying the EMT and might be responsible for tumor cell spread [15]. Dissemination of invasive ductal breast cancer cells through hematogenous or lymphomatous vessels was studied by Kalinkova et al. The authors interrogated the correlation between several miRNAs and EMT genes. As a result, they demonstrated the downregulation of miR-205-5p in CD45-depleted circulating tumor cell-positive tumor fraction and a negative correlation between miR-205-5p and *ZEB1* expression. These findings can potentially deliver markers for the metastatic behavior of disseminated tumor cells originating from invasive ductal carcinoma [16].

Cancer has long been regarded as a problem solely of cancer cells. However, the development and metastasis involve cross-talk between epithelial and stromal compartments mediated by paracrine signals and extracellular matrix [17]. Immune and non-immune cells control anti-metastatic defense or metastasis-supportive responses [18]. Cancer and stromal cell signaling influence one another, and this communication may co-evolve during the course of tumor progression. The maturity stage of mesenchymal stromal cells involved in tissue regeneration, immune modulation, and secretion of angiogenic molecules, cytokines, and paracrine factors was studied by Manocha et al. [19]. The authors demonstrated that in fat tissue, CD146-expressing cells might represent a more mature pericyte subpopulation having higher efficacy in controlling and stimulating vascular regeneration and stabilization than their CD146-negative counterparts.

Through their cargo, consisting of various molecules, including DNA, miRNA, siRNA, and proteins, extracellular vesicles are important mediators of cell-to-cell communication. In recent years, many studies have focused on exosomes and their role in cancer progression and metastasis [20]. The potential of carboxypeptidase E (CPE) as an exosomal bioactive molecule driving the growth and invasion of low-metastatic hepatocellular carcinoma cells was studied by Hareendran et al. [21]. The authors showed that CPE is a key player in the exosome-based delivery of CPE-shRNA, which offers a potential treatment for hepatocellular carcinoma and utility as a liquid biopsy tool.

In many cancers, surgical resection of the primary tumor is followed by a period without evidence of disease followed by aggressive metastatic growth. The study by Lin et al. identified gene expression signatures able to predict 100% of brain-metastasizing lung adenocarcinoma tumors with a 91% specificity, thus facilitating the detection of patients at the highest risk of brain metastasis by analyzing primary tumors [22]. These findings demonstrate that cancer-glia/neuron interaction may play a fundamental role in developing lung cancer brain metastasis.

As mentioned earlier, during tumorigenesis, cancer cells face a variety of intrinsic and extrinsic stresses, forcing the activation of several mechanisms, including autophagy which is often characterized as a double-edged sword, and its role is still under investigation [23]. Zaarour et al. explained why waterpipe smokers with lung adenocarcinoma and an increase in autophagy-activating genes, higher mutation burden, and CD8+ T-cell levels respond better to immunotherapy, despite a lack of differences in immune checkpoint gene PD-1, PD-L1, PD-L2 and CTLA-4 expression [24].

We believe that deciphering the role of genetic and epigenetic changes and their regulatory mechanisms in cancer progression will be crucial for the further molecular understanding of the metastatic process. Epigenetic therapies targeting epigenetic regulators could have a major clinical impact on the development of next-generation drugs, especially when combined with new preclinical patient-derived preclinical models. In addition, given the potential of novel generations of epigenetic inhibitors, the characterization of specific epigenetic subtypes may lead to better patient stratification. Targeting epigenetic modifiers and modifications represents an innovative strategy for treating disease and delaying or preventing resistance to other anticancer therapies in solid tumors [25].

Author Contributions: Conceptualization, B.S., J.E. and A.K.; writing—original draft preparation, B.S.; writing—review and editing, J.E. and A.K. All authors have read and agreed to the published version of the manuscript.

Funding: This research was funded by the European Union's Horizon 2020 research and innovation program under grant agreement No 857381/VISION, the Spanish Biomedical Research Network in Cancer CIBERONC (CB16/12/00446), from the Slovak Research and Development Agency (APVV-21-0197, APVV-20-0143) and TRANSCAN-2 program ERA-NET JTC 2017 "Translational research on rare cancers" within the project NExT.

Conflicts of Interest: The authors declare no conflict of interest.

References

1. Waddington, C.H. The Epigenotype. *Int. J. Epidemiol.* **2011**, *41*, 10–13. [CrossRef] [PubMed]
2. Peschansky, V.J.; Wahlestedt, C. Non-coding RNAs as direct and indirect modulators of epigenetic regulation. *Epigenetics* **2014**, *9*, 3–12. [CrossRef] [PubMed]
3. Quintanal-Villalonga, Á.; Chan, J.M.; Yu, H.A.; Pe'er, D.; Sawyers, C.L.; Sen, T.; Rudin, C.M. Lineage plasticity in cancer: A shared pathway of therapeutic resistance. *Nat. Rev. Clin. Oncol.* **2020**, *17*, 360–371. [CrossRef] [PubMed]
4. Siegel, R.L.; Miller, K.D.; Jemal, A. Cancer statistics, 2019. *CA Cancer J. Clin.* **2019**, *69*, 7–34. [CrossRef] [PubMed]
5. Denny, S.K.; Yang, D.; Chuang, C.H.; Brady, J.J.; Lim, J.S.; Grüner, B.M.; Chiou, S.H.; Schep, A.N.; Baral, J.; Hamard, C.; et al. Nfib Promotes Metastasis through a Widespread Increase in Chromatin Accessibility. *Cell* **2016**, *166*, 328–342. [CrossRef] [PubMed]
6. Hu, Z.; Li, Z.; Ma, Z.; Curtis, C. Multi-cancer analysis of clonality and the timing of systemic spread in paired primary tumors and metastases. *Nat. Genet.* **2020**, *52*, 701–708. [CrossRef] [PubMed]
7. Reiter, J.G.; Makohon-Moore, A.P.; Gerold, J.M.; Heyde, A.; Attiyeh, M.A.; Kohutek, Z.A.; Tokheim, C.J.; Brown, A.; DeBlasio, R.M.; Niyazov, J. Minimal functional driver gene heterogeneity among untreated metastases. *Science* **2018**, *361*, 1033–1037. [CrossRef] [PubMed]
8. Lu, Y.; Chan, Y.-T.; Tan, H.-Y.; Li, S.; Wang, N.; Feng, Y. Epigenetic regulation in human cancer: The potential role of epi-drug in cancer therapy. *Mol. Cancer* **2020**, *19*, 79. [CrossRef]
9. Ruscitto, F.; Roda, N.; Priami, C.; Migliaccio, E.; Pelicci, P.G. Beyond Genetics: Metastasis as an Adaptive Response in Breast Cancer. *Int. J. Mol. Sci.* **2022**, *23*, 6271. [CrossRef]
10. Benhassine, M.; Le-Bel, G.; Guérin, S.L. Contribution of the STAT Family of Transcription Factors to the Expression of the Serotonin 2B (HTR2B) Receptor in Human Uveal Melanoma. *Int. J. Mol. Sci.* **2022**, *23*, 1564. [CrossRef]
11. Shibue, T.; Weinberg, R.A. EMT, CSCs, and drug resistance: The mechanistic link and clinical implications. *Nat. Rev. Clin. Oncol.* **2017**, *14*, 611–629. [CrossRef]

12. Jolly, M.K.; Somarelli, J.A.; Sheth, M.; Biddle, A.; Tripathi, S.C.; Armstrong, A.J.; Hanash, S.M.; Bapat, S.A.; Rangarajan, A.; Levine, H. Hybrid epithelial/mesenchymal phenotypes promote metastasis and therapy resistance across carcinomas. *Pharmacol. Ther.* **2019**, *194*, 161–184. [CrossRef] [PubMed]
13. Lim, S.K.; Khoo, B.Y. An overview of mesenchymal stem cells and their potential therapeutic benefits in cancer therapy. *Oncol. Lett.* **2021**, *22*, 785. [CrossRef] [PubMed]
14. Kitz, J.; Lefebvre, C.; Carlos, J.; Lowes, L.E.; Allan, A.L. Reduced Zeb1 Expression in Prostate Cancer Cells Leads to an Aggressive Partial-EMT Phenotype Associated with Altered Global Methylation Patterns. *Int. J. Mol. Sci.* **2021**, *22*, 12840. [CrossRef]
15. Urbanova, M.; Buocikova, V.; Trnkova, L.; Strapcova, S.; Kajabova, V.H.; Melian, E.B.; Novisedlakova, M.; Tomas, M.; Dubovan, P.; Earl, J. DNA Methylation Mediates EMT Gene Expression in Human Pancreatic Ductal Adenocarcinoma Cell Lines. *Int. J. Mol. Sci.* **2022**, *23*, 2117. [CrossRef] [PubMed]
16. Kalinkova, L.; Nikolaieva, N.; Smolkova, B.; Ciernikova, S.; Kajo, K.; Bella, V.; Kajabova, V.H.; Kosnacova, H.; Minarik, G.; Fridrichova, I. miR-205-5p Downregulation and ZEB1 Upregulation Characterize the Disseminated Tumor Cells in Patients with Invasive Ductal Breast Cancer. *Int. J. Mol. Sci.* **2021**, *23*, 103. [CrossRef] [PubMed]
17. Plaks, V.; Kong, N.; Werb, Z. The cancer stem cell niche: How essential is the niche in regulating stemness of tumor cells? *Cell Stem Cell* **2015**, *16*, 225–238. [CrossRef] [PubMed]
18. Janssen, L.M.E.; Ramsay, E.E.; Logsdon, C.D.; Overwijk, W.W. The immune system in cancer metastasis: Friend or foe? *J. Immunother. Cancer* **2017**, *5*, 79. [CrossRef]
19. Manocha, E.; Consonni, A.; Baggi, F.; Ciusani, E.; Cocce, V.; Paino, F.; Tremolada, C.; Caruso, A.; Alessandri, G. CD146+ Pericytes Subset Isolated from Human Micro-Fragmented Fat Tissue Display a Strong Interaction with Endothelial Cells: A Potential Cell Target for Therapeutic Angiogenesis. *Int. J. Mol. Sci.* **2022**, *23*, 5806. [CrossRef]
20. Li, I.; Nabet, B.Y. Exosomes in the tumor microenvironment as mediators of cancer therapy resistance. *Mol. Cancer* **2019**, *18*, 32. [CrossRef]
21. Hareendran, S.; Albraidy, B.; Yang, X.; Liu, A.; Breggia, A.; Chen, C.C.; Loh, Y.P. Exosomal Carboxypeptidase E (CPE) and CPE-shRNA-Loaded Exosomes Regulate Metastatic Phenotype of Tumor Cells. *Int. J. Mol. Sci.* **2022**, *23*, 3113. [CrossRef] [PubMed]
22. Lin, Y.-Y.; Wang, Y.-C.; Yeh, D.-W.; Hung, C.-Y.; Yeh, Y.-C.; Ho, H.-L.; Mon, H.-C.; Chen, M.-Y.; Wu, Y.-C.; Chou, T.-Y. Gene Expression Profile in Primary Tumor Is Associated with Brain-Tropism of Metastasis from Lung Adenocarcinoma. *Int. J. Mol. Sci.* **2021**, *22*, 13374. [CrossRef] [PubMed]
23. Chavez-Dominguez, R.; Perez-Medina, M.; Lopez-Gonzalez, J.S.; Galicia-Velasco, M.; Aguilar-Cazares, D. The double-edge sword of autophagy in cancer: From tumor suppression to pro-tumor activity. *Front. Oncol.* **2020**, *10*, 578418. [CrossRef] [PubMed]
24. Zaarour, R.F.; Sharda, M.; Azakir, B.; Hassan Venkatesh, G.; Abou Khouzam, R.; Rifath, A.; Nizami, Z.N.; Abdullah, F.; Mohammad, F.; Karaali, H.; et al. Genomic Analysis of Waterpipe Smoke-Induced Lung Tumor Autophagy and Plasticity. *Int. J. Mol. Sci.* **2022**, *23*, 6848. [CrossRef] [PubMed]
25. Morel, D.; Jeffery, D.; Aspeslagh, S.; Almouzni, G.; Postel-Vinay, S. Combining epigenetic drugs with other therapies for solid tumours—Past lessons and future promise. *Nat. Rev. Clin. Oncol.* **2020**, *17*, 91–107. [CrossRef]

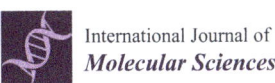

Article

DNA Methylation and Gene Expression of the Cysteinyl Leukotriene Receptors as a Prognostic and Metastatic Factor for Colorectal Cancer Patients

Souvik Ghatak *, Shakti Ranjan Satapathy and Anita Sjölander *

Cell and Experimental Pathology, Department of Translational Medicine, Lund University, 205 02 Malmö, Sweden
* Correspondence: souvik.ghatak@med.lu.se (S.G.); anita.sjolander@med.lu.se (A.S.)

Abstract: Colorectal cancer (CRC), one of the leading causes of cancer-related deaths in the western world, is the third most common cancer for both men and women. As a heterogeneous disease, colon cancer (CC) is caused by both genetic and epigenetic changes. The prognosis for CRC is affected by a variety of features, including late diagnosis, lymph node and distant metastasis. The cysteinyl leukotrienes (CysLT), as leukotriene D_4 and C_4 (LTD_4 and LTC_4), are synthesized from arachidonic acid via the 5-lipoxygenase pathway, and play an important role in several types of diseases such as inflammation and cancer. Their effects are mediated via the two main G-protein-coupled receptors, $CysLT_1R$ and $CysLT_2R$. Multiple studies from our group observed a significant increase in $CysLT_1R$ expression in the poor prognosis group, whereas $CysLT_2R$ expression was higher in the good prognosis group of CRC patients. Here, we systematically explored and established the role of the CysLTRs, cysteinyl leukotriene receptor 1(*CYSLTR1*) and cysteinyl leukotriene receptor 2 (*CYSLTR2*) gene expression and methylation in the progression and metastasis of CRC using three unique in silico cohorts and one clinical CRC cohort. Primary tumor tissues showed significant *CYSLTR1* upregulation compared with matched normal tissues, whereas it was the opposite for the *CYSLTR2*. Univariate Cox proportional-hazards (CoxPH) analysis yielded a high expression of *CYSLTR1* and accurately predicted high-risk patients in terms of overall survival (OS; hazard ratio (HR) = 1.87, p = 0.03) and disease-free survival [DFS] Hazard ratio [HR] = 1.54, p = 0.05). Hypomethylation of the *CYSLTR1* gene and hypermethylation of the *CYSLTR2* gene were found in CRC patients. The M values of the CpG probes for *CYSLTR1* are significantly lower in primary tumor and metastasis samples than in matched normal samples, but those for *CYSLTR2* are significantly higher. The differentially upregulated genes between tumor and metastatic samples were uniformly expressed in the high-*CYSLTR1* group. Two epithelial–mesenchymal transition (EMT) markers, E-cadherin (*CDH1*) and vimentin (*VIM*) were significantly downregulated and upregulated in the high-*CYSLTR1* group, respectively, but the result was opposite to that of *CYSLTR2* expression in CRC. *CDH1* expression was high in patients with less methylated *CYSLTR1* but low in those with more methylated *CYSLTR2*. The EMT-associated observations were also validated in CC SW620 cell-derived colonospheres, which showed decreased E-cadherin expression in the LTD_4 stimulated cells, but not in the $CysLT_1R$ knockdown SW620 cells. The methylation profiles of the CpG probes for CysLTRs significantly predicted lymph node (area under the curve [AUC] = 0.76, p < 0.0001) and distant (AUC = 0.83, p < 0.0001) metastasis. Intriguingly, the CpG probes cg26848126 (HR = 1.51, p = 0.03) for *CYSLTR1*, and cg16299590 (HR = 2.14, p = 0.03) for *CYSLTR2* significantly predicted poor prognosis in terms of OS, whereas the CpG probe cg16886259 for *CYSLTR2* significantly predicts a poor prognosis group in terms of DFS (HR = 2.88, p = 0.03). The *CYSLTR1* and *CYSLTR2* gene expression and methylation results were successfully validated in a CC patient cohort. In this study, we have demonstrated that CysLTRs' methylation and gene expression profile are associated with the progression, prognosis, and metastasis of CRC, which might be used for the assessment of high-risk CRC patients after validating the result in a larger CRC cohort.

Keywords: *CYSLTR1*; *CYSLTR2*; methylation; prognosis; metastasis; colorectal cancer; EMT

Citation: Ghatak, S.; Satapathy, S.R.; Sjölander, A. DNA Methylation and Gene Expression of the Cysteinyl Leukotriene Receptors as a Prognostic and Metastatic Factor for Colorectal Cancer Patients. *Int. J. Mol. Sci.* **2023**, *24*, 3409. https://doi.org/10.3390/ijms24043409

Academic Editors: Bozena Smolkova, Julie Earl and Agapi Kataki

Received: 5 January 2023
Revised: 19 January 2023
Accepted: 31 January 2023
Published: 8 February 2023

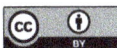

Copyright: © 2023 by the authors. Licensee MDPI, Basel, Switzerland. This article is an open access article distributed under the terms and conditions of the Creative Commons Attribution (CC BY) license (https://creativecommons.org/licenses/by/4.0/).

1. Introduction

Colorectal cancer (CRC) is one of the leading causes of cancer-related deaths, ranking third for both men and women [1,2]. A decreasing trend in the metastatic CRC (mCRC) has been observed during the last years after the introduction of screening programs. However, the treatment strategies are still complicated due to the large number of patients detected with lymph node or distant metastasis. Metastasis is one of the most serious issues that reduce the survival of CRC patients and the effectiveness of their treatment. The median disease-free survival (DFS) and overall survival (OS) of patients with lymph node or distant mCRC have significantly increased because of late diagnosis or implementation of combined chemotherapy and drug treatment. Hence, there is a need to identify potentially related genes and their roles in the metastasis development. In addition, identifying robust predictive and prognostic markers to be validated in population-based cohorts could improve survival for mCRC patients.

Leukotrienes are inflammatory lipid mediators produced in different cells type from arachidonic acid via the 5-lipoxygenase pathway [3]. The two main cysteinyl leukotrienes (CysLTs) are LTC_4, and LTD_4, well known for their inflammatory effect caused by the CysLTs in cancer [3–5]. There has been an emerging role for CysLTs in cancer [6–8]. The roles of the two cysteinyl leukotriene receptors, $CysLT_1R$ and $CysLT_2R$, have been well-reported for different types of cancer [6–8]. $CysLT_1R$ and $CysLT_2R$ are the high-affinity receptors for LTD_4 and LTC_4, respectively [4,5]. Montelukast and zafirlukast, $CysLT_1R$ antagonists, were found to possess dose-dependent chemopreventive effects against several cancers [9]. Moreover, $CysLT_1R$ overexpression has been observed in different types of cancers, including colorectal cancer, breast cancer, prostate cancer, urothelial transitional cell carcinoma and renal cell carcinoma [10–17]. The expression of $CysLT_1R$ and $CysLT_2R$ varies in various human tissues, including the respiratory and gastrointestinal systems and the brain [3,6–9]. The expression of $CysLT_2R$, compared with that of $CysLT_1R$, has been found to be higher in normal mucosa compared to its matched cancer tissues; however, $CysLT_1R$ expression was higher than $CysLT_2R$ expression in tumor samples [6]. A recurrent, hotspot mutation, p.Leu129Gln in *CYSLTR2*, an oncogene driver in uveal melanoma and leptomeningeal melanocytic tumors, leads to the activation of endogenous Gαq signaling and contributes to tumor progression in vivo [18,19]. To our knowledge, no reported evidence exists for genetic alterations of these receptors, resulting in good prognosis for CRC patients with low $CysLT_1R$ and high $CysLT_2R$ expressions.

A crucial step in cancer invasion and metastasis is the epithelial–mesenchymal transition (EMT). Cell adhesion molecules, such as E-cadherin, must be suppressed in order for EMT to occur. Furthermore, EMT results in the decline in E-cadherin and the increase in mesenchymal markers such as vimentin [20]. E-cadherin is decreased by LTD_4 in CC cell lines [21]. Whereas MMP-9 is a metallopeptidase known to induce EMT in breast cancer cells, it is also induced by LTD_4 in SW480 CC cells [22]. In a recent study, under basal conditions, *Cysltr1*$^{-/-}$ mice had higher expression of E-cadherin mRNA than wild-type mice [23]. Furthermore, in an earlier report from our group, a significant reduction in E-cadherin levels was observed in HCT-116 CC cells after LTD_4 stimulation and GSK-3ß inhibition [21].

DNA methylation is a common and early epigenetic event that controls gene expression without changing genomic DNA sequences, and it consists of the attachment of methyl groups primarily to cytosines in the context of CpG dinucleotides. Multiple studies have proven that DNA methylation plays a key role in disease development by controlling driver gene expression [24], especially in cancers [25–28]. It is generally believed that the promoter regions of tumor suppressor genes (TSGs) are hypermethylated and repressed, whereas oncogenes are hypomethylated and abnormally active in cancer cells [29]. Furthermore, differentially methylated CpG probes could be used as biomarkers for the prognosis, metastasis prediction and treatment response of different cancers [25,30]. For patients presenting with a secondary tumor or metastases, DNA methylation markers can also be used to predict the origin of primary tumors [31]. Moreover, tissue- and disease-specific gene expression is also associated with DNA methylation differences in CpG islands [32].

Although several studies have investigated the DNA methylation profile of CRC [33], no sensitive or specific biomarkers have been identified for the prognosis of mCRC.

Building upon this evidence, we performed a systematic and comprehensive analysis of the methylation and expression of the *CYSLTR1* and *CYSLTR2* genes in the TCGA-COADREAD cohort, and the results were validated in two independent in silico cohorts (GSE77955 cohort from the GEO database and E-MTAB-8148 from the EMBL—EBI). We demonstrate the role of $CysLT_1R$ and $CysLT_2R$ in colorectal cancer progression and metastasis. Furthermore, we performed a comprehensive analysis of the methylation status of the *CYSLTR1* and *CYSLTR2* genes, which serve as drivers for CRC prognosis and metastasis development and could be used as prognostic markers for CRC patients.

2. Results

The Cancer Genome Atlas for colorectal cancer (TCGA-COADREAD) contains a gene expression profile from the Illumina HiSeq 2000 RNA sequencing platform and a DNA methylation profile from Illumina Infinium HumanMethylation450 platform with 416 primary colorectal cancer (COAD n = 284, READ n = 91) and matched normal (n = 41) samples (see Table 1 and study plan). Both the CysLT receptor (*CYSLTR1* and *CYSLTR2*) genes were expressed in the CRC samples, confirming their potential disease relevance. The differentially global methylated CpGs in TCGA-COADREAD dataset with $\delta|\beta| > 0.25$ and adjusted $p < 0.05$ is visualized in Supplementary Figure S1. There were 16,122 hyper-methylated and 8736 hypomethylated CpGs observed in the TCGA-COADREAD dataset. Among the three CpG probes (cg00813999, cg10091155 and cg26848126) for the *CYSLTR1* gene, two CpG probes (cg00813999 and cg26848126) exhibited a methylation profile, whereas, among the five CpG probes (cg06038701, cg06322064, cg16299590, cg16886259 and cg18236297) for the *CYSLTR2* gene, two CpG probes (cg16299590 and cg16886259) exhibited a methylation profile for CRC.

CYSLTR1 and *CYSLTR2* expression were significantly differentially regulated between CRC tumor tissues and corresponding normal tissues in the TCGA-COADREAD cohort. *CYSLTR1* expression was significantly upregulated in CRC tumor tissues compared with matched normal tissues ($p = 0.0004$, paired t-test, Figure 1A). Likewise, *CYSLTR2* expression was significantly decreased in CRC tumor tissues compared with corresponding normal tissues ($p \leq 0.00001$, paired t-test, Figure 1B). These data are significant, as high *CYSLTR1* expression was correlated with poor prognosis in CRC patients. *CYSLTR1* expression significantly separated the good and poor prognosis groups for overall survival in the TCGA-COADREAD cohort with a hazard ratio (HR) of 1.87 (95% CI = 1.04–3.37, $p = 0.03$, Figure 1C). Low expression of *CYSLTR2* was not significantly correlated with the poor prognosis group in CRC patients (Figure 1D).

Table 1. Distribution of clinical and pathological covariates of in silico and clinical datasets. N—matched normal; AD—adenoma; PT—primary tumor; ME—distant metastasis; CC—Colon cancer; FF—Fresh frozen; FFPE—Formalin fixed paraffin embedded.

Datasets	Sample Type	Tissue Types	Data Types	Platform	Age (Mean ± SD)	Gender			Anatomical Location			TNM Stage			
						Male (n)	Female (n)	Missing (n)	Left (n)	Right (n)	Missing (n)	Stage I	Stage II	Stage III	Stage IV
TCGA COADREAD cohort	N (n = 41)	FF	Tissue mRNA and DNA methylation	RNA-seq and HumanMethylation450k	63.64 ± 13.83	22	19	-	20	16	5	-	-	-	-
	PT (n = 375)				63.56 ± 13.92	207	168	-	187	163	25	57	143	123	52
	N (n = 13)				52.46 ± 10.64	5	5	2	5	5	3	-	-	-	-
GSE77955 cohort	PT (n = 17) AD (n = 17)	FF	Tissue mRNA and DNA methylation	Gene expression Microarray and HumanMethylation450k	64.55 ± 11.38	11	6	-	11	6	-	-	-	-	17
	ME (Liver, n = 10 Ovary, n = 1)				53.26 ± 8.53	7	8	2	5	7	5	-	-	-	-
E-MTAB-8148 cohort	N (n = 32)	FF	Tissue mRNA and DNA methylation	RNA-seq and HumanMethylation450k	66.28 ± 11.24	6	26	-	-	-	-	-	-	-	-
	PT (n = 216)				68.92 ± 16.55	100	116	-	Missing			Missing			
Malmö-CC cohort	N (n = 20)	FFPE	Tissue mRNA and DNA methylation	qRT-PCR and quantitative methylation-specific PCR	66.24 ± 13.10	14	6	-	9	8	3	-	-	-	-
	PT (n = 20)				65.73 ± 12.73	14	6	-	9	8	3	-	5	13	2

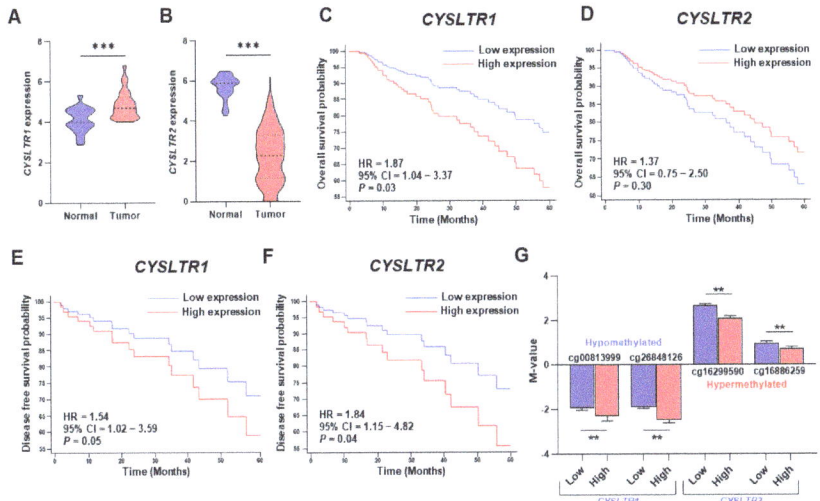

Figure 1. Violin plot of the relative expression and Kaplan–Meier survival plot of the *CYSLTR1* and *CYSLTR2* genes in the TCGA-COADREAD cohort. Relative expression of *CYSLTR1* (**A**) and *CYSLTR2* (**B**) between normal and tumor samples. Five-year Kaplan–Meier overall survival plots for *CYSLTR1* (**C**) and *CYSLTR2* (**D**). Five-year Kaplan–Meier disease-free survival plots for *CYSLTR1* (**E**) and *CYSLTR2* (**F**). (**G**) Correlation of M-values for CpG probes with *CYSLTR1* (cg00813999, cg26848126) and *CYSLTR2* (cg16299590, cg16886259) gene expression in tumor samples. ** $p < 0.01$; *** $p < 0.001$.

On the other hand, high *CYSLTR1* expression was also significantly correlated with poor prognosis, with an HR of 1.54 (95% CI = 1.02–3.59, $p = 0.05$, Figure 1E) for disease-free survival (DFS). In accordance with the overall survival for *CYSLTR2* expression, the DFS Kaplan–Meier curve exhibited the opposite result; a high expression of *CYSLTR2* was significantly correlated with poor prognosis in the TCGA-COADREAD cohort (HR = 1.84, 95% CI = 1.15–4.82, $p = 0.04$, Figure 1F). After correlating the M-values for the CpG probes of *CYSLTR1* (cg00813999 and cd26848126) and *CYSLTR2* (cg16886259 and cg16299590) with *CYSLTR1* and *CYSLTR2* gene expression, we observed a significant reduction in negative M-values for high expression of the *CYSLTR1* gene and a significant increase in positive M-values for low expression of the *CYSLTR2* gene. Hence, the *CYSLTR1* and *CYSLTR2* genes were hypomethylated and hypermethylated in CRC tumors, respectively, and significantly controlled the associated gene expression (Figure 1G).

There was a significant decrease in the negative M values for the two CpG probes for *CYSLTR1* in colon tumors (cg00813999 and cd26848126, Figure 2A,B) and rectal tumors (cg16886259 and cg16299590, Figure 2C,D) compared with matched normal samples. However, a significant decrease in positive M-values for the CpG probe cg16886259 (Figure 2E,G) and an increase in positive M-values for the CpG probe cg16299590 (Figure 2F,H) for *CYSLTR2* were observed in the colon and rectal tumors compared with matched normal samples. On the other hand, the M-values for cg00813999 and cd16299590 probes were significantly decreased and increased in the late TNM stages (stage III and IV) compared with early TNM stages (stage I and II), respectively (Figure 2I,L), but the other two probes (cg026848126 and cg16886259) did not achieve a significant level (Figure 2J,K).

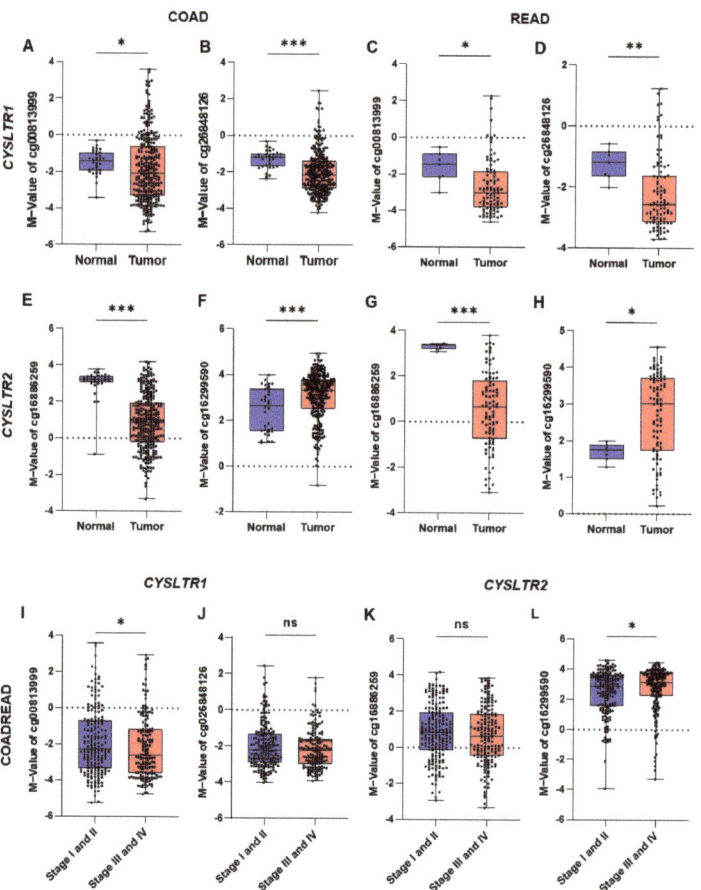

Figure 2. Box-and-whisker plots of the M−value distribution for CpG probes between normal and tumor samples in the TCGA−COADREAD cohort. The M−value distribution between normal and tumor samples for cg00813999 (**A**,**C**) and cg26848126 (**B**,**D**) in colon (COAD) and rectal (READ) cancer. The M−value distribution between normal and tumor samples for cg16886259 (**E**,**G**) and cg16299590 (**F**,**H**) in colon (COAD) and rectal (READ) cancer. The M−value distribution between early and advanced stages for cg00813999 (**I**), cg26848126 (**J**), cg16886259 (**K**) and cg16299590 (**L**) in colorectal (COADREAD) cancer. * $p < 0.05$; ** $p < 0.01$; *** $p < 0.001$; ns = not significant.

There was a significant correlation between the mRNA expression of the EMT (epithelial-mesenchymal transition) markers *CDH1* (E-cadherin) and *VIM* (vimentin) and high *CYSLTR1* gene expression in tumor samples. *CDH1* and *VIM* gene expression were significantly reduced and increased, respectively, in tumor samples with high *CYSLTR1* gene expression (Figure 3A). However, the opposite was true for *CYSLTR2* gene expression (Figure 3B). *CDH1* and *VIM* gene expression were significantly decreased and increased in the low M-value groups for both CpG probes of *CYSLTR1* (cg00813999 and cd26848126, Figure 3C,D). Interestingly, the opposite result was obtained for both CpG probes of *CYSLTR2* (cg16886259 and cg16299590, Figure 3E,F). Hence, these results indicate a positive association between CpG probe methylation and *CYSLTR1* and *CYSLTR2* gene expression to control EMT markers in CRC. Next, we checked the prediction ability of lymph node metastasis (LNM, Stages II and III) and distant metastasis (ME Stage IV), we performed ROC–AUC (receiver operating curve–area under the curve) analysis using the multivariate logistic regression probability scores of the four probes. Surprisingly, we achieved a significantly high AUC value for both models (for LNM, AUC = 0.769, Figure 3G; and for ME, AUC = 0.831, Figure 3H) with high sensitivity.

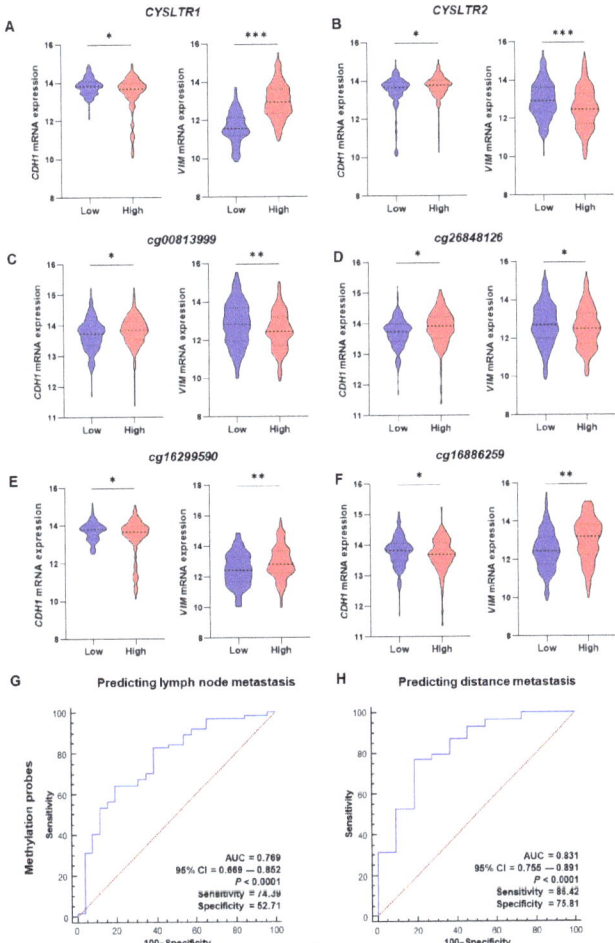

Figure 3. Correlation of EMT marker (*CDH1* and *VIM*) expression and *CYSLTR1* and *CYSLTR2* gene expression and their CpG probes in the TCGA-COADREAD cohort. (**A**) Correlation between *CDH1* and *VIM* gene expression with high and low *CYSLTR1* gene expression. (**B**) Correlation between *CDH1* and *VIM* gene expression with high and low *CYSLTR2* gene expression. (**C**–**F**) Correlation between *CDH1* and *VIM* gene expression with high and low M values for the CpG probes of *CYSLTR1* (cg00813999 and cg26848126) and *CYSLTR2* (cg16299590 and cg16886259) genes. ROC–AUC curve for the prediction of lymph node metastasis (**G**) and distant metastasis (**H**) using the M values for CpG probes of *CYSLTR1* and *CYSLTR2* genes. * $p < 0.05$; ** $p < 0.01$; *** $p < 0.001$.

To validate our results from the TCGA-COADREAD datasets, we used the GEO database (GSE77955 dataset) with adenoma, matched normal, primary tumor and distant metastasis tissues. Interestingly, the negative M-value for the CpG probe for *CYSLTR1* genes was significantly lower for primary tumors than for adenoma and matched normal tissues. Moreover, it was further decreased in the metastatic specimens compared with the primary tumor (Figure 4A,B). The result was similar for the CpG probe cg16886259

(Figure 4C) for the *CYSLTR2* gene, but the other probe, cg16299590 (Figure 4D), exhibited the opposite result to that observed in the TCGA-COADREAD cohort.

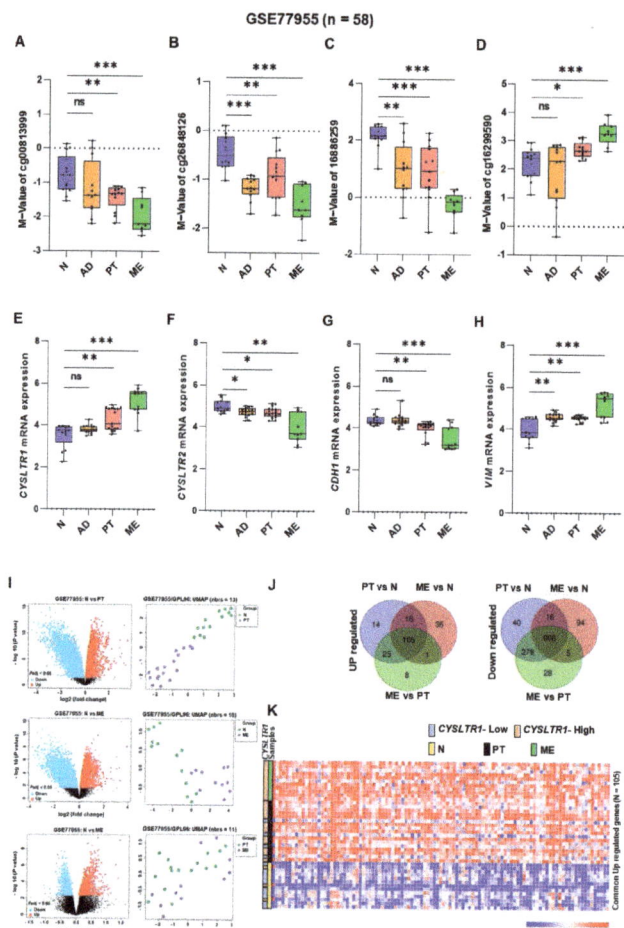

Figure 4. M-value distribution for the CpG probes of the *CYSLTR1* and *CYSLTR2* genes and their expression in matched normal (N), adenoma (AD), primary tumor (PT) and distant metastasis (ME) samples in the GSE77955 CRC cohort. (**A–D**) M-value distribution for the CpG probes in the N, AD, PT and ME samples. Relative expression of *CYSLTR1* (**E**) and *CYSLTR2* (**F**) genes between the N, AD, PT and ME samples. Relative expression of *CDH1* (**G**) and *VIM* (**H**) genes between the N, AD, PT and ME samples. (**I**) Volcano plots and UMAP plots for the differentially expressed genes (DEGs) between PT vs. N, ME vs. N and ME vs. PT samples. (**J**) Venn diagram for the up-and downregulated genes from the DEGs between PT vs. N, ME vs. N and ME vs. PT samples. (**K**) Heatmap for the commonly upregulated gene expression in N, PT and ME samples. * $p < 0.05$; ** $p < 0.01$; *** $p < 0.001$.

CYSLTR1 and *CYSLTR2* expression were significantly higher and lower in the primary tumor samples than in the adenoma and normal samples, but it was higher and lower in the metastatic specimens than in the primary tumor samples, respectively (Figure 4E,F). Whereas *CDH1* expression was gradually decreased in primary tumor and metastasis specimens compared with adenoma and normal samples, the opposite was true for *VIM* expression (Figure 4G,H). Hence, *CYSLTR1* and *CYSLTR2* expression influenced tumor metastasis through the alteration of EMT marker expression (*CDH1* and *VIM*). *CYSLTR1/2* gene expression was controlled by the methylation of CpG probes, specifically cg00813999 and cg26848126 for *CYSLTR1* and cg16299590 for *CYSLTR2*.

We found 13 983, 12 925 and 5 169 genes from the differential gene expression (DGE) analysis between primary tumor vs. normal (PT vs. N), distant metastasis vs. normal (ME vs. N) and distant metastasis vs. primary tumor (ME vs. PT) samples, respectively (cutoff: adjusted $p \leq 0.05$ and log fold change more than ± 1) (Figure 4I). The UMAP plots for normal vs. tumor and normal vs. metastasis exhibited two distinct separate clusters for the group of samples used for DGE, but the tumor vs. metastasis group did not separate the samples distinctly (Figure 4I). We found 105 upregulated and 966 downregulated genes that are common between PT vs. N, ME vs. N and ME vs. PT by the DGE analysis (Figure 4J). *CYSLTR1* gene expression was significantly high in tumor and metastasis samples, and the 105 common upregulated genes were also significantly high in these groups; hence, the expression of these genes was positively correlated with *CYSLTR1* expression (Figure 4K, Supplementary Table S1).

We achieved a significant hazard ratio (HR) in the overall survival analysis for the CpG probe cg26848126 (HR = 1.51, 95% CI = 1.03–3.44, $p = 0.03$), whereas the other CpG probe (cg00813999) for *CYSLTR1* did not achieve a significant p value (Figure 5A,B). The low M-value significantly separated the poor prognosis group for five years of OS prediction. On the other hand, the HR was not significant for five years of DFS for either CpG probe, although the low M-value of cg26848126 could separate the poor prognosis group with a $p = 0.06$ (Figure 5C,D). Interestingly, we observed the opposite trend for the CpG probe of *CYSLTR2*. A high M-value for both probes (cg16299590 and cg16886259) was positively correlated with poor prognosis in five years of overall survival; although cg16299590 achieved a significant HR (HR = 2.14, 95% CI = 1.11–4.12, $p = 0.03$, Figure 5E), the other probe did not achieve a significant p value (HR = 0.77, 95% CI = 0.44–1.14, $p = 0.09$, Figure 5F). In the case of the five-year DFS prediction, a high M-value of the CpG probes of the *CYSLTR2* gene was positively correlated with poor prognosis (Figure 5G,H), although cg16886259 was only significant for DFS assessment (HR = 2.88, 95% CI = 1.07–5.76, $p = 0.03$, Figure 5H).

The *CYSLTR1* and *CYSLTR2* gene expressions and methylation were validated in an additional in silico cohort (E-MTAB), with the transcriptome and genome-wide methylation sequencing for primary tumor and normal samples (Figure 6A–J). In tumor samples, *CYSLTR1* (Figure 6A) was significantly upregulated, but the opposite was true for *CYSLTR2* (Figure 6F) expression. The M values of cg00813999 (Figure 6B) and cg26848126 (Figure 6C) CpG probes were significantly lower in the tumor samples than normal. Conversely, *CDH1* (Figure 6D) and *VIM* (Figure 6E) expression were low and high in patients with high *CYSLTR1* gene expression, respectively. The M values of cg16299590 (Figure 6G) and cg16886259 (Figure 6H) CpG probes for the *CYSLTR2* gene were significantly high in tumor samples than in normal areas. Interestingly, *CYSLTR2* gene expression was low in patients with low *CDH1* (Figure 6I) and high *VIM* (Figure 6J) expression.

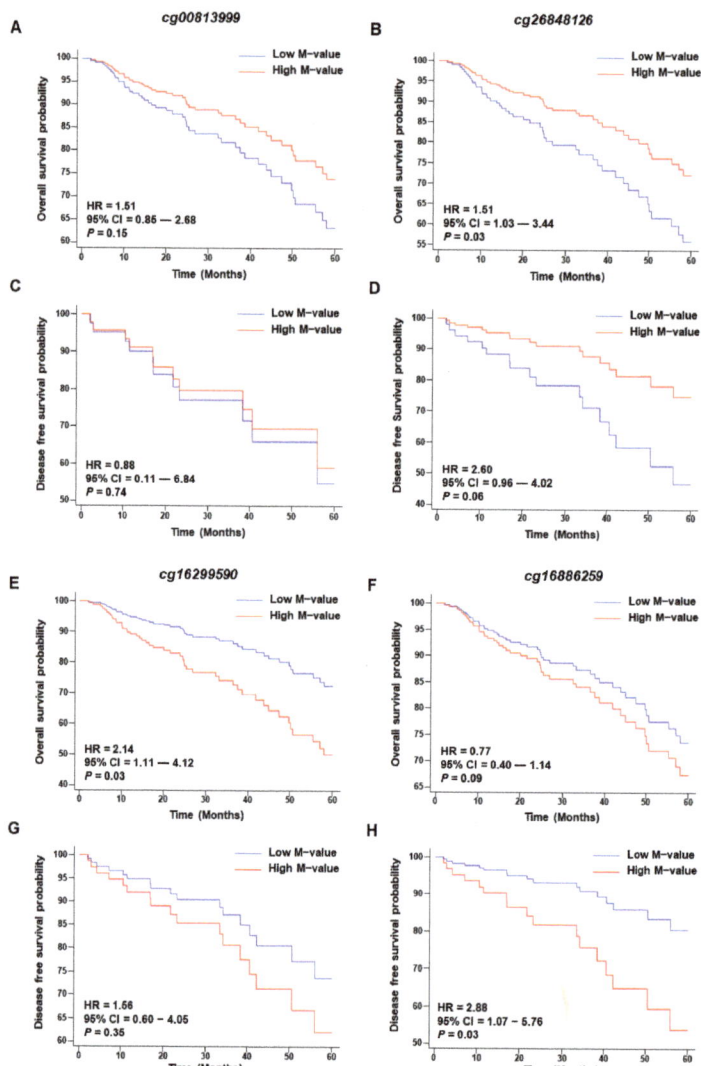

Figure 5. Kaplan–Meier plot for the CpG probes. Five-year overall and disease-free survival plots for CpG probes cg00813999 (**A**,**C**) and cg26848126 (**B**,**D**) for the *CYSLTR1* gene. Five-year overall and disease-free survival plots for CpG probes cg16299590 (**E**,**G**) and cg16886259 (**F**,**H**) for the *CYSLTR2* gene.

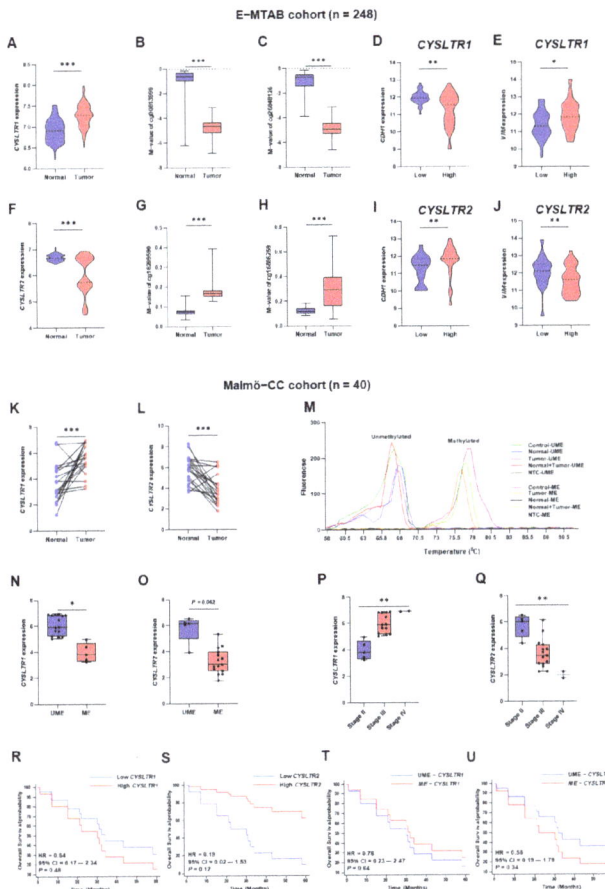

Figure 6. Expression and DNA methylation of *CYSLTR1* and *CYSLTR2* genes in the E-MTAB in silico and Malmö-CC clinical cohort. Relative expression of *CYSLTR1* (**A**) and M-value distribution of cg00813999 (**B**) and cg26848126 (**C**) between normal and tumor samples, *CDH1* (**D**), *VIM* (**E**) gene expressions in low- and high-expressed *CYSLTR1* groups of patients in E-MTAB cohort. Relative expression of *CYSLTR2* (**F**) and M-value distribution of cg16299590 (**G**) and cg16886259 (**H**) between normal and tumor samples, *CDH1* (**I**), *VIM* (**J**) gene expressions in low- and high-expressed *CYSLTR2* groups of patients in E-MTAB cohort. Relative expression of *CYSLTR1* (**K**) and *CYSLTR2* (**L**) gene expression between normal (N) and primary tumor (PT) samples in the Malmö cohort. (**M**) Quantitative methylation-specific PCR melting curve analysis in N and PT samples from the Malmö cohort. *CYSLTR1* (**N**) and *CYSLTR2* (**O**) gene expressions in unmethylated and methylated (*CYSLTR1* and *CYSLTR2*) patient groups in the Malmö cohort. *CYSLTR1* (**P**) and *CYSLTR2* (**Q**) gene expression in different stage (stage II, III and IV) tumor samples in the Malmö cohort. Five year overall survival plots for *CYSLTR1* (**R**), *CYSLTR2* (**S**), *CYSLTR1*—unmethylated and methylated (**T**) and *CYSLTR2*—unmethylated and methylated (**U**) patient samples in the Malmö cohort. HR—hazard ratio, CI—confidence interval, UME—Unmethylated, ME—Methylated, * $p < 0.05$; ** $p < 0.01$; *** $p < 0.001$.

The results were validated in a CC patient cohort (Malmö-CC) [14], consisting of twenty paraffin-embedded normal tissues and twenty matched primary tumor tissues. The *CYSLTR1* gene was significantly upregulated in tumors and the *CYSLTR2* gene was significantly downregulated in tumors compared with normal samples (Figure 6K,L). The promotor region methylation status of the *CYSLTR1* and *CYSLTR2* genes were validated using quantitative methylation-specific melting curve analysis and agarose gel electrophoresis using a specific set of primers (Figure 6M, Supplementary Figure S2A,B). *CYSLTR1* and *CYSLTR2* gene expressions were higher in unmethylated samples than in methylated samples in the Malmö-CC cohort (Figure 6N,O). Interestingly, the CC samples from the high-risk group based on the *CYSLTR1* gene expression were unmethylated and highly expressed; however, the CC samples in the high-risk group based on *CYSLTR2* gene expression were methylated and less expressed. The *CYSLTR1* and *CYSLTR2* gene expressions gradually increased and decreased in stage II, III and IV primary tumor samples, respectively (Figure 6P,Q). The Malmö-CC cohort demonstrated high expression of *CYSLTR1* (Figure 6R) and low expression of *CYSLTR2* (Figure 6S), while unmethylated *CYSLTR1* (Figure 6T) and methylated *CYSLTR2* (Figure 6U) genes were observed in the poor prognosis group, although at a statistically non-significant level. *CDH1* gene expression was significantly downregulated in the tumor samples compared to normal areas, while *VIM* expression did not differ between tumors and normal areas (Figure 7A,B). Interestingly, *CDH1* expression was lower and *VIM* expression was higher in the tumor samples with high *CYSLTR1* expression, although the statistical significance was not achieved, possibly due to the smaller number of patients (Figure 7C,D). On the other hand, *CDH1* and *VIM* expression were higher in tumor samples with high expression of the *CYSLTR2* gene (Figure 7E,F). We next used CC SW620 cell-derived colonospheres with or without CysLT$_1$R expression. The colonospheres showed a decrease in E-cadherin expression after LTD$_4$ stimulation, which was not observed in the CysLT$_1$R, knockdown cells. No significant changes were observed of the mesenchymal marker vimentin (Supplementary Figure S3A–C).

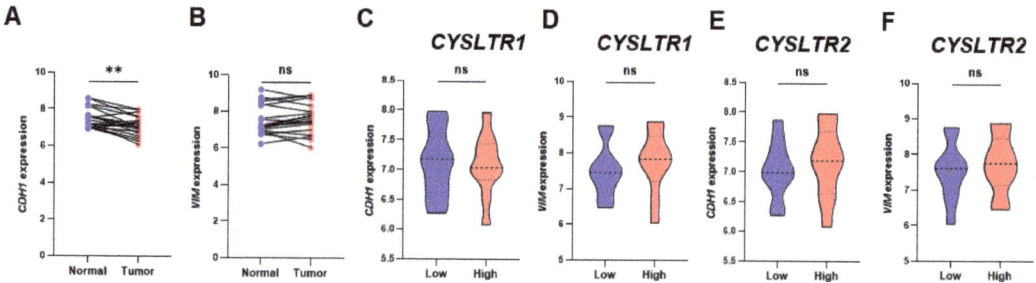

Figure 7. Expression of the EMT markers *CDH1* and *VIM* in patient samples with low and high expression of *CYSLTR1* and *CYSLTR2* genes in the Malmö–CC clinical cohort. Relative expression of *CDH1* (**A**) and *VIM* (**B**) genes between normal and primary tumor samples. *CDH1* (**C**) and *VIM* (**D**) gene expressions in low and high *CYSLTR1* groups of patients. *CDH1* (**E**) and *VIM* (**F**) gene expressions in low and high *CYSLTR2* group of patients. ** $p < 0.01$; ns = non-significant.

3. Discussion

Our goal was to determine the influence of the methylation profile of the CysLTRs receptors on their gene expression and their association with prognosis and metastasis development in CRC patients. We successfully identified methylated CpG probes for CysLTRs that could influence gene expression in CRC. Furthermore, the gene expression and methylation profiles for the CysLTRs are one of the strongest prognostic indicators and metastasis predictors for CRC patients in the TCGA-COADREAD cohort. To further highlight the clinical significance of our findings, we validated the results using the well-structured GSE77955 cohort with normal tissue, primary tumor and distant metastasis samples. The results were further validated using an additional in silico cohort (EMBL—EBI, E-MTAB-8148), which included normal tissues and primary tumors and FFPE tissue-based CC clinical cohort (Malmö-CC), which includes both normal tissues and primary tumors.

The role of CysLTRs (CysLT$_1$R and CysLT$_2$R) has been well reported for the development and metastasis of different types of cancer [34]. We previously showed that high CysLT$_1$R expression in CRC patients was associated with poor prognosis and was positively correlated with nuclear β-catenin and negatively correlated with membrane β-catenin, which is associated with poor prognosis for CRC patients [14]. Although previous studies have demonstrated the involvement of CysLTRs in various cancers, their precise role in cancer pathogenesis and the molecular mechanisms underlying their methylation profile remain unclear. We identified that CRC tumors exhibited higher *CYSLTR1* gene expression than matched normal tissues, whereas the opposite was true for *CYSLTR2* expression. This is supported by the result from Magnusson et al. that the expression of CysLT$_1$R was higher in colon tumor tissues than in matched normal mucosa [14]. TCGA-COADREAD data also suggests that high expression of the *CYSLTR1* gene and low expression of the *CYSLTR2* gene are associated with a poor prognosis in CRC patients. This finding was supported by the data generated from our earlier publications at the protein level using the patient CRC tumor microarray (TMA), which showed that high protein expression of CysLT$_1$R was associated with poor prognosis and that low protein expression of CysLT$_2$R was positively correlated with poor prognosis in CRC patients [14]. Notably, high expression of CysLT$_1$R was associated with poor prognosis in CRC patients and reduced survival and stemness in colorectal and breast cancer [14,16,17], while CysLT$_2$R has been reported to have an antitumorigenic effect in CRC patients and cell lines [14,35].

Our study is the first to show that the methylation and gene expression profiles for *CYSLTR1*/*CYSLTR2* receptors together to investigate their role in colorectal cancer progression and metastasis using three independent in silico datasets and one clinical cohort. DNA CpG methylation is usually associated with a closed state of chromatin and has been well-accepted as an important mechanism for maintaining gene expression and pathway alteration in diseases [36,37]. Usually, DNA methylation and gene expression are negatively correlated with each other, but very few genes have been reported, and the correlation direction is both positive and negative [38]. It is important to determine the influence of methylation profiles on cancer-associated gene expression. To prove this hypothesis for CysLTRs, we used three independent CRC datasets (TCGA-COADREAD, GSE77955 and E-MTAB-8148), which included methylation and gene expression profiles for each patient.

Here, we investigated the interplay between CpG methylation and gene expression for CysLTRs in CRC progression, metastasis, and patient prognosis. We used the GSE77955 dataset genome-wide deep sequencing to compare the methylomes and transcriptomes of primary CRCs and CRC liver metastases. The methylation profile for *CYSLTR1* genes was used only to establish lung function in asthmatic individuals exposed to traffic-related air pollution and not for any cancer [39]. Although the role of CysLTRs in relation to the development and metastasis of different cancers has been well established, it is important to determine the effect of the methylation profile of CpG probes for CysLTRs on gene expression, cancer progression and metastasis. Interestingly, the high expression of the *CYSLTR1* gene was positively correlated with the more hypomethylated patient group, and the low expression of the *CYSLTR2* gene was significantly correlated with the more hypomethylated patient group.

Based on the annotations from UCSC, the CpG probes for CRC were located on the CpG island (promoter region) and the shore of the *CYSLTR1* and *CYSLTR2* genes, respectively (Supplementary Figure S4). Among all the clinicopathological factors, a history of colon polyps was significantly correlated with *CYSLTR1* gene expression in CRC patients, but the sample type (metastasis, normal and primary tumor) was significantly correlated with *CYSLTR1* and *CYSLTR2* gene expression in colon and rectal cancer patients (Supplementary Figure S4). We observed a significant number of mutations in the *CYSLTR1* and *CYSLTR2* genes in CC, whereas the *CYSLTR1* gene was not mutated in rectal cancer patients. CysLTRs expression was negatively correlated with copy number variation in CRC patients.

The M-values for the CpG probes of *CYSLTR1* (cg00813999 and cg16299590) were significantly decreased and increased, respectively, for advanced-stage patients compared with early-stage patients. Hence, these CpG probes were significantly associated with CRC progression. The activation of LTD_4–$CysLT_1R$ signaling is well-reported to promote cell proliferation and survival through multiple pathways [7,40]. Furthermore, our previous findings showed increased expression of $CysLT_1R$ in patients with CC and the inhibition of LTD_4 signaling by blocking $CysLT_1R$ receptor-induced apoptosis in CC cells [12,41–43]. However, the methylation profile of CysLTRs has not been studied for cancer progression and metastasis. Hence, it is necessary to fill this gap to establish the role of CysLTRs in cancers. Among the most widely used drugs that block the actions of CysLTRs are also those commonly used to treat allergic asthma [44,45]. In addition to its role in asthma, the leukotriene pathway is known to contribute to cancers and tumor-mediated immune suppression [46]. Furthermore, a comprehensive study from Taiwan with two million subjects reported that the use of a $CysLT_1R$ antagonist in asthma patients is associated with a significantly decreased risk of cancer in a dose-dependent manner [9]. A recent study from the United States with more than five million asthma patients (with or without $CysLT_1R$ antagonist treatment) concluded that antagonists reduced the risk of lung cancer by 22% [47].

The disturbance of the E-cadherin–catenin adhesion complex is one of the main events in the early and late stages of cancer [48]. The inhibition of GSK-3β leads to the downregulation of E-cadherin, which can also lead to the cytoplasmic mobilization of β-catenin [49,50]. Relatively little is known about the ability of leukotrienes to regulate tumor cell migration and invasion, but LTB_4 was shown to inhibit metastatic spread to the liver and other organs in an in vivo study of pancreatic cancer [51], and previous results from our laboratory suggested that LTD_4 could induce the cell invasion via modulating the expression of EMT markers [22]. As a result of LTD_4 treatment, E-cadherin (*CDH1*) was downregulated in the plasma membrane, and cell–cell contacts were reduced, whereas montelukast restored the E-cadherin expression to the control levels [22]. Lukic et al., demonstrated that exosomes prepared from lung cancer patient pleura exudates promoted the migration of both A549 lung cancer cells and primary lung cancer cells via CysLTs, whereas the $CysLT_1R$ antagonist montelukast blocked this migration [52]. Interestingly, we observed a significant reduction in E-cadherin in CRC patients with high expression of *CYSLTR1* and low expression of *CYSLTR2*, while *VIM* expression showed the opposite trend. Moreover, *CDH1* and *VIM* expression was significantly increased and decreased, respectively, in the methylated *CYSLTR1* gene. However, it was oppositely regulated for the methylated *CYSLTR2* gene. Hence, EMT might be regulated through the methylation of CysLTRs, ultimately controlling their expression. E-cadherin expression was significantly increased after inhibiting the LTD_4 signaling pathway and β-catenin expression in a SW480 CC cell line, followed by a reduction in cancer cell migration [53]. In this study, we successfully estimated the prediction ability for lymph node metastasis (Figure 3G) and distant metastasis (Figure 3F) in a group of patients using the methylation of the CysLTRs. Therefore, CpG probe methylation of CysLTRs could be a valuable marker for detecting a group of CRC patients with lymph node and distant metastasis. Moreover, in another report, the direct association of $CysLT_1R$ with CRC metastasis was established in a zebrafish model, with less metastatic foci found in the montelukast-treated group compared to the only-LTD_4-treated group [54].

We found a similar trend for methylation and expression of CysLTRs for the metastasis group of patients in the GSE77955 patient cohort. Thus, the distant metastasis samples exhibited reduced methylation and high expression of $CysLT_1R$ and high methylation and reduced expression of $CysLT_2R$. This finding provides direct evidence of the relationship between CysLTRs and metastasis in CRC patients. Moreover, E-cadherin was significantly lower, and vimentin was higher in metastasis samples than in primary tumors for this cohort. Interestingly, the differentially upregulated common genes for the T vs. N, M vs. N and M vs. N groups exhibited higher expression of *CYSLTR1* in primary tumors than in matched normal samples, whereas it was further increased for distant metastasis samples. Therefore, *CYSLTR1* expression might control the expression of other genes involved in the development of metastasis in CRC patients. The methylation profile for CpG probes for CysLTRs also significantly predicted the OS and DFS of CRC patients. The OS curves for cg26848126 (*CYSLTR1*) and cg16299590 (*CYSLTR2*) were significant, and the DFS curves for cg16886259 (*CYSLTR2*) were significant for CRC patients in the TCGA-COADREAD cohort. Hence, the methylation of the *CYSLTR1* and *CYSLTR2* genes could influence OS and DFS in CRC patients, respectively.

Due to the small number of samples in the Malmö–CC clinical cohort, there was no significant correlation between *CDH1* and *VIM* expression and *CYSLTR1* and *CYSLTR2* expression. However, the LTD_4-treated SW620 CC cell-derived colonospheres model exhibited less expression of E-cadherin ($p \leq 0.01$), and *CYSLTR1* knockdown did not significantly increase the E-cadherin expression (Supplementary Figure S3A,B), whereas the expression of vimentin was not significantly changed after LTD_4 treatment or *CYSLTR1* knockdown. As we reported in our previous publications, E-cadherin was decreased by LTD_4 in HCT-116 CC cells [21], and one of the EMT markers, MMP-9, was also induced by LTD_4 in SW480 CC cells [22]. Considering the complexity of the epithelial-to-mesenchymal transition state in cancer, our observations provide some insights into the involvement of methylation and gene expression of $CysLT_1R$ in preparing cells for the transition state without controlling the whole phenomenon.

4. Materials and Methods

4.1. Patient Cohorts

This study included four CRC patient cohorts with a total of 762 patients. These cohorts included patients from three public datasets—the in silico discovery cohort from the Cancer Genome Atlas [TCGA-COADREAD; primary tumor (PT) = 375 and matched normal (N) = 41], the two in silico validation cohorts from the Gene Expression Omnibus (GEO; GSE77955; N = 13; PT = 17; matched distant metastasis, ME = 11 and adenoma from separate patients, AD = 17) and the European Molecular Biology Laboratory—European Bioinformatics Institute (EMBL—EBI, E-MTAB-8148, N = 32 and PT = 216) and one patient-based clinical validation cohort from the Malmö—colon cancer (Malmö-CC; N = 20; PT = 20). All the in silico cohorts are unique because of the availability of genome-wide methylation and transcriptome profiles for all the patients in these cohorts (Table 1).

4.2. Analysis of DNA Methylation in the Cancer Genome TCGA and GSE Cohort

DNA methylation and clinical data for colorectal cancer (COADREAD) were collected from TCGA (International Cancer Genome Consortium) [55]. The data were downloaded from UCSC Xena (http://xena.ucsc.edu, accessed on 23 April 2022) [56]. The DNA methylation profile was measured experimentally using the Illumina Infinium HumanMethylation 450k platform (Illumina, San Diego, CA, USA), which contains 485 577 CpG sites. The methylation level was expressed as β and M-values. Poorly performing probes, cross-reactive probes, and SNP probes were excluded from our data processing. The R function "BMIQ type-II probe normalization" was used to normalize the data between arrays. For validation, the methylation profiles of 58 matched normal, primary tumor and distant metastasis samples were collected from the GSE77955 datasets [57]. The β values of methylation sites with more than 10% missing values were deleted. The remaining missing values were estimated by the k-nearest neighbor (KNN) estimation method. The "limma" package [58] was used to calculate the methylation difference. The sites with an FDR < 0.05 and an absolute β value difference > 0.2 were considered to be differentially methylated. For the correlation analysis of DNA methylation and gene expression, we used the R package "ChAMP" to map the sites assigned to a gene. The Pearson correlation test was used (a correlation coefficient > 0.3 and a $p < 0.05$ were considered to be significant). The correlation coefficients of DMSs were obtained by the Pearson correlation test, and the R package "corplot" was used to plot the correlation between DMSs. The average β and M-values in the promoter and body regions of each gene were calculated (Figure 6A). Positive M values = more molecules methylated than unmethylated, while negative M values are the opposite.

4.3. Analysis of Gene Expression in the Cancer Genome TCGA and GSE Cohorts

Gene expression and clinical data for colorectal cancer (COADREAD) were collected from TCGA. The data were downloaded from UCSC Xena (http://xena.ucsc.edu, accessed on 23 April 2022) [56]. The gene expression profile was measured experimentally using the Illumina HiSeq 2000 RNA sequencing platform (Illumina, San Diego, CA, USA). The mRNA expression levels, measured by reads per million mRNA mapped (RPM), were first log2 transformed. We checked the expression of genes that reached significance ($p \leq 0.05$) and log2 fold change >±1. The differentially regulated genes were represented as upregulated and downregulated in the volcano plot for the GSE77955 dataset. The validation cohort was used to identify differentially regulated cancer and metastasis-related genes in the three groups, matched normal (N) vs. primary tumor samples (PT), PT vs. distant metastasis (ME) and N vs. ME, in CRC patients after performing the "limma"-based differential gene expression (DGE) analysis. Finally, the associated CpG probes and the gene expression profile for the *CYSLTR1* and *CYSLTR2* genes were filtered and used for further analysis (Figure 8A). A detailed flowchart for study designing, included with the analysis and sample information for each cohort are explained in Figure 8B. Two cancer-related receptor genes for CysLT were selected based on gene ontology and cancer hallmark databases (Figure 8C).

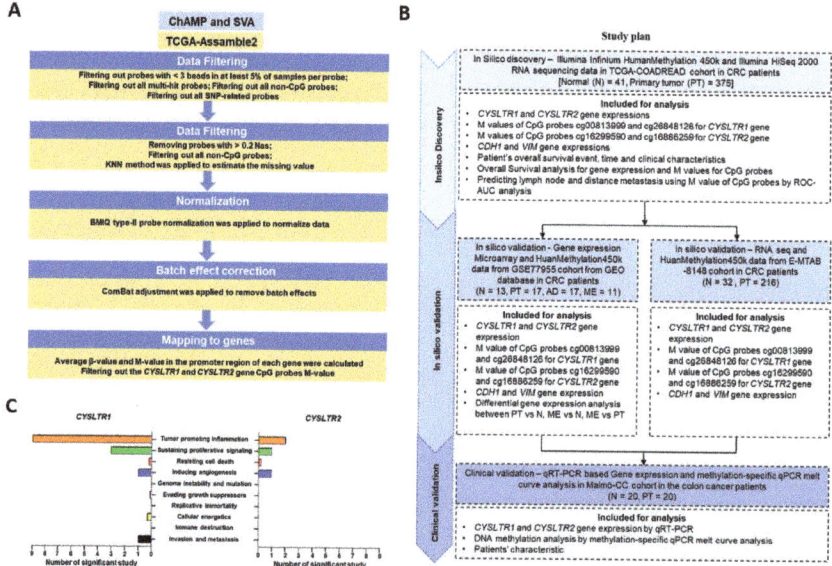

Figure 8. (**A**) Flowchart for CRC-specific DNA methylation data collection from TCGA-COADREAD dataset. (**B**) Flowchart for study designing, normal—N, adenoma—AD, primary tumor—PT and distant metastasis—ME. (**C**) The role of *CYSLTR1* and *CYSLTR2* in different cancer hallmarks based on different datasets and publications (based on the Cancer Hallmarks Analytics Tool (CHAT); http://chat.lionproject.net, accessed on 8 February 2022).

4.4. MSP Primers Designing for DNA Methylation Analysis

CpG sites were studied via the synthesis of oligonucleotide fragments (primers) representing the bisulfite-modified *CYSLTR1* and *CYSLTR2* gene sequences from Integrated DNA Technologies (Supplementary Table S2). Specifically designed primers using the

MethPrimer tool (Li Lab, Dongcheng, Beijing, China) [59] for melt curve analysis amplified methylated as well as unmethylated bisulfite-modified DNA, but not unmodified DNA. To increase the likelihood of amplification of only bisulfite modified template, the primer contained at least one T corresponding to a non-CpG C at the 3'-end of the forward primers. As far as possible, CpGs were avoided, but, when necessary, should be placed at the 5'-end of the primer with a degenerate base. These allow both methylated and unmethylated template amplification. Primers had limited self-complementarity between pairs which was analyzed using OligoAnalyzer™ Tool (https://eu.idtdna.com/pages/tools/oligoanalyzer, accessed on 14 August 2022).

4.5. DNA/RNA Extraction from FFPE Tissue and Bisulfite Modification of Extracted DNA

Nucleic acids (DNA and RNA) were extracted from formalin-fixed paraffin-embedded (FFPE) matched normal and tumor specimens using the previously published protocol after some modifications [60]. Extracted genomic DNA (1 µg) was bisulfite modified using the Epitect Fast Bisulfite Conversion kit (Qiagen, Hilden, Germany). Extracted RNA (1 µg) was converted to cDNA using the RevertAid H Minus First Strand cDNA Synthesis Kit (Thermo Fisher Scientific Inc., Rochester, NY, USA).

4.6. DNA Methylation by qPCR and Melt Curve Analysis

Melt curve analysis was used to identify methylated *CYSLTR1* and *CYSLTR2* genes using the previously published protocol after some modifications [61]. Bisulfite-modified DNA (2 µL) was amplified using Maxima SYBR Green/ROC qPCR master Kit (Thermo Fisher Scientific, Inc. Rochester, NY, USA) containing a final concentration of 0.5 µM of each primer in a final reaction volume of 15 µL. Both primers and PCR conditions were specific for bisulfite-modified DNA and did not produce amplification of unmodified DNA. Every run included fully methylated, fully unmethylated, and no template control. The PCR was performed using a Stratagene Mx3005P qPCR (Agilent Technologies, Santa Clara, CA, USA) with a 95 °C activation step for 10 min; 95 °C for 30 s, 55 °C for 60 s for 40 cycles; and a final extension step of 72 °C for 5 min. In order to melt the PCR product, we increased the temperature from 58 to 92 °C in increments of 0.5 °C, waited for 30 s at the first step and for 5 s at each subsequent step, and acquired fluorescence for each temperature increment.

4.7. qPCR for CYSLTR1, CYSLTR2, CDH1 and VIM Gene Expression

qPCR was used to evaluate the expression profiles of *CYSLTR1* and *CYSLTR2* genes using the Maxima Probe/ROX qPCR Master Mix (Thermo Fisher Scientific Inc., Rochester, NY, USA) and Maxima SYBR Green/ROC qPCR master Kit (Thermo Fisher Scientific Inc., Rochester, NY, USA). TaqMan probes (Thermo Fisher Scientific Inc., Rochester, NY, USA) for the following genes were used in this study: *CYSLTR1* (Hs00929113_m1), *CYSLTR2* (Hs00252658_s1), and *HPRT1* (Hs99999909_m1) and primers for SYBR Green-based qPCR of *CDH1*, *VIM* and *GAPDH* genes are listed in Supplementary Table S2. Normalization was performed using the endogenous housekeeping gene *HPRT1* for TaqMan probes and *GAPDH* for SYBR Green. MxPro software (Agilent Technologies, Santa Clara, CA, USA) was used to quantify fold changes using the $2^{-\Delta\Delta Ct}$ method.

4.8. CRISPR-Cas9 Based Knockdown of CysLT$_1$R

CRISPR-Cas9 based knockdown of *CYSLTR1* in SW620 CC cells was achieved using the protocol from Satapathy et al. [54]. Briefly, after transfection of cells with either *Cas9-CTRL* or *CRISPR-CYSLTR1* using lipofectamine, 2000, cells were subjected to antibiotic selection. *Cas9-CTRL* (sc-418922; Control *CRISPR/Cas9* Plasmid); *CRISPR-Cas9* for *CYSLTR1* (sc-416516; Santacruz Biotechnology, Heidelberg, Germany) were used for the *CYSLTR1* knockdown. Selected colonies were expanded and used for the colonosphere formation.

4.9. SW620 Cells Colonosphere Formation and Western Blot Analysis

SW620 CC cell-derived colonospheres were formed using the protocol described earlier [53,61]. Briefly, cells were counted after trypsinization and approximately 1000 cells were seeded per well in ultra-low attachment round bottom plates (7007; Corning Inc., Corning, NY, USA). For the formation of colonospheres, DMEM-F12 medium supplemented with L-glutamine and antibiotics was used. After 3 weeks colonospheres were collected from each well and protein was extracted using RIPA lysis buffer. Extracted protein was used for western blot analysis of the following proteins: E-Cadherin (#3195, Cell Signaling Technology, Danvers, MA, USA); vimentin (#5741, Cell Signaling Technology, Danvers, MA, USA); CysLT$_1$R (NBP2-92396; Novus Biologicals, Centennial, CO, USA). α-Tubulin (sc-8035; Santa Cruz Biotechnology, Heidelberg, Germany) antibodies were used for western blot experiment [54,62].

4.10. Statistical Analysis and Data Visualization

Statistical analyses were performed using IBM SPSS version 20 (IBM, Chicago, IL, USA), MedCalc version 18 (MedCalc Software Ltd., Ostend, Belgium), GraphPad Prism version 8.0 (La Jolla, CA, USA) and R 3.2.4 (The R Foundation, Indianapolis, IN, United States). Statistical differences between mRNAs and various clinicopathologic factors were determined by the χ^2 test. The Benjamini–Hochberg method was used to correct for multiple hypothesis testing wherever applicable. All statistical tests were two-sided, and a $p \leq 0.05$ was considered significant. OS was defined from the day of surgery to death or the end of follow-up and was analyzed by the log-rank test. We performed receiver operating characteristic (ROC) curve analysis to evaluate the predictive power of the selected gene signature. mRNA expression values for *CYSLTR1* and *CYSLTR2* derived from the transcriptome datasets were used to build an overall survival classifier (OSC) using Cox proportional hazard regression. The risk scores derived from the five-gene OSC Cox model were used to plot the area under the curve (AUC). The risk scores were calculated using the formula derived from the Cox model. To evaluate the association of gene expression and methylation status in CRC samples with OS, univariate and multivariate Cox proportional hazard regression models were applied, and hazard ratios (HRs) together with 95% confidence intervals (CIs) were calculated to determine the risk of death or cancer recurrence. The multivariate model was adjusted for established prognostic factors such as age, sex, lymph node metastasis (LNM) tumor-node-metastasis (TNM) stage, and tumor size. All patients with incomplete or missing clinical information were excluded from the analysis. To plot the Kaplan–Meier curves, we dichotomized the patients into low- and high-risk groups based on Youden index-derived cutoff values (X-tile software 3.6.1, Rimm Lab, Yale School of Medicine, New Haven, CT, USA). The differences in mRNA levels between normal, tumor and metastasis samples from CRC patients were assessed using a t-test for paired and unpaired data. We performed ROC curve analysis to evaluate the predicted values for lymph node and distant metastasis. M-values for all four CpG sites were used to build a signature for the lymph node and distant metastasis group classifier using a logistic regression model. The risk scores derived from the four-CpG-probe M-values and a logistic model were used to plot the AUCs. Venn diagrams for significant DEGs and heatmaps were generated using the "VennDiagram" and "Plotly" packages, respectively.

5. Conclusions

In conclusion, this study first elucidates the oncogenic role of hypomethylation- and hypermethylation-mediated regulation of *CYSLTR1* and *CYSLTR2* expression in CRC, respectively. Moreover, our discovery of *CYSLTR1* and *CYSLTR2* as novel prognostic, lymph node and distant metastasis predictive markers provides important evidence for the clinical significance of the expression and methylation profile of these two CysLTRs in patients with CRC. Further validation of these results in multicenter CRC cohorts could lead to the development of affordable, noninvasive prognostic and predictive markers and population screening assays for CRC patients.

Supplementary Materials: The following supporting information can be downloaded at: https://www.mdpi.com/article/10.3390/ijms24043409/s1.

Author Contributions: Conceptualization, S.G., S.R.S. and A.S.; methodology, S.G. and S.R.S.; writing—original draft preparation, S.G., S.R.S. and A.S.; writing—review and editing, S.G., S.R.S. and A.S.; supervision, A.S.; funding acquisition, A.S. All authors have read and agreed to the published version of the manuscript.

Funding: This work was supported by grants to A.S. from the Swedish Cancer Foundation, Sweden (Grant number: CAN 21 1453), the Malmö University Hospital Cancer Foundation, and by Governmental Funding of Clinical Research within the national health services and grants to S.G. and S.R.S. from the Royal Physiographic Society in Lund, Sweden.

Institutional Review Board Statement: Not applicable.

Informed Consent Statement: Not applicable.

Data Availability Statement: The datasets used and/or analyzed during the current study are available from the corresponding author on request.

Acknowledgments: We would like to acknowledge the Swedish Cancer Foundation, Sweden; and the Foundations at Skåne University Hospital, Sweden, for funding.

Conflicts of Interest: The authors declare no conflict of interest.

References

1. Siegel, R.L.; Miller, K.D.; Fuchs, H.E.; Jemal, A. Cancer statistics. *CA Cancer J. Clin.* **2022**, *72*, 7–33. [CrossRef] [PubMed]
2. Miller, K.D.; Nogueira, L.; Devasia, T.; Mariotto, A.B.; Yabroff, K.R.; Jemal, A.; Kramer, J.; Siegel, R.L. Cancer treatment and survivorship statistics, 2022. *CA Cancer J. Clin.* **2022**, *72*, 409–436. [CrossRef] [PubMed]
3. Luo, M.; Lee, S.; Brock, T.G. Leukotriene synthesis by epithelial cells. *Histol. Histopathol.* **2003**, *118*, 587–595. [CrossRef]
4. Tian, W.; Jiang, X.; Kim, D.; Guan, T.; Nicolls, M.R.; Rockson, S.G. Leukotrienes in Tumor-Associated Inflammation. *Front. Pharmacol.* **2020**, *11*, 1289. [CrossRef] [PubMed]
5. Yokomizo, T.; Nakamura, M.; Shimizu, T. Leukotriene receptors as potential therapeutic targets. *J. Clin. Investig.* **2018**, *128*, 2691–2701. [CrossRef] [PubMed]
6. Slater, K.; Hoo, P.S.; Buckley, A.M.; Piulats, J.M.; Villanueva, A.; Portela, A.; Kennedy, B.N. Evaluation of oncogenic cysteinyl leukotriene receptor 2 as a therapeutic target for uveal melanoma. *Cancer Metastasis Rev.* **2018**, *37*, 335–345. [CrossRef]
7. Burke, L.; Butler, C.T.; Murphy, A.; Moran, B.; Gallagher, W.M.; O'Sullivan, J.; Kennedy, B.N. Evaluation of Cysteinyl Leukotriene Signaling as a Therapeutic Target for Colorectal Cancer. *Front. Cell Dev. Biol.* **2016**, *4*, 103. [CrossRef] [PubMed]
8. Duah, E.; Teegala, L.R.; Kondeti, V.; Adapala, R.K.; Keshamouni, V.G.; Kanaoka, Y.; Austen, K.F.; Thodeti, C.K.; Paruchuri, S. Cysteinyl leukotriene 2 receptor promotes endothelial permeability, tumor angiogenesis, and metastasis. *Proc. Natl. Acad. Sci. USA* **2019**, *116*, 199–204. [CrossRef] [PubMed]
9. Tsai, M.-J.; Wu, P.-H.; Sheu, C.-C.; Hsu, Y.-L.; Chang, W.-A.; Hung, J.-Y.; Yang, C.-J.; Yang, Y.-H.; Kuo, P.-L.; Huang, M.-S. Cysteinyl Leukotriene Receptor Antagonists Decrease Cancer Risk in Asthma Patients. *Sci. Rep.* **2016**, *6*, 23979. [CrossRef]
10. Kawahito, Y.; Sano, H.; Nakatani, T.; Yoshimura, R.; Naganuma, T.; Funao, K.; Matsuyama, M. The cysteinylLT1 receptor in human renal cell carcinoma. *Mol. Med. Rep.* **2008**, *1*, 185–189. [CrossRef]
11. Matsuyama, M.; Funao, K.; Kawahito, Y.; Sano, H.; Chargui, J.; Touraine, J.-L.; Nakatani, T.; Yoshimura, R. Expression of cysteinylLT1 receptor in human testicular cancer and growth reduction by its antagonist through apoptosis. *Mol. Med. Rep.* **2009**, *2*, 163–167. [CrossRef] [PubMed]
12. Matsuyama, M.; Funao, K.; Hayama, T.; Tanaka, T.; Kawahito, Y.; Sano, H.; Takemoto, Y.; Nakatani, T.; Yoshimura, R. Relationship Between Cysteinyl-Leukotriene-1 Receptor and Human Transitional Cell Carcinoma in Bladder. *Urology* **2009**, *73*, 916–921. [CrossRef] [PubMed]
13. Nielsen, C.K.; Öhd, J.F.; Wikström, K.; Massoumi, R.; Paruchuri, S.; Juhas, M.; Sjölander, A. The Leukotriene Receptor CYSLT1 And 5- Lipoxygenase Are Upregulated In Colon Cancer. *Adv. Exp. Med. Biol.* **2003**, *525*, 201–204. [CrossRef] [PubMed]
14. Magnusson, C.; Mezhybovska, M.; Lörinc, E.; Fernebro, E.; Nilbert, M.; Sjölander, A. Low expression of CysLT1R and high expression of CysLT2R mediate good prognosis in colorectal cancer. *Eur. J. Cancer* **2010**, *46*, 826–835. [CrossRef]
15. Mehrabi, S.F.; Ghatak, S.; Mehdawi, L.M.; Topi, G.; Satapathy, S.R.; Sjölander, A. Brain-Derived Neurotrophic Factor, Neutrophils and Cysteinyl Leukotriene Receptor 1 as Potential Prognostic Biomarkers for Patients with Colon Cancer. *Cancers* **2021**, *13*, 5520. [CrossRef]
16. Magnusson, C.; Liu, J.; Ehrnström, R.; Manjer, J.; Jirström, K.; Andersson, T.; Sjölander, A. Cysteinyl leukotriene receptor expression pattern affects migration of breast cancer cells and survival of breast cancer patients. *Int. J. Cancer* **2011**, *129*, 9–22. [CrossRef]

17. Bellamkonda, K.; Satapathy, S.R.; Douglas, D.; Chandrashekar, N.; Selvanesan, B.C.; Liu, M.; Savari, S.; Jonsson, G.; Sjölander, A. Montelukast, a CysLT1 receptor antagonist, reduces colon cancer stemness and tumor burden in a mouse xenograft model of human colon cancer. *Cancer Lett.* **2018**, *437*, 13–24. [CrossRef]
18. Moore, A.R.; Ceraudo, E.; Sher, J.J.; Guan, Y.; Shoushtari, A.N.; Chang, M.T.; Zhang, J.Q.; Walczak, E.G.; Kazmi, M.A.; Taylor, B.S.; et al. Recurrent activating mutations of G-protein-coupled receptor CYSLTR2 in uveal melanoma. *Nat. Genet.* **2016**, *48*, 675–680. [CrossRef]
19. Van de Nes, J.A.; Koelsche, C.; Gessi, M.; Möller, I.; Sucker, A.; Scolyer, R.A.; Buckland, M.E.; Pietsch, T.; Murali, R.; Schadendorf, D.; et al. Activating CYSLTR2 and PLCB4 Mutations in Primary Leptomeningeal Melanocytic Tumors. *J. Investig. Dermatol.* **2017**, *137*, 2033–2035. [CrossRef]
20. Ye, Z.; Zhou, M.; Tian, B.; Wu, B.; Li, J. Expression of lncRNA-CCAT1, E-cadherin and N-cadherin in colorectal cancer and its clinical significance. *Int. J. Clin. Exp. Med.* **2015**, *8*, 3707–3715.
21. Salim, T.; Sand-Dejmek, J.; Sjölander, A. The inflammatory mediator leukotriene D4 induces subcellular β-catenin translocation and migration of colon cancer cells. *Exp. Cell Res.* **2014**, *321*, 255–266. [CrossRef] [PubMed]
22. Vinnakota, K.; Zhang, Y.; Selvanesan, B.C.; Topi, G.; Salim, T.; Sand-Dejmek, J.; Jönsson, G.; Sjölander, A. M2-like macrophages induce colon cancer cell invasion via matrix metalloproteinases. *J. Cell. Physiol.* **2017**, *232*, 3468–3480. [CrossRef] [PubMed]
23. McGovern, T.; Goldberger, M.; Chen, M.; Allard, B.; Hamamoto, Y.; Kanaoka, Y.; Austen, K.F.; Powell, W.S.; Martin, J.G. CysLT1 Receptor Is Protective against Oxidative Stress in a Model of Irritant-Induced Asthma. *J. Immunol.* **2016**, *197*, 266–277. [CrossRef] [PubMed]
24. Jin, Z.; Liu, Y. DNA methylation in human diseases. *Genes Dis.* **2018**, *5*, 1–8. [CrossRef] [PubMed]
25. Hao, X.; Luo, H.; Krawczyk, M.; Wei, W.; Wang, W.; Wang, J.; Flagg, K.; Hou, J.; Zhang, H.; Yi, S.; et al. DNA methylation markers for diagnosis and prognosis of common cancers. *Proc. Natl. Acad. Sci. USA* **2017**, *114*, 7414–7419. [CrossRef]
26. Díez-Villanueva, A.; Sanz-Pamplona, R.; Carreras-Torres, R.; Moratalla-Navarro, F.; Alonso, M.H.; Pare, L.; Aussó, S.; Guinó, E.; Solé, X.; Cordero, D.; et al. DNA methylation events in transcription factors and gene expression changes in colon cancer. *Epigenomics* **2020**, *12*, 1593–1610. [CrossRef]
27. Zhang, H.; Sun, X.; Lu, Y.; Wu, J.; Feng, J. DNA-methylated gene markers for colorectal cancer in TCGA database. *Exp. Ther. Med.* **2020**, *19*, 3042–3050. [CrossRef]
28. Wajed, S.A.; Laird, P.W.; Demeester, T.R. DNA Methylation: An Alternative Pathway to Cancer. *Ann. Surg.* **2001**, *234*, 10–20. [CrossRef]
29. Zhang, J.; Huang, K. Pan-cancer analysis of frequent DNA co-methylation patterns reveals consistent epigenetic landscape changes in multiple cancers. *BMC Genom.* **2017**, *18*, 1045. [CrossRef]
30. Ding, W.; Chen, G.; Shi, T. Integrative analysis identifies potential DNA methylation biomarkers for pan-cancer diagnosis and prognosis. *Epigenetics* **2019**, *14*, 67–80. [CrossRef]
31. Tang, W.; Wan, S.; Yang, Z.; Teschendorff, A.E.; Zou, Q. Tumor origin detection with tissue-specific miRNA and DNA methylation markers. *Bioinformatics* **2018**, *34*, 398–406. [CrossRef] [PubMed]
32. Irizarry, R.A.; Ladd-Acosta, C.; Wen, B.; Wu, Z.; Montano, C.; Onyango, P.; Cui, H.; Gabo, K.; Rongione, M.; Webster, M.; et al. The human colon cancer methylome shows similar hypo- and hypermethylation at conserved tissue-specific CpG island shores. *Nat. Genet.* **2009**, *41*, 178–186. [CrossRef] [PubMed]
33. Feng, Z.; Liu, Z.; Peng, K.; Wu, W. A Prognostic Model Based on Nine DNA Methylation-Driven Genes Predicts Overall Survival for Colorectal Cancer. *Front. Genet.* **2021**, *12*, 779383. [CrossRef] [PubMed]
34. Tsai, M.-J.; Chang, W.-A.; Chuang, C.-H.; Wu, K.-L.; Cheng, C.-H.; Sheu, C.-C.; Hsu, Y.-L.; Hung, J.-Y. Cysteinyl Leukotriene Pathway and Cancer. *Int. J. Mol. Sci.* **2022**, *23*, 120. [CrossRef]
35. Mehdawi, L.M.; Satapathy, S.R.; Gustafsson, A.; Lundholm, K.; Alvarado-Kristensson, M.; Sjölander, A. A potential anti-tumor effect of leukotriene C4 through the induction of 15-hydroxyprostaglandin dehydrogenase expression in colon cancer cells. *Oncotarget* **2017**, *8*, 35033–35047. [CrossRef]
36. Lande-Diner, L.; Cedar, H. Silence of the genes—mechanisms of long-term repression. *Nat. Rev. Genet.* **2005**, *6*, 648–654. [CrossRef]
37. Zaidi, S.K.; Van Wijnen, A.J.; Lian, J.B.; Stein, J.L.; Stein, G.S. Targeting deregulated epigenetic control in cancer. *J. Cell. Physiol.* **2013**, *228*, 2103–2108. [CrossRef]
38. Lee, K.; Moon, S.; Park, M.-J.; Koh, I.-U.; Choi, N.-H.; Yu, H.-Y.; Kim, Y.J.; Kong, J.; Kang, H.G.; Kim, S.C.; et al. Integrated Analysis of Tissue-Specific Promoter Methylation and Gene Expression Profile in Complex Diseases. *Int. J. Mol. Sci.* **2020**, *21*, 5056. [CrossRef]
39. Rabinovitch, N.; Jones, M.J.; Gladish, N.; Faino, A.V.; Strand, M.; Morin, A.M.; MacIsaac, J.; Lin, D.T.S.; Reynolds, P.R.; Singh, A.; et al. Methylation of cysteinyl leukotriene receptor 1 genes associates with lung function in asthmatics exposed to traffic-related air pollution. *Epigenetics* **2021**, *16*, 177–185. [CrossRef]
40. Öhd, J.F.; Nielsen, C.K.; Campbell, J.; Landberg, G.; Löfberg, H.; Sjölander, A. Expression of the leukotriene D4 receptor CysLT1, COX-2, and other cell survival factors in colorectal adenocarcinomas. *Gastroenterology* **2003**, *124*, 57–70. [CrossRef]
41. Nielsen, C.K.; Campbell, J.I.; Öhd, J.F.; Mörgelin, M.; Riesbeck, K.; Landberg, G.; Sjölander, A. A Novel Localization of the G-Protein-Coupled CysLT1 Receptor in the Nucleus of Colorectal Adenocarcinoma Cells. *Cancer Res.* **2005**, *65*, 732–742. [CrossRef] [PubMed]

42. Matsuyama, M.; Hayama, T.; Funao, K.; Kawahito, Y.; Sano, H.; Takemoto, Y.; Nakatani, T.; Yoshimura, R. Overexpression of cysteinyl LT1 receptor in prostate cancer and CysLT1R antagonist inhibits prostate cancer cell growth through apoptosis. *Oncol. Rep.* **2007**, *18*, 99–104. [CrossRef] [PubMed]
43. Savari, S.; Chandrashekar, N.K.; Osman, J.; Douglas, D.; Bellamkonda, K.; Jönsson, G.; Juhas, M.; Greicius, G.; Pettersson, S.; Sjölander, A. Cysteinyl leukotriene 1 receptor influences intestinal polyp incidence in a gender-specific manner in the ApcMin/+mouse model. *Carcinogenesis* **2016**, *37*, 491–499. [CrossRef]
44. Szabo, E.; Mao, J.T.; Lam, S.; Reid, M.E.; Keith, R.L. Chemoprevention of Lung Cancer: Diagnosis and management of lung cancer, 3rd ed: American College of Chest Physicians evidence-based clinical practice guidelines. *Chest* **2013**, *143*, e40S–e60S. [CrossRef] [PubMed]
45. Scott, J.P.; Peters-Golden, M. Antileukotriene Agents for the Treatment of Lung Disease. *Am. J. Respir. Crit. Care Med.* **2013**, *188*, 538–544. [CrossRef]
46. Wang, D.; DuBois, R.N. Eicosanoids and cancer. *Nat. Rev. Cancer* **2010**, *10*, 181–193. [CrossRef] [PubMed]
47. Sutton, S.S.; Magagnoli, J.; Cummings, T.H.; Hardin, J.W. Leukotriene inhibition and the risk of lung cancer among U.S. veterans with asthma. *Pulm. Pharmacol. Ther.* **2021**, *71*, 102084. [CrossRef]
48. Wijnhoven, B.P.L.; Dinjens, W.N.M.; Pignatelli, M. E-cadherin—Catenin cell—Cell adhesion complex and human cancer. *Br. J. Surg.* **2000**, *87*, 992–1005. [CrossRef]
49. McCubrey, J.A.; Steelman, L.S.; Bertrand, F.E.; Davis, N.M.; Sokolosky, M.; Abrams, S.L.; Montalto, G.; D'Assoro, A.B.; Libra, M.; Nicoletti, F.; et al. GSK-3 as potential target for therapeutic intervention in cancer. *Oncotarget* **2014**, *5*, 2881–2911. [CrossRef]
50. Zhou, B.P.; Deng, J.; Xia, W.; Xu, J.; Li, Y.M.; Gunduz, M.C.; Hung, M.-C. Dual regulation of Snail by GSK-3β-mediated phosphorylation in control of epithelial–mesenchymal transition. *Nat. Cell Biol.* **2004**, *6*, 931–940. [CrossRef]
51. Hennig, R.; Ventura, J.; Segersvärd, R.; Ward, E.; Ding, X.-Z.; Rao, S.M.; Jovanovic, B.D.; Iwamura, T.; Talamonti, M.S.; Bell, R.H., Jr.; et al. LY293111 Improves Efficacy of Gemcitabine Therapy on Pancreatic Cancer in a Fluorescent Orthotopic Model in Athymic Mice. *Neoplasia* **2005**, *7*, 417–425. [CrossRef] [PubMed]
52. Lukic, A.; Wahlund, C.J.; Gómez, C.; Brodin, D.; Samuelsson, B.; Wheelock, C.E.; Gabrielsson, S.; Rådmark, O. Exosomes and cells from lung cancer pleural exudates transform LTC4 to LTD4, promoting cell migration and survival via CysLT1. *Cancer Lett.* **2019**, *444*, 1–8. [CrossRef] [PubMed]
53. Park, S.Y.; Lee, S.-J.; Cho, H.J.; Kim, T.W.; Kim, J.-T.; Kim, J.W.; Lee, C.-H.; Kim, B.-Y.; Yeom, Y.I.; Lim, J.-S.; et al. Dehydropeptidase 1 promotes metastasis through regulation of E-cadherin expression in colon cancer. *Oncotarget* **2016**, *7*, 9501–9512. [CrossRef]
54. Satapathy, S.R.; Sjölander, A. Cysteinyl leukotriene receptor 1 promotes 5-fluorouracil resistance and resistance-derived stemness in colon cancer cells. *Cancer Lett.* **2020**, *488*, 50–62. [CrossRef] [PubMed]
55. The Cancer Genome Atlas Research Network; Weinstein, J.N.; Collisson, E.A.; Mills, G.B.; Shaw, K.R.M.; Ozenberger, B.A.; Ellrott, K.; Shmulevich, I.; Sander, C.; Stuart, J.M. The Cancer Genome Atlas Pan-Cancer analysis project. *Nat. Genet.* **2013**, *45*, 1113–1120. [CrossRef] [PubMed]
56. Goldman, M.J.; Craft, B.; Hastie, M.; Repečka, K.; McDade, F.; Kamath, A.; Banerjee, A.; Luo, Y.; Rogers, D.; Brooks, A.N.; et al. Visualizing and interpreting cancer genomics data via the Xena platform. *Nat. Biotechnol.* **2020**, *38*, 675–678. [CrossRef]
57. Qu, X.; Sandmann, T.; Frierson, H., Jr.; Fu, L.; Fuentes, E.; Walter, K.; Okrah, K.; Rumpel, C.; Moskaluk, C.; Lu, S.; et al. Integrated genomic analysis of colorectal cancer progression reveals activation of EGFR through demethylation of the EREG promoter. *Oncogene* **2016**, *35*, 6403–6415. [CrossRef]
58. Tjärnberg, A.; Mahmood, O.; Jackson, C.A.; Saldi, G.-A.; Cho, K.; Christiaen, L.A.; Bonneau, R.A. Optimal tuning of weighted kNN- and diffusion-based methods for denoising single cell genomics data. *PLOS Comput. Biol.* **2021**, *17*, e1008569. [CrossRef]
59. Li, L.-C.; Dahiya, R. MethPrimer: Designing primers for methylation PCRs. *Bioinformatics* **2002**, *18*, 1427–1431. [CrossRef]
60. Ghatak, S.; Sanga, Z.; Pautu, J.L.; Kumar, N.S. Coextraction and PCR Based Analysis of Nucleic Acids from Formalin-Fixed Paraffin-Embedded Specimens. *J. Clin. Lab. Anal.* **2015**, *29*, 485–492. [CrossRef]
61. Smith, E.; Jones, M.E.; Drew, P.A. Quantitation of DNA methylation by melt curve analysis. *BMC Cancer* **2009**, *9*, 123. [CrossRef] [PubMed]
62. Satapathy, S.R.; Topi, G.; Osman, J.; Hellman, K.; Ek, F.; Olsson, R.; Sime, W.; Mehdawi, L.M.; Sjölander, A. Tumour suppressor 15-hydroxyprostaglandin dehydrogenase induces differentiation in colon cancer via GLI1 inhibition. *Oncogenesis* **2020**, *9*, 74. [CrossRef] [PubMed]

Disclaimer/Publisher's Note: The statements, opinions and data contained in all publications are solely those of the individual author(s) and contributor(s) and not of MDPI and/or the editor(s). MDPI and/or the editor(s) disclaim responsibility for any injury to people or property resulting from any ideas, methods, instructions or products referred to in the content.

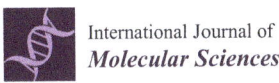

Article

Genomic Analysis of Waterpipe Smoke-Induced Lung Tumor Autophagy and Plasticity

Rania Faouzi Zaarour [1], Mohak Sharda [2,3], Bilal Azakir [4], Goutham Hassan Venkatesh [1], Raefa Abou Khouzam [1], Ayesha Rifath [1], Zohra Nausheen Nizami [1], Fatima Abdullah [1], Fatin Mohammad [1], Hajar Karaali [4], Husam Nawafleh [1], Yehya Elsayed [5] and Salem Chouaib [1,6,*]

1. Thumbay Research Institute for Precision Medicine, Gulf Medical University, Ajman 4184, United Arab Emirates; dr.rania@gmu.ac.ae (R.F.Z.); gouthamhv@gmail.com (G.H.V.); dr.raefa@gmu.ac.ae (R.A.K.); ayesha@gmu.ac.ae (A.R.); zohranausheennizami@gmail.com (Z.N.N.); 2017bm10@mygmu.ac.ae (F.A.); 2017bm07@mygmu.ac.ae (F.M.); husam@gmu.ac.ae (H.N.)
2. National Center for Biological Sciences, Tata Institute of Fundamental Research, Bangalore 560065, India; mohaks@ncbs.res.in
3. School of Life Science, The University of Trans-Disciplinary Health Sciences & Technology (TDU), Bangalore 560064, India
4. Molecular and Translational Medicine Laboratory, Faculty of Medicine, Beirut Arab University, Beirut 11072809, Lebanon; b.azakir@bau.edu.lb (B.A.); hajar.karaali@hotmail.com (H.K.)
5. Department of Biology, Chemistry and Environmental Sciences (BCE), American University of Sharjah, Sharjah 26666, United Arab Emirates; yehyaelsayed@gmail.com
6. Inserm Umr 1186, Integrative Tumor Immunology and Immunotherapy, Gustave Roussy, Faculty of Medicine, University Paris-Saclay, 94805 Villejuif, France
* Correspondence: salem.chouaib@gmu.ac.ae

Abstract: The role of autophagy in lung cancer cells exposed to waterpipe smoke (WPS) is not known. Because of the important role of autophagy in tumor resistance and progression, we investigated its relationship with WP smoking. We first showed that WPS activated autophagy, as reflected by LC3 processing, in lung cancer cell lines. The autophagy response in smokers with lung adenocarcinoma, as compared to non-smokers with lung adenocarcinoma, was investigated further using the TCGA lung adenocarcinoma bulk RNA-seq dataset with the available patient metadata on smoking status. The results, based on a machine learning classification model using Random Forest, indicate that smokers have an increase in autophagy-activating genes. Comparative analysis of lung adenocarcinoma molecular signatures in affected patients with a long-term active exposure to smoke compared to non-smoker patients indicates a higher tumor mutational burden, a higher CD8+ T-cell level and a lower dysfunction level in smokers. While the expression of the checkpoint genes tested—PD-1, PD-L1, PD-L2 and CTLA-4—remains unchanged between smokers and non-smokers, B7-1, B7-2, IDO1 and CD200R1 were found to be higher in non-smokers than smokers. Because multiple factors in the tumor microenvironment dictate the success of immunotherapy, in addition to the expression of immune checkpoint genes, our analysis explains why patients who are smokers with lung adenocarcinoma respond better to immunotherapy, even though there are no relative differences in immune checkpoint genes in the two groups. Therefore, targeting autophagy in lung adenocarcinoma patients, in combination with checkpoint inhibitor-targeted therapies or chemotherapy, should be considered in smoker patients with lung adenocarcinoma.

Keywords: autophagy; tumor mutational burden; tumor microenvironment; waterpipe smoke; lung cancer

1. Introduction

Lung cancer is the second most common diagnosed type of cancer in men and women, after prostate and breast cancers, respectively [1]. The greatest number of deaths are due to cancers of the lung, which account for 25% of all cancer-related deaths [1]. Tobacco smoking is the most common cause for lung cancer [2]. One type of tobacco smoking is waterpipe smoking (WPS), where the smoke of the tobacco passes through water prior to being inhaled. WP use is on the rise globally [3], and there is a strong link between WPS and lung cancer [4,5]. Because of the toxicants present in WPS, smokers are exposed to a large amount and variety of chemicals, including many carcinogens [6,7]. WPS has been shown to result in the generation of free radicals, reactive oxygen species (ROS) and inflammation [8–10].

Previous studies have shown that WPS condensate (WPSC) treatment of lung cancer cell lines modulates cell plasticity. WPSC induced epithelial to mesenchymal transition (EMT), cancer stem cell (CSC) features, and an increase in inflammation and DNA damage [11,12]. The consequences of DNA damage depend on the cell type and on the extent and intensity of the stress and could activate senescence, autophagy, or cell death programs. Apoptosis functions to suppress tumor growth, while autophagy can be activated in different cells at different stages of tumor growth and has paradoxical roles as it can suppress or promote tumor growth depending on the type and stage of the tumor [13]. While apoptosis fulfills its role through dismantling damaged or unwanted cells, autophagy maintains cellular homeostasis through recycling selective intracellular organelles and molecules. Autophagy is activated by different metabolic stressors in the tumor microenvironment (TME), including hypoxia, nutrient deprivation, and inflammation. In the context of WPS, nicotine present in WPS and in cigarette smoke has been shown to induce bronchial epithelial cell apoptosis, senescence, and autophagy impairment in normal lung epithelial cells post treatment for up to 6 h [14–16].

The molecular switch between cell death and cell survival is a key determinant of cell fate and cancer progression. Tumor mutational burden (TMB) rises because of DNA damage response and repair gene alterations, which have direct implications on the immune cells' landscape. An increase in TMB is associated with a favorable response to immune checkpoint inhibitors (ICI) [17] as this can increase immunogenic neoantigen production and its subsequent presentation by antigen-presenting cells, such as dendritic cells (DCs), to CD8+ T-cells, thus promoting their anticancer activity [18]. ICI have been increasingly used in the treatment of non-small cell lung cancer (NSCLC), enhancing response rates and long-term survival but only in a fraction of treated patients [19,20]. The most used ICI-based therapy is anti-PD-1 or anti-PD-L1, which work to block the inhibitory signaling between PD-1, present on the surface of activated T cells, and its ligand PD-L1, expressed on tumor cells [21]. The aim is to revitalize the immune response and eliminate tumor cells. Currently, the application of ICI in NSCLC is determined based on high microsatellite instability (MSI), TMB, PD-L1 expression, and disease burden [20]. These determinants are clearly insufficient to ensure patient response, and other factors in the TME could additionally be involved. Indeed, the TME is a collection of cellular components, including tumor, immune, and endothelial cells, as well as non-cellular components, such as extracellular matrix and signaling factors, cytokines, and chemokines, all of which are functioning together in acidic, hypoxic and nutrient-deprived conditions [22]. Tumor-promoting immune cells, such as myeloid-derived suppressor cells (MDSCs), M2 macrophages and regulatory T cells (Tregs), tend to thrive in such an environment, while tumor antagonizing-cells, including CD8+ T cells and natural killer (NK) cells, tend to be inhibited or even excluded from the tumor site [22]. A better understanding of how these features merge in lung adenocarcinoma patients exposed to smoke is needed to better delineate their response rates following immunotherapy.

Our study addresses the role of WPS on autophagy, on TMB in lung cancer cell lines and using TCGA datasets of lung adenocarcinoma patients with a history of smoking. We further investigated the immunological landscape in these datasets. In vitro, we observed an increase in apoptosis at early exposure times followed by an activation of autophagy at longer treatment duration. Long-term exposure up to 6 months in lung cancer cell lines identified an increase in TMB that was also depicted in our analysis of TCGA datasets. Further analysis of the immune landscape of lung adenocarcinoma patients identified no change in immune checkpoint inhibitors between smokers and non-smokers. We also observed an increase in NK cells and CD8+ T cells, coupled by lower T-cell dysfunction. However, there were lower dendritic cell numbers. The current studies point to autophagy as a potential target for treatment of lung adenocarcinoma patients with a history of smoking. Our results are suggestive of better prognosis of smokers with lung adenocarcinoma post immunotherapy treatment.

2. Results

2.1. Waterpipe Smoke Condensate Increases Apoptosis and Activates Autophagy in Lung Cancer Cell Lines

We first investigated the cytotoxic effects of waterpipe smoke condensate (WPSC) and its impact on autophagy. For this purpose, both A549 and H460 lung cancer cell lines were treated with 0.5% WPSC. This WPSC concentration was previously found to cause only a small fraction of A549 and H460 cells to die [11]. Cell viability using the MTT assay at 24, 48 and 72 h was measured. As depicted in Figure 1A,B, A549 cells displayed reduced viability in response to WPSC, whereas H460 cells did not up till 72 h of treatment. The vacuolar (H+) ATPase (V-ATPase) inhibitor Bafilomycin A1 (BafA1) was used to inhibit autophagy [23]. We observed a decrease in cell viability in response to 100 nM of BafA1 in both cell lines. The concomitant treatment of BafA1 and WPSC resulted in an additive negative effect on cell viability that was significant at 72 h, indicating that autophagy pathways could be contributing to cell survival following WPSC treatment.

Autophagy and apoptosis are both important in maintaining cellular homeostasis. Stress-inducing signals influence both apoptosis and autophagy, and while functionally distinct, a crosstalk between the two could play an important role in pathological processes, including cancer. As we observed a decrease in cell viability following WPSC treatment, we asked whether apoptosis was activated. Treating A549 and H460 cells with 0.5% WPSC up to 5 days (120 h) resulted in a decrease in cell viability with a gradual increase in apoptosis as measured by an increase in Annexin V/PI positive cells (Figure 1C–F).

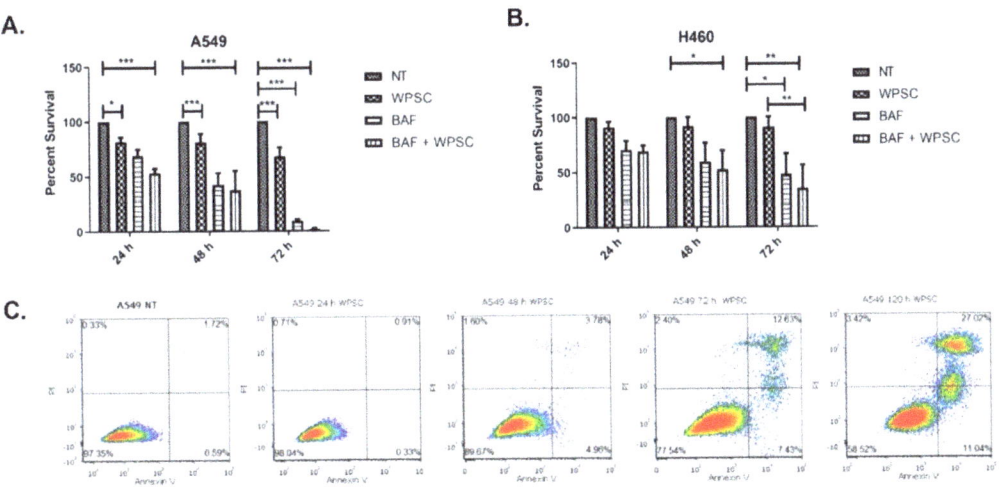

Figure 1. *Cont.*

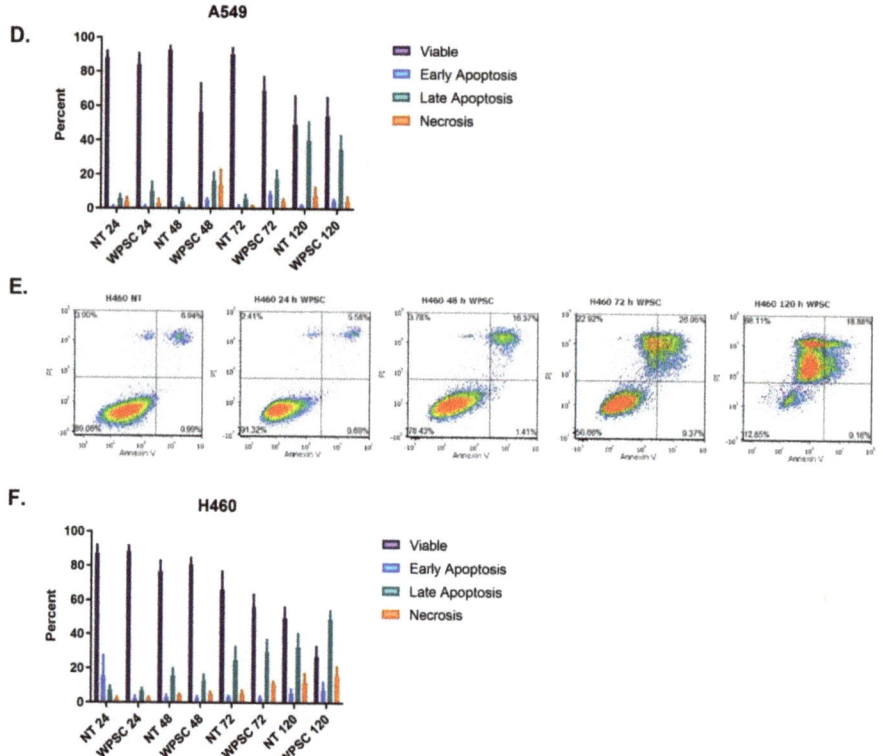

Figure 1. WPSC increases apoptosis and autophagy in lung cancer cell lines. Cell viability in response to 0.5% WPSC was measured using MTT assay in A549 (**A**) and H460 (**B**) cell lines at 24, 48 and 72 h. Apoptosis was measured by flow cytometry. Cells were stained with a combination of Annexin V-FITC, propidium iodide (PI) following WPSC treatment, in A549 (**C**,**D**) and H460 (**E**,**F**). Results represent means of three independent experiments, and data represent mean ± standard error of mean. * $p \leq 0.05$, ** $p \leq 0.01$ and *** $p \leq 0.001$.

Despite the increase in apoptotic cells, a large percentage of the cells survived the WPSC treatment; up to 60% of A549 and 30% of H460 cells remained viable following 5-day exposure. We therefore examined whether autophagy was activated following WPSC treatment. One method for detecting autophagic flux is by measuring differences in the amounts of LC3-II in the presence of an autophagy inhibitor; we thus analyzed the increase in the ratio of LC3-II to LC3-I by western blot with and without BafA1. The amount of LC3-II in WPSC-treated cells increased further in the presence of BafA1, which indicates an enhancement of autophagic flux starting at 8 h and up to 24 h (Figure 2A,B). The ubiquitin-associated protein p62, which binds to LC3, is also used to monitor autophagic flux; as such, we analyzed the expression levels of p62 following WPSC treatment. Immunofluorescence indicated an increase in p62 puncta, and western blots demonstrated an increase in p62 levels (Figure 2B). Because autophagy could promote cell survival, we analyzed whether WPSC in combination with autophagy inhibitors would result in a further increase in cell death. Pretreating the cells with BafA1 prior to WPSC exposure in A549 cells resulted in a slight increase in late apoptotic cells at 48 h when compared to BafA1-alone-treated cells. In H460 cells, the number of late apoptotic cells increased at 24 h, and necrotic cell death was more prominent at 48 h (Figure 2F). This result indicates that both cell lines are susceptible to stress-induced cell death, and that autophagy is important in maintaining the surviving cells. Therefore, manipulating pathways of apoptosis, necrosis and autophagy in cancer cells could skew cell fate decisions. We next sought to investigate if this autophagy response is specific to smokers with lung adenocarcinoma, as compared to non-smokers with lung adenocarcinoma. We analyzed the TCGA lung adenocarcinoma bulk RNA-seq dataset with the available patient metadata on smoking status. Using random-forest-based multivariate modeling implemented in GeneSrF, we obtained the top 14 autophagy genes as the best predictors of smoking status [24]. We compared the fold change in expression of all autophagy genes between smokers and non-smokers (Figure 2G). We also implemented our own random forest modeling using the randomForest package in R (model accuracy = 0.65, sensitivity = 0.96, and precision = 0.60; see methods). Using two feature importance techniques, meanDecreaseAccuracy and meanDecreaseGini, we found that there were four genes that were consistently reported as the top predictors of smoking status (Figure 2H). The results showed an activation of autophagy in smokers, and among the differentially expressed genes, BNIP3 (Wilcoxon rank sum test, p-value = 2.16×10^{-5}) was significantly up-regulated in smokers, and SESN2 (Wilcoxon rank sum test, p-value = 1.67×10^{-5}), TRIM22 (Wilcoxon rank sum test, p-value = 2.9×10^{-7}) and TNFSF10 (Wilcoxon rank sum test, p-value = 1.74×10^{-6}) were significantly down-regulated in smokers (Figure 2G). The list of additional top predicted genes can be found in Supplementary File S1 (see Supplementary Materials).

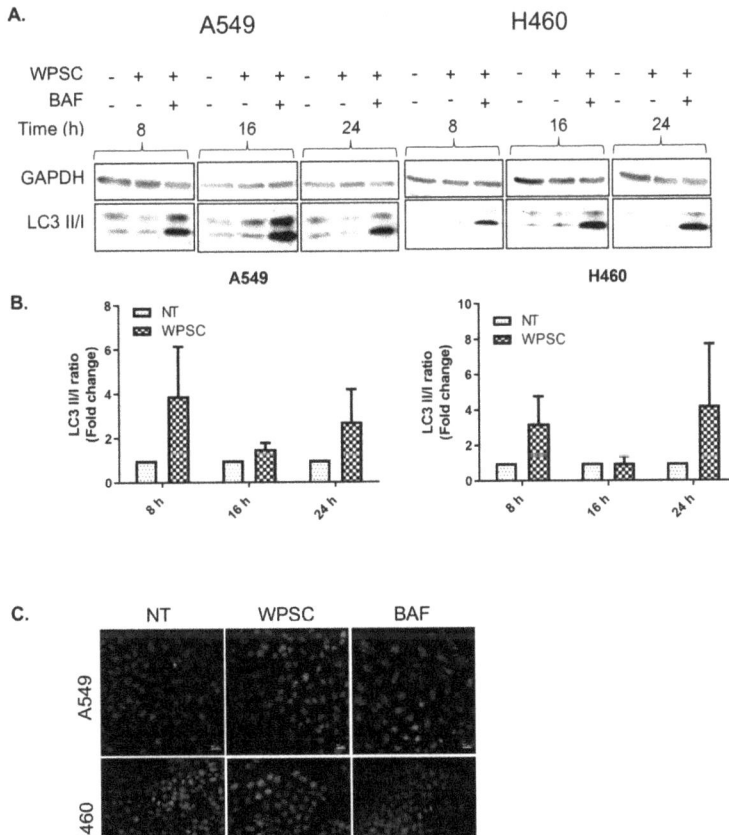

Figure 2. Cont.

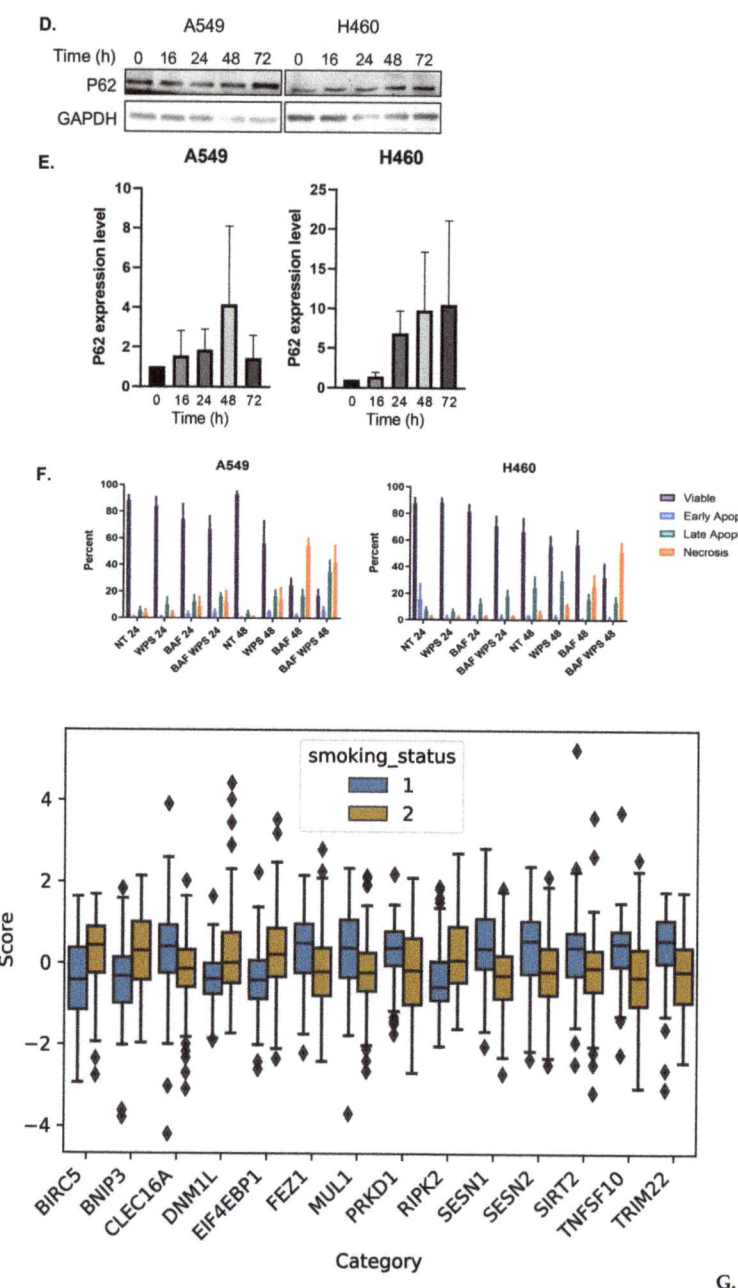

Figure 2. Cont.

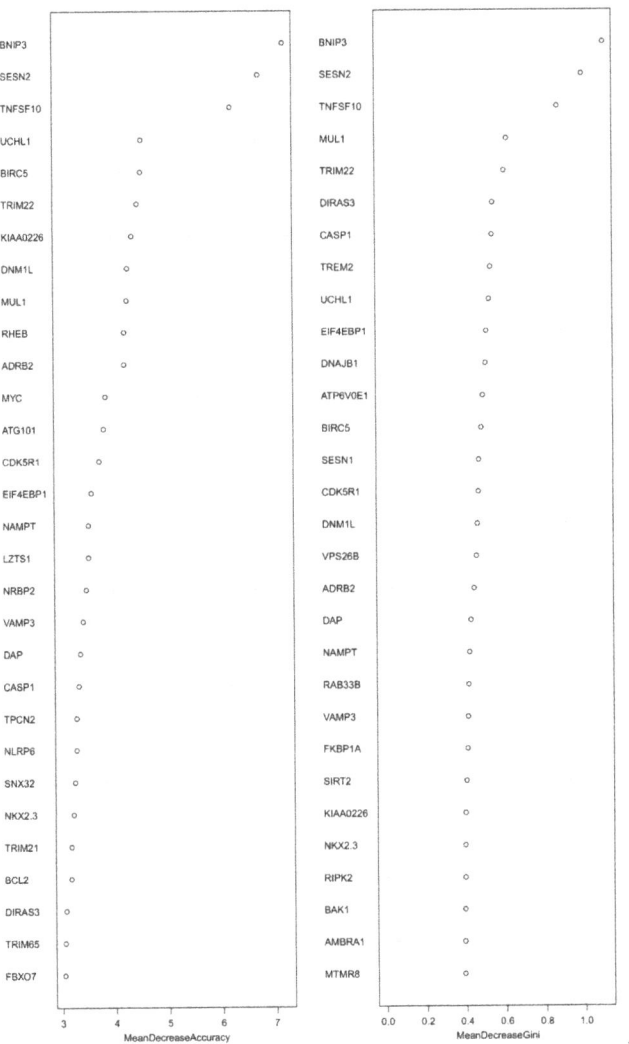

Figure 2. WPSC induces autophagy in lung cancer cell lines. A549 and H460 cell lines were treated with 0.5% WPSC for 24 h. LC3I/II levels were monitored by western blotting using standard procedures with anti-LC3 and GAPDH as a loading control for (**A**) band intensity was quantified in (**B**). The immunofluorescence analysis of p62 protein was performed following 72 h WPSC treatment; cells were treated with 100 nM Baf-A1 for 24 h as positive control (**C**). Western blotting for p62 protein was performed by standard procedures with anti-p62, and anti-GAPDH as a loading control (**D**) band intensity was quantified in (**E**). Cells were stained with a combination of Annexin V-FITC and propidium iodide (PI) to measure apoptosis, following 100nM Baf-A1 pre-treatment and WPSC treatment for the indicated time points, in both cell lines (**F**). TCGA lung adenocarcinoma bulk RNA-seq datasets of all autophagy genes between smokers and non-smokers (**G**). Two feature importance techniques were used—meanDecreaseAccuracy and meanDecreaseGini—to classify the top predictors of the autophagy-related genes with smoking status (**H**). Representative images of confocal microscopic analysis of p62 (green) and DAPI (blue) are shown. Scale bar, 10 μm. Results represent means of three independent experiments, and data represent mean ± standard error of mean.

2.2. Temporal Changes in Mutational Landscape of Long-Term Exposure to Waterpipe Smoke in Lung Cancer Cell Lines Genomes

While high-throughput sequencing studies have previously reported whole-genome analysis at the genomic, transcriptomic and proteomic levels in samples from smokers compared to non-smokers [25–30], as well as in samples from lung cancer [31,32], to date, the genomic landscape in long-term WPS-exposed lung cancer cell lines remains unknown.

We used NGS-based whole genome sequencing to analyze mutational burden in A549 and H460 cell lines exposed to 0.5% WPSC for up to 6 months. Our results indicate an overall increase in TMB (per Mb) in 3-month-treated samples that increased further in 6-month-treated samples ($1 < $ medianTMB $ < 4$; p-value < 0.05, Wilcoxon Rank Sum test) (Figure 3A). We observed that there were more missense mutations and frameshift insertions, compared to frameshift deletions and nonsense mutations in both cell lines. An overall increase in the frame shift insertions in the 6-month-treated samples was observed compared to 3-month-treated samples; these were limited to 1 to 4 bps insertions of C or T of homopolymer lengths. No insertions of >1bp as repeats were found for either of the cell lines (Figure S1, A549 and Figure S2 H460). When we analyzed missense mutations, we observed a greater number of transitions compared to transversions, specifically C -> T and T -> C mutations (Figure 3B–E); these are not enriched at APOBEC target sites (the TCW motif). Finally, we analyzed the distribution of single nucleotide variants (SNV) across different chromosomes as a function of $\log_{10}$(inter SNV event distance). This allowed us to look for patterns of localized hypermutations or Kataegis, known to be implicated in various cancer types. We observed an increase in Kataegis on chromosome 19 in 6-month-treated A549 and chromosome 1 in 6-month-treated H460 when compared to the respective three month treated samples (Figure S3A–D). Together, these data indicate that WPSC exposure over time leads to an increase in tumor mutational burden.

Mutations in cancer genes have been shown to occur at certain hot spots, providing an adaptive advantage to the cells and thereby getting positively selected during clonal evolution. We analyzed the genes that are mutated in response to WPS treatment in both cell lines. We investigated gene mutations with a large spatial clustering using clusterScore at z-score >2 and FDR < 0.01 (see Section 4). A clusterScore of 1 indicates the presence of reported mutations within clusters across all samples. In A549, ZNF99, PCDHB5, GPRIN2 and LILRB1 had clusterScores > 0.7 (cluster numbers: ≥ 5, 2, 2 and ≥ 1). In H460, FLG, PCDHA10, GPRIN2 and PCDHB13 had clusterScores > 0.7 (cluster numbers: ≥ 25, ≥ 1, >2 and ≥ 1). A complete breakdown of the clustering can be found in the Tables S1–S4.

Next, we performed pathway analysis to identify differentially mutated oncogenic genes following long-term WPSC exposure. We identified genes in the MYC and NOTCH pathways that were mutated in 6-month-treated H460 samples but not in 3-month-treated samples (Figure 4); these were MYC (mutation rate 50%) and PDE4DIP (mutation rate 75%), due to frameshift insertions and nonsense mutations. Mutations in these genes have not been reported previously as per the variant effect predictor (VEP) database. Genes that were differentially mutated in 6-month-treated A549 samples were PRX and RYR1 (75% mutation rate each) due to missense and nonsense mutations, and frameshift insertions. One missense mutation observed in PRX gene-rs268673: Ile921Met had already been reported in the dbSNP database, with a known moderate impact; however, all the additional mutations we observed in PRX and RYR1 genes have not been reported previously to the best of our knowledge. Additional differentially mutated genes can be found in Figure S4.

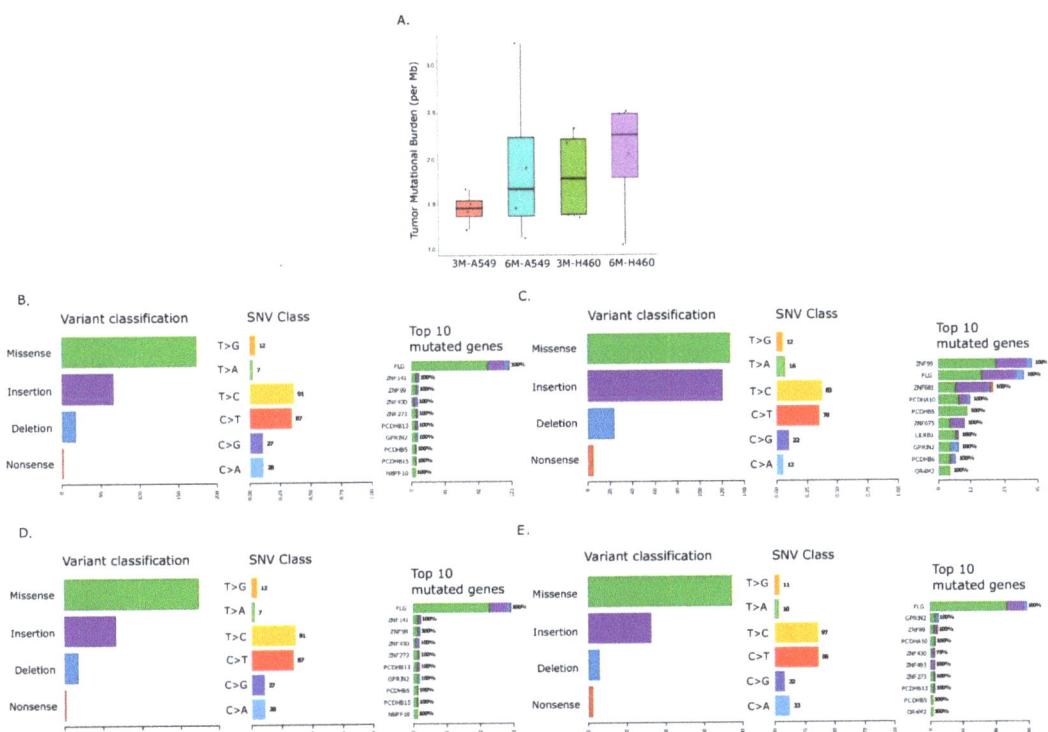

Figure 3. Mutational analysis of long-term WPSC treatment of lung cancer cell lines. WPSC treatment led to an increase in the tumor mutational burden (TMB), represented as an increase in total mutations per megabase in both A549 and H460 cell lines (**A**). Summary of mutations in A549 and H460 cell lines, respectively, treated with WPSC for 3 months (**B**,**D**) and 6 months (**C**,**E**).

In sum, we found an increase in TMB in six-month, WPS-treated cancer cell lines, with an increase in C to T and T to C transitions and frameshift insertions of 1–4 bp homopolymer lengths. We identified genes with an adaptive potential, with GPRIN2 being common across both cell lines. Finally, we found differentially mutated genes in response to the long-term exposure of WPS, including genes from the MYC and NOTCH pathways.

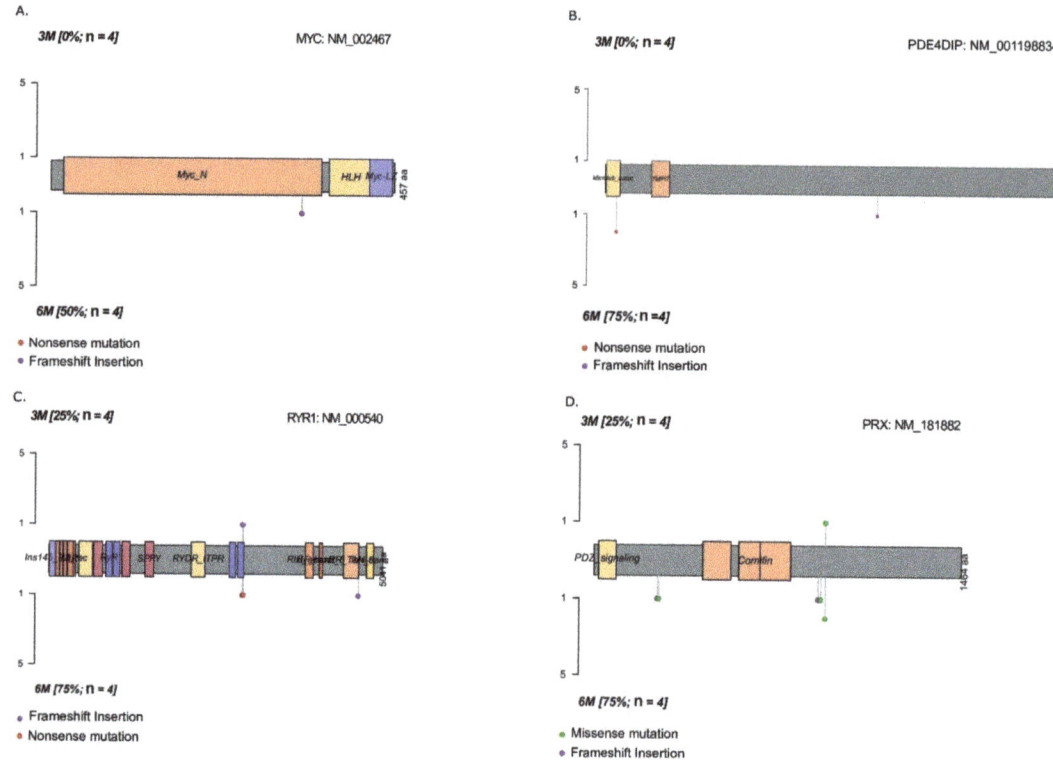

Figure 4. Mutational landscape of long-term WPSC treatment of lung cancer cell lines. Genes differentially mutated in 6-month-treated H460 samples were MYC (mutation rate 50%) and PDE4DIP (mutation rate 75%) (**A**,**B**), and genes differentially mutated in 6-month-treated A549 samples were RYR1 and PRX (75% mutation rate each) (**C**,**D**).

2.3. Smoking Is a Key Determinant of TMB of Lung Adenocarcinoma Patients

Although cancer cell lines are widely used as an in vitro experimental model in cancer studies, they do not constitute an ideal model for primary tumors due to differences in the microenvironment [33]. Furthermore, studies using smoke extract on cell lines do not parallel human smoking parameters because of variabilities in concentration and in the cell-to-smoke exposure interface in vivo vs. in vitro. In line with this, studying primary lung tumors and their microenvironment in smokers and non-smokers at a molecular level assumes a level of importance. We thus investigated lung adenocarcinoma (LUAD) molecular signatures in affected patients with long-term active exposure to smoke and compared them to patients who had not had any active exposure to smoke in their life. Because there are no studies on patients solely consuming WPS, as which would have been most relevant to our study, we took advantage of the large-scale TCGA molecular dataset on LUADs to compare the differences in molecular signatures in lifelong non-smokers versus tobacco smokers.

We divided the patients into two groups based on their smoking status: (1) life-long non-smokers and (2) smokers. We first compared the TMB in smokers and non-smokers affected with LUAD. A higher TMB was observed in smokers compared to non-smokers

$$\text{medianTMB}_{\text{smokers}} = 4.5, \text{medianTMB}_{\text{non-smokers}} = 1.09$$

p-value = 4.13 × 10^{-10} Wilcoxon Rank Sum test with continuity correction) (Figure 5A). In addition to the smoking status, several factors such as age, gender, tumor stage and metastasis status could affect the overall TMB state. We used two random-forest-model-based feature importance techniques, Increase in Mean Square Error (IncMSE) and Increase in Node Purity (IncNodePurity), to assess the effect of smoking status alone while controlling for these confounding factors. We observed that smoking status remained among the top three important features that are important for TMB prediction with IncMSE = 4.5 and IncNodePurity = 161 (Figure 5B).

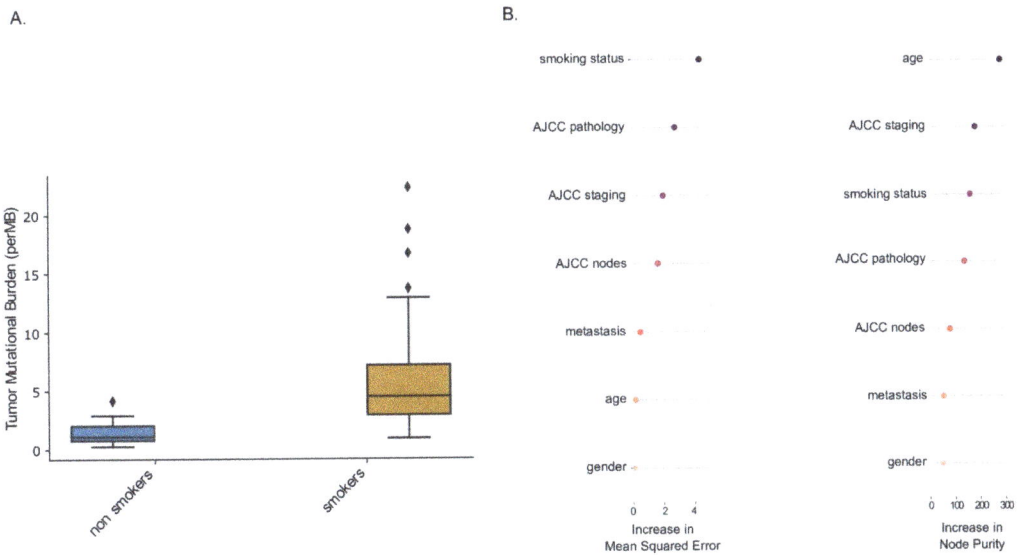

Figure 5. Tumor mutational burden increases in smokers affected with lung adenocarcinoma. (**A**) Analysis of the TCGA molecular dataset on lung adenocarcinoma patients was performed comparing molecular signatures in lifelong non-smokers versus tobacco smokers. A higher TMB was observed in smokers compared to non-smokers (median$TMB_{smokers}$ = 4.5, median$TMB_{non-smokers}$ = 1.09; p-value = 4.13 × 10^{-10} Wilcoxon Rank Sum test with continuity correction). (**B**) Random forest model-based feature importance technique was performed to assess the effect of smoking status alone while controlling for the listed confounding factors.

2.4. Smoke Exposure Is Associated with a Reprogramed Tumor Immune Microenvironment

The immune microenvironment could have a key role in determining immunotherapy outcomes. To better understand these microenvironmental factors, we focused on four major signatures: (1) immune cell fractions associated with immunotherapy response, (2) the success of T-cell infiltration into tumors, (3) T-cell dysfunction within the tumor microenvironment and (4) the expression of immune checkpoint genes.

The digital cytometer CIBERSORTx was first applied to examine immune cell fractions residing in smokers vs. non-smokers (Figure 6). When compared to smokers, non-smokers had a higher fraction of the antigen-presenting dendritic cells (Wilcoxon rank sum test, p-value = 9.369 × 10^{-5}). However, they also had a higher fraction of the immunosuppressive M2-polarized macrophages (Wilcoxon rank sum test, p-value = 0.0048). Regarding smokers, they displayed higher cell fractions of anti-tumor M1 macrophages (Wilcoxon rank sum test, p-value = 0.05), as well as NK cells (Wilcoxon rank sum test, p-value = 0.017). Finally, we observed a higher cell fraction of Cytotoxic T lymphocytes in smokers when compared to non-smokers (Wilcoxon rank sum test, p-value = 0.04). No differences were found in other B-cell and T-cell fractions, including T-regulatory cells, with the latter being associated with immunosuppressive effects.

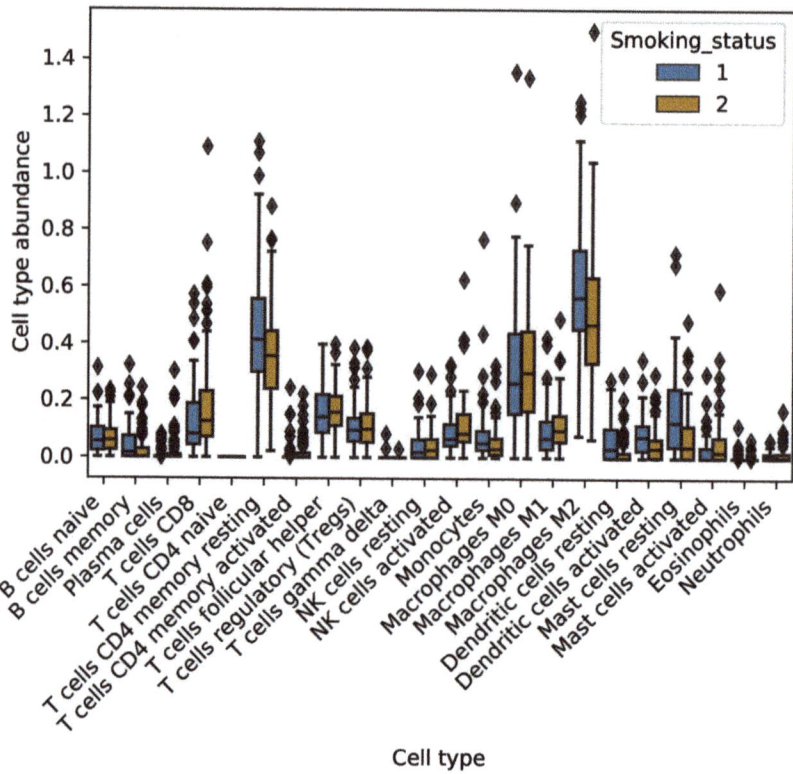

Figure 6. Immune profile of smokers affected with lung adenocarcinoma. Various immune cells profiles were analyzed in non-smokers (1) compared to smokers (2).

To evaluate the functional state of infiltrating CTLs and their degree of exclusion from the tumor microenvironment, the TIDE (Tumor Immune Dysfunction and Exclusion) algorithm, TIDEPY, was utilized (Figure 7). First, we observed a higher score of Cytotoxic T lymphocytes in smokers when compared to non-smokers (Wilcoxon rank sum test, p-value = 0.0036). This was calculated using five genes, CD8A, CD8B, granzyme A, granzyme B and Perforin expression. This effect remains after controlling for confounding factors such as age and gender using a multiple linear regression (MLR) model fit (coefficient$_{\text{smoking status}}$ = 0.67, 95% confidence interval = (0.22, 1.12), p-value = 0.003). Of interest, a lower read out for T-cell dysfunction score was observed in smokers as compared to non-smokers (Wilcoxon rank sum test, p-value: 0.0096). Regarding T-cell exclusion, which was based on the presence of immune-inhibitory cells (Cancer Associated Fibroblasts (CAFs), myeloid-derived suppressor cells (MDSCs) and M2 macrophages), no differences could be observed between smokers and non-smokers (Wilcoxon rank sum test, p-value = 0.1). Other markers such as microsatellite instability (MSI) and interferon gamma (IFN-γ) were also analyzed for differential expression between the two groups. There was no difference in IFN-γ levels between smokers and non-smokers (Wilcoxon rank sum test, p-value = 0.3). Furthermore, a higher median score of MSI, a result of defective mismatch DNA repair, was observed in non-smokers than smokers (Wilcoxon rank sum test, p-value = 0.028), albeit the distributions were broad.

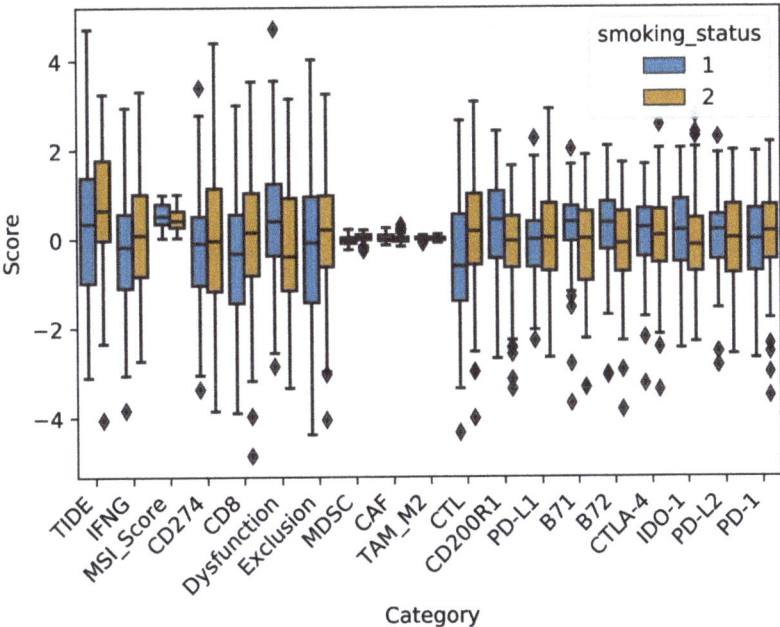

Figure 7. Functional state of infiltrating CTLs and Immune checkpoint genes expression. The functional state of infiltrating CTLs and their degree of exclusion from the tumor microenvironment were evaluated using TIDE. Furthermore, expression of eight immune checkpoint genes was analyzed in LADC patients with a history of smoking. (1) non-smokers; (2) smokers.

Finally, the expression of immune checkpoint genes (ICGs) in both groups was analyzed (Figure 7). Expression was measured in terms of z-score (see Section 4. for details). While there was no difference in the expression levels of PD-1 (Wilcoxon rank sum test, p-value = 0.24), PD-L1 (Wilcoxon rank sum test, p-value = 0.32), PD-L2 (Wilcoxon rank sum test, p-value = 0.66) and CTLA-4 (Wilcoxon rank sum test, p-value = 0.52) between smokers and non-smokers, higher expression levels of co-inhibitory molecules B7-1 (Wilcoxon rank sum test, p-value = 0.0025) and B7-2 (Wilcoxon rank sum test, p-value = 0.0174) were observed in non-smokers. Similarly, other suppressors of antitumor responses had higher expression in non-smokers than smokers, namely, IDO1 (Indoleamine 2, 3-dioxygenase 1) (Wilcoxon rank sum test, p-value = 0.27) and CD200R1 (Wilcoxon rank sum test, p-value = 0.001). Our analyses of TCGA data provide support for smoking in modulating lung adenocarcinoma patient's tumor microenvironment resulting in immune cell landscape variations. These would constitute potential key targets in therapy modalities.

3. Discussion

Accumulated evidence indicates that smoke plays a central role in the evolution of tumor ecosystem and immune escape mechanisms by tumor cells through its impact on immune plasticity and tumor heterogeneity. In this regard, we had previously observed that treating lung cancer cell lines with WPSC resulted in an increase in DNA damage [11]. Here, we asked whether WPSC interferes with the autophagic process and how this may influence the immune landscape in the lung of smokers. Our current data indicate an increase in apoptosis at early WPSC exposure times, confirming other published works [14,34–37]. Furthermore, we noted an activation of autophagy following WPSC treatment. Autophagy inhibition resulted in an increase in apoptosis, highlighting a role for autophagy in sustaining cancer cell survival. The cells that escape apoptosis can either undergo autophagy or senescence. While elevated levels of autophagy induce cell death, inadequate autophagy can trigger cellular senescence [38], which we have previously shown is also induced following 8-day treatment with the same concentrations of WPSC [11]. While DNA damage potentiates different repair mechanisms to restore the damaged DNA, which, if unrepaired, would lead to the activation of cell death programs [39], autophagy has been shown to function in delaying apoptotic cell death in cancers as autophagy inhibition sensitizes cancer cells to chemotherapeutic drugs and/or ionizing radiation [32,40–43] and is also shown to play a role in the inhibition of the immune response in cancers with high TMB [44]. In WPSC-treated cells, we measured an increase in TMB in vitro; TMB has been observed in several cancers with DNA damage repair gene mutations [45–47]. While we did not analyze the DNA damage repair gene status in our study, we did observe an increase in TMB in cell lines exposed to WPSC from 3 to 6 months exposure. Our analysis of the TCGA LUAD dataset reaffirms our results, where we saw an increase in TMB in patients with an active smoking status. Other studies have also addressed the effects of tobacco smoking on normal as well as lung cancer and found this to be associated with an increase in TMB [48–50]. We analyzed the genes that were affected with mutations and divided them into two categories: (1) genes with specific mutational hotspots that arise because of the treatment across all samples and (2) differentially mutated genes that only get mutated as the mutational burden increases in the 6-month-treated samples. Genes such as zinc finger protein 99 (ZNF99), a gene found to be mutated in NSCLC with resistance to etoposide [51], and FLG, a highly mutated driver gene found in lung cancer [52], GPRIN2 and PCDHB13 that has been found to be downregulated in NCSLC and that negatively correlated with pathological grade [53], were mutated in all treated samples in both cell lines with a 100% mutation rate. In addition, discrepancies in the results obtained in our study with respect to WPS exposure to cell lines and patients' data could be due to the significant role of the TME in modulating cancer cell behavior.

WPS exposure could be modulating several biological pathways that would act upstream of DNA damage. Exposure to WPS induces significant alterations in inflammatory cytokines and oxidative stress markers in mice [8–10,54,55]. WPS exposure also induces hypoxia [56]. Reactive oxygen species (ROS) could also be generated because of an increase in apoptotic cell death [57], which could generate a positive feed-back to further activate autophagy pathways [58].

Upon modeling-based analysis of TCGA lung adenocarcinoma RNA-seq datasets, we found an activation of autophagy in smokers. The most significantly affected genes were BNIP3, SESN2, TRIM22 and TNFSF10. BNIP3 expression results in the initiation of autophagy by disrupting the beclin1/Bcl-2 complex [59], and BNIP3 protein has been reported to be overexpressed in several cancer types and to participate in enhanced tumor growth [60]. SESN2/Sestrin 2 is a stress-inducible protein that is induced under hypoxic conditions and is reported to be associated with oxidative-stress-induced autophagy [61,62]; indeed, the occurrence of cancers is associated with significant downregulation of SESN2 [63]. Interestingly, TRIM22 stimulates autophagy by promoting BECLIN 1 expression [64] and has also been shown to play a role in driving tumor growth and progression [65]. TNFSF10/TRAIL could induce autophagy in certain cancer cells [66]. Our results suggest that the genes predicted by our model can correctly classify smokers as smokers but could also misclassify non-smokers as smokers. This low accuracy of 0.65 (C.I:(0.5,0.78)) is due to excluding non-autophagy related genes in our analysis. Nevertheless, future treatment interventions based on the autophagy genes could be designed for smokers with a higher confidence than for non-smokers. The limitation of our analysis is that this dataset was analyzed for gene expression in smokers of any devices (cigarettes and others), due to the non-availability of studies that include patients consuming WPS alone.

Several studies have shown evidence for the significant role for autophagy in the response to therapeutic treatments in cancers [67]. Because autophagy induction could be associated with resistance to therapy, concomitant targeting of autophagy pathways synergizes with cancer therapeutic drugs to enhance cell death [67–69]. On the other hand, pro-autophagic drugs have been used successfully to enhance apoptosis in resistant cells [67]. This is due to the turning on of autophagic cell death mechanisms. Our in vitro data support the mechanism that autophagy is important to maintain cell survival, however the plastic nature of tumor cells and their continuous plasticity in response to their microenvironment may require regular monitoring to assess more effective treatment strategies. How WPS alone affects the autophagy response and the genetic landscape in lung adenocarcinoma patients compared to non-WP smoker patients has yet to be fully elucidated.

Unraveling the changes in the immune microenvironment in lung adenocarcinoma patients with a history of smoking could enhance our understanding of factors that could contribute to predicting response to immune checkpoint inhibitors. While various biomarkers of response have been validated and are being used in the clinic, the absence of efficacy in a fraction of patients underlines the need for further studies. We thus investigated the immunological landscape in LUAD patients with a history of smoking. We found a higher TMB, NK-cell infiltration, CD8+ T-cell fraction and lower dysfunction level in smokers as compared to non-smokers, even after controlling for various confounding factors. On the other hand, non-smokers seemed to display a more immunosuppressed state, with a higher infiltration of M2 pro-tumor macrophages. Our findings are in agreement with a recent study that showed that NSCLC patients who are previous or current smokers had a higher TMB and neoantigen load, accompanied by a higher infiltration of immune cells, compared to those classified as never-smokers [70]. However, unlike previous studies similar to ours, using statistical models like Random Forest and Multiple Linear Regression, we report for the first time that these results are not affected by, and are not a sole artifact of, other confounding factors; at least for the dataset that we analyze in the present study. Moreover, in accordance with our results, they also reported following mass cytometry (CyTOF) analysis of fresh NSCLC tissues, that smokers have a more immune-activated TME, while the TME of non-smokers is in an immunosuppressed or resting state [70]. Our findings further suggest a more complex relationship between smoking status and immune infiltration. A higher fraction of the immunosuppressive MDSC was present in smokers compared to non-smokers who displayed a higher infiltration of DCs and a higher level of MSI, which is a positive predictor of response to ICI. Considering other markers of response, no differences could be detected in expression levels of PD-L1, among other immune checkpoint genes. Autophagy activation has been shown to decrease the expression of histone deacetylases that downregulate PD-L1 expression [48], validating our findings. Interestingly however, B7-1, B7-2, IDO1 and CD200R1 had higher expression levels in non-smokers relative to smokers. Immune checkpoint inhibitors against IDO1, which negatively impacts T-cell differentiation, are currently being investigated in clinical trials [20]. Our results would suggest better efficacy of such agents in non-smokers compared to smokers. It is important to note that our findings are all based on in silico analysis of a single dataset and would require further validation in independent cohorts of lung adenocarcinoma. Nonetheless, they help shed light on the complexity that is the tumor immune microenvironment in smokers vs nonsmokers with LUAD and supplement the perspective that smoking is only a putative biomarker of response to immunotherapy.

Our results provide the first comprehensive analysis, to the best of our knowledge, that would help plan better treatment interventions targeted at LUAD patients with a history of smoking. We also call out the need for carrying similar TCGA studies including information specifically on patients exposed to WPS alone. Studying tumor microenvironment in patients with a history of smoking with a focus on autophagy could provide a stepping stone for novel directed immunotherapy approaches.

4. Materials and Methods

4.1. Waterpipe Smoke Sampling and Analysis

Waterpipe smoke sampling and analysis was described previously [11].

4.2. Cell Culture

A549 (gift from Prof Fathia Mami Chouaib, Gustave Roussy, Villejuif Cedex, France) and H460 cells (AddexBio C0016003 RRID:CVCL_0023, San Diego, CA, USA) were grown in complete RPMI 1640 Medium, (Gibco 61870010, Life Technologies, Warrington, UK) supplemented with 10% Heat Inactivated Fetal Bovine Serum (Gibco 10270-106 Life Technologies, UK), 1% Penicillin-Streptomycin (Gibco 15140-122, Life Technologies, UK) and 1% sodium pyruvate (Gibco 11360-039, Life Technologies, UK). We tested and confirmed that all the cell lines were mycoplasma-free.

4.3. MTT Assay

MTT was obtained from Abcam (MTT Assay Kit, Abcam ab211091, Cambridge, UK). A549 and H460 cells were seeded at a density of $0.5-1 \times 10^4$ cells/mL in 96 well plates. The plates were then treated with concentrations of 0.2% WPSC for 24, 48 and 72 h. 200 µM hydrogen peroxide treatment was used as a positive control for 25 min. Cells were treated with 100 nM Bafilomycin A1 (Cell Signaling, 54645, Danvers, MA, USA), where indicated for 1 h prior to WPSC treatment. 20 µL of MTT solution (5 mg/mL) was added to each well and the cells were cultured for another 2 h. The treatment medium was then discarded and 50 µL of serum-free media and 50 µL of MTT Reagent were added together into each well and the plate was incubated at 37 °C for 3 h. Following incubation, 150 µL of MTT solvent was added to each well. The plate was covered in foil and agitated on an orbital shaker for 15 min then read at 590 nm using a microplate reader (BioTek Epoch 2, Winooski, VT, USA). Cell proliferation rates were calculated by comparing with the control cells.

4.4. Flow Cytometry

Apoptosis assays were performed using APC Annexin V Apoptosis Detection Kit with Propidium Iodide (PI) (Biolegend, 640914 San Diego, CA, USA). Briefly, cells were plated at a density of 100,000 cells per dish in 35 mm dishes (Eppendorf 0030 700.112, Hamburg, Germany). Following WPSC treatment, the cells were collected at the indicated timepoints by trypsinization and subsequently washed with $1\times$ PBS prior to labeling with Annexin V-APC and PI following the manufacturer's protocol. Acquisitions of 20,000 cells were performed using a Biorad S3E Cell Sorter and data processed using the FCS Express flow cytometry program (De Novo Software, Pasadena, CA, USA). Annexin V-positive cells were classified as apoptotic.

4.5. Statistical Analysis

Statistical analyses were carried out using GraphPad Prism Software version 9.3.1 (GraphPad Software, Inc, San Diego, CA, USA). All data are expressed as means ± SEM. Significant differences were found using two-way analysis of variance (ANOVA) followed by correction for multiple comparison using Tukey test.

4.6. Antibodies Used in This Study

Mouse anti-human SQSTM1/p62 (D5L7G) (Cell Signaling, Danvers, 88588, MA, USA), rabbit anti-human GAPDH (Cell Signaling 2118, MA, USA) and rabbit anti-human LC3A/B (Cell Signaling 4108, MA, USA).

4.7. Immunoblotting

Cells grown in 6-well dishes were washed once with ice cold PBS $1\times$ and lysed in 100 µL of RIPA (150 mM NaCl, 0.1% TX-100, 0.5% NaDOC, 0.1% SDS, and 50 mM Tris-HCl pH 8.0) with protease inhibitor cocktail (Sigma P2714, Burlington, MA, USA). Proteins were quantified following brief sonication, by Pierce BCA protein assay kit (Thermo Fisher 23225, Rockford, IL, USA), and 15–20 µg of proteins were loaded on 10% or 12% SDS-PAGE and transferred onto a nitrocellulose membrane (Sigma GE10600004, Burlington, MA, USA) at 80 Volts for 3 h. After blocking with 5% BSA in TBST (10 mM Tris, pH 8.0, 150 mM NaCl, and 0.5 % Tween 20) for 60 min, the membrane was washed once with TBST and incubated with the listed antibodies according to their data sheets.

4.8. Immunofluorescence

Cells were fixed in 4% paraformaldehyde (ThermoFisher Scientific 28906, Waltham, MA, USA) in 1× PBS for 10 min at room temperature. Cells were then washed with 1× PBS and permeabilized with 0.1% TX-100 in PBS for 15 min at room temperature. Prior to staining, cells were blocked in 2% BSA in 1× PBS for 1 h at RT. Cells were then stained with a primary and secondary antibody as per the data sheets followed by three 5 min washes after each antibody staining. Cells were then mounted on glass slides using Prolong gold antifade reagent (ThermoFisher Scientific P36930, MA, USA) and visualized on Zeiss LSM 800 with Airyscan.

4.9. Whole Exome Sequencing Variant Analysis

Whole exome sequencing (WES) was carried out for two non-small cell lung cancer cell lines A549 and H460. Each cell line was treated with water pipe smoke (WPS) and cultured for six months in two sets of biological replicates. Furthermore, two technical replicates were set up for a given biological replicate. Samples for sequencing for each set were collected at 3 months and 6 months. Untreated cancer cells were used as a control.

The QiaAmp DNA Mini Kit was used to extract genomic DNA (Qiagen, Hilden, Germany). Exome libraries were prepared from 100 ng of genomic DNA using Ion AmpliSeq™ Exome RDY kit (ThermoFisher Scientific, A38264, MA, USA). With 293'903 total amplicons, this kit covers almost 97 percent of the exonic regions. The samples were barcoded using Ion Xpress Barcode Adapter 1–16 kit (ThermoFisher Scientific, 4474009, MA, USA). The libraries were purified using CleanPCR (Clean NA, GC Biotech, Waddinxveen, The Netherlands). Library quantification was performed using the Ion Library TaqMan Quantitation Kit (ThermoFisher Scientific, 4468802, MA, USA). The libraries were loaded onto the chips using Ion Chef System (ThermoFisher Scientific, 4484177, MA, USA) by utilizing Ion 540 Chef Reagents. Two samples per chip were loaded in equimolar concentrations (40 picomolar) and were sequenced on Ion S5 XL sequencer (ThermoFisher Scientific, MA, USA). The raw data were aligned with the hg19 version of the genome using Ion Torrent Suite (TS) software, and the bam files were processed for variant calling using low-stringency somatic variant and indel calling.

VCF files were obtained as an output of the Torrent Variant Caller. The sample IDs in the vcf header column were changed to ensure uniformity in the downstream analysis. These files were indexed and merged using the respective commands bcftools index and bcftools merge from the package bcftools v1.10.2 [71]. The merging was done in order to create a treated condition and an untreated control pair file. The vcf2maf.pl perl script was used with –remap-chain, vcf-tumor-id, vcf-normal-id, –tumor-id and –normal-id options to obtain the Mutation Annotation Format or MAF files. The –remap-chain option allowed us to remap variants from hg19 to GRCh37 assembly. This was important to successfully run the variant effect predictor (VEP) v102.0 for annotating variants [72]. The id options helped distinguish which sample out of the pair obtained in the previous step was the control. The preprocessing pipeline till this point was automated in Python 3.7.9.

The maf files were further analyzed using the R package maftools v2.6.05 [73]. The analyses were carried out after normalizing the variants called in the treated cancer cells against the untreated cancer cells used as the control. This allowed us to focus on only those variants that emerged in the cancer cells post-stress treatment. Sigprofiler was used to report Indel types across all samples [74].

4.10. TCGA Analyses

TCGA Firehose Legacy bulk RNA-seq Expression profiles were downloaded from cBioportal for Lung Adenocarcinoma (LUAD) with ~500 patient samples per dataset. Patient populations were segregated based on their smoking status. Six ordinal categories represented the following meta-data: (1) lifelong non-smoker, (2) current smoker, (3) current reformed smoker for ≥ 15 years, (4) current reformed smoker for ≤ 15 years, (5) current reformed smoker (duration not specified) and (6) smoking history not documented. We carried out the entire analysis, which follows below, using two categories: (1) lifelong non-smokers and (2) current smokers.

4.11. Tumor Mutational Burden (TMB) Analysis

The maf format files were segregated into smokers and non-smokers. The tumor mutational burden was calculated using the maftools package in R. To assess the feature importance, we used two metrics: (1) "increase in Mean Squared Error" or IncMSE, and (2) "increase in Node Purity" or IncNodePurity. They were used since the model was trained using the Random Forest Regressor in the R package randomForest. Seven features were included for this analysis: smoking status, age, gender, metastasis state, AJCC staging, AJCC pathology and AJCC nodes.

4.12. Immune Cell Abundance Analysis

Tumor deconvolution or immune cell abundance analysis was carried out using CIBERSORTx [75]. LM22 was used as the signature matrix, and B-mode batch correction (bulk mode) was applied. Quantile normalization was disabled. The analyses were run for 100 permutations, each with an absolute mode. Immune cell fraction distributions were compared across patients with different smoking statuses. The non-parametric Wilcoxon rank sum test was used to check for statistical significance. Multiple hypothesis tests were carried out using the false discovery rate (FDR) < 0.05.

4.13. TIDEPY Analysis

The python package TIDEPY (https://github.com/jingxinfu/TIDEpy, accessed on 12 May 2021) [76] was used to calculate the tumor immune dysfunction and exclusion for two groups, smokers and non-smokers, with lung adenocarcinoma (same dataset as mentioned above). Normalization was carried out using $\log 2(x + 1)$ transformation followed by average subtraction across all samples.

4.14. Immune Checkpoint Analysis

Eight immune checkpoint genes were included in the analysis: PD-1, PD-L1, PD-L2, B7-1, B7-2, CTLA-4, IDO-1 and CD200R1, based on the two recent studies [77,78] highlighting the most responsive ICGs in lung adenocarcinomas as compared to normal tissues. The log(TPM) values were extracted for patients with confirmed status of being either smokers or nonsmokers, and Z-scores were calculated for each gene:

$$\text{Z-score} = \log(\text{TPM})_{\text{GeneX, PatientX}} - \text{Mean} - \log(\text{TPM})_{\text{GeneX}}$$

$$\text{Standard-deviation} - \log(\text{TPM})_{\text{GeneX}}$$

Z-score ranges from -1 to $+1$. A negative value indicates downregulation, and a positive value indicates upregulation.

4.15. Autophagy Modeling Analysis

A list of 370 genes involved in autophagy was curated from Fang et al. [24]. To fish out the autophagy genes that were highly predictive of smoking status based on their differential expression, we used a random forest regression model approach. For this, we used GeneSrF (varSelRF) [79], a python-based utility, to predict the top autophagy genes. We also applied our own random forest model testing using the R package randomForest with two hyperparameter values, ntree = 1500 and mtry = 19, obtained such that the Out-of-bag error rate was minimized to 22%. We used three performance metrics for our model: accuracy, precision and recall. Feature importance was calculated using MeanDecreaseAccuracy and

MeanDecreaseGini. Autophagy gene expression distributions were compared using the Z-score as described above.

Supplementary Materials: The following supporting information can be downloaded at: https://www.mdpi.com/article/10.3390/ijms23126848/s1.

Author Contributions: Conceptualization S.C. and significantly guided in the design, analysis and interpretation of the findings of this study. R.F.Z., B.A., M.S., G.H.V., R.A.K., A.R., Z.N.N., F.A., F.M., H.K. and H.N. conceived and designed experiments and acquired and interpreted data. R.A.K. and G.H.V. performed the NGS- experiments, M.S. performed the NGS- and TCGA-related bioinformatics analysis, H.N. performed confocal imaging, Y.E. performed the WPSC generation and analysis. Writing—original draft preparation R.F.Z., B.A., M.S., G.H.V., R.A.K. and S.C. All authors have read and agreed to the published version of the manuscript.

Funding: The present study was supported by Al Jalila Foundation (AJF 2018009) to Zaarour. The smoke sampling and analysis research were funded by the office of Research and Graduate Studies at the American University of Sharjah (FRG19-L-S11).

Institutional Review Board Statement: Not applicable.

Informed Consent Statement: Patient consent was waived due to the data of the article being obtained from the public database (TCGA), and informed consent statements had been applied.

Data Availability Statement: The code employed in carrying out the entire analysis, along with supporting files and information, can be found at https://github.com/Mohak91/Waterpipe_smoke_lung_cancer_study (accessed on 1 June 2022).

Conflicts of Interest: The authors declare no conflict of interest.

References

1. Siegel, R.L.; Miller, K.D.; Fuchs, H.E.; Jemal, A. Cancer Statistics, 2021. *CA Cancer J. Clin.* **2021**, *71*, 7–33. [CrossRef] [PubMed]
2. Islami, F.; Goding Sauer, A.; Miller, K.D.; Siegel, R.L.; Fedewa, S.A.; Jacobs, E.J.; McCullough, M.L.; Patel, A.V.; Ma, J.; Soerjomataram, I.; et al. Proportion and number of cancer cases and deaths attributable to potentially modifiable risk factors in the United States. *CA Cancer J. Clin.* **2018**, *68*, 31–54. [CrossRef] [PubMed]
3. Maziak, W. The global epidemic of waterpipe smoking. *Addict. Behav.* **2011**, *36*, 1–5. [CrossRef] [PubMed]
4. Awan, K.H.; Siddiqi, K.; Patil, S.; Hussain, Q.A. Assessing the Effect of Waterpipe Smoking on Cancer Outcome—A Systematic Review of Current Evidence. *Asian Pac. J. Cancer Prev.* **2017**, *18*, 495–502. [CrossRef]
5. Jabra, E.; Al-Omari, A.; Haddadin, F.; Alam, W.; Ammar, K.; Charafeddine, M.; Alrawashdeh, M.; Kasasbeh, N.; Habis, C.; Mukherji, D.; et al. Waterpipe Smoking among Bladder Cancer Patients: A Cross-Sectional Study of Lebanese and Jordanian Populations. *J. Smok. Cessat.* **2021**, *2021*, 6615832. [CrossRef]
6. Elsayed, Y.; Dalibalta, S.; Abu-Farha, N. Chemical analysis and potential health risks of hookah charcoal. *Sci. Total Environ.* **2016**, *569*, 262–268. [CrossRef]
7. Schubert, J.; Muller, F.D.; Schmidt, R.; Luch, A.; Schulz, T.G. Waterpipe smoke: Source of toxic and carcinogenic VOCs, phenols and heavy metals? *Arch. Toxicol.* **2015**, *89*, 2129–2139. [CrossRef]
8. Arazi, H.; Taati, B.; Rafati Sajedi, F.; Suzuki, K. Salivary Antioxidants Status Following Progressive Aerobic Exercise: What Are the Differences between Waterpipe Smokers and Non-Smokers? *Antioxidants* **2019**, *8*, 418. [CrossRef]
9. Khabour, O.F.; Alzoubi, K.H.; Bani-Ahmad, M.; Dodin, A.; Eissenberg, T.; Shihadeh, A. Acute exposure to waterpipe tobacco smoke induces changes in the oxidative and inflammatory markers in mouse lung. *Inhal. Toxicol.* **2012**, *24*, 667–675. [CrossRef]
10. Golbidi, S.; Li, H.; Laher, I. Oxidative Stress: A Unifying Mechanism for Cell Damage Induced by Noise, (Water-Pipe) Smoking, and Emotional Stress-Therapeutic Strategies Targeting Redox Imbalance. *Antioxid. Redox Signal.* **2018**, *28*, 741–759. [CrossRef]
11. Zaarour, R.F.; Prasad, P.; Venkatesh, G.H.; Khouzam, R.A.; Amirtharaj, F.; Zeinelabdin, N.; Rifath, A.; Terry, S.; Nawafleh, H.; El Sayed, Y.; et al. Waterpipe smoke condensate influences epithelial to mesenchymal transition and interferes with the cytotoxic immune response in non-small cell lung cancer cell lines. *Oncol. Rep.* **2021**, *45*, 879–890. [CrossRef]
12. Alsaad, A.M.; Al-Arifi, M.N.; Maayah, Z.H.; Attafi, I.M.; Alanazi, F.E.; Belali, O.M.; Alhoshani, A.; Asiri, Y.A.; Korashy, H.M. Genotoxic impact of long-term cigarette and waterpipe smoking on DNA damage and oxidative stress in healthy subjects. *Toxicol. Mech. Methods* **2019**, *29*, 119–127. [CrossRef]
13. Su, M.; Mei, Y.; Sinha, S. Role of the Crosstalk between Autophagy and Apoptosis in Cancer. *J. Oncol.* **2013**, *2013*, 102735. [CrossRef]
14. Bodas, M.; Van Westphal, C.; Carpenter-Thompson, R.; Mohanty, D.K.; Vij, N. Nicotine exposure induces bronchial epithelial cell apoptosis and senescence via ROS mediated autophagy-impairment. *Free Radic. Biol. Med.* **2016**, *97*, 441–453. [CrossRef]

15. Shivalingappa, P.C.; Hole, R.; Westphal, C.V.; Vij, N. Airway Exposure to E-Cigarette Vapors Impairs Autophagy and Induces Aggresome Formation. *Antioxid. Redox Signal.* **2016**, *24*, 186–204. [CrossRef]
16. Tran, I.; Ji, C.; Ni, I.; Min, T.; Tang, D.; Vij, N. Role of Cigarette Smoke-Induced Aggresome Formation in Chronic Obstructive Pulmonary Disease-Emphysema Pathogenesis. *Am. J. Respir. Cell Mol. Biol.* **2015**, *53*, 159–173. [CrossRef]
17. Samstein, R.M.; Lee, C.H.; Shoushtari, A.N.; Hellmann, M.D.; Shen, R.; Janjigian, Y.Y.; Barron, D.A.; Zehir, A.; Jordan, E.J.; Omuro, A.; et al. Tumor mutational load predicts survival after immunotherapy across multiple cancer types. *Nat. Genet.* **2019**, *51*, 202–206. [CrossRef]
18. Pilie, P.G.; Tang, C.; Mills, G.B.; Yap, T.A. State-of-the-art strategies for targeting the DNA damage response in cancer. *Nat. Rev. Clin. Oncol.* **2019**, *16*, 81–104. [CrossRef]
19. Reck, M.; Rodriguez-Abreu, D.; Robinson, A.G.; Hui, R.; Csoszi, T.; Fulop, A.; Gottfried, M.; Peled, N.; Tafreshi, A.; Cuffe, S.; et al. Five-Year Outcomes with Pembrolizumab Versus Chemotherapy for Metastatic Non-Small-Cell Lung Cancer with PD-L1 Tumor Proportion Score $\geq$ 50. *J. Clin. Oncol.* **2021**, *39*, 2339–2349. [CrossRef]
20. Mamdani, H.; Matosevic, S.; Khalid, A.B.; Durm, G.; Jalal, S.I. Immunotherapy in Lung Cancer: Current Landscape and Future Directions. *Front. Immunol.* **2022**, *13*, 823618. [CrossRef]
21. Pardoll, D.M. The blockade of immune checkpoints in cancer immunotherapy. *Nat. Rev. Cancer* **2012**, *12*, 252–264. [CrossRef] [PubMed]
22. Abou Khouzam, R.; Zaarour, R.F.; Brodaczewska, K.; Azakir, B.; Venkatesh, G.H.; Thiery, J.; Terry, S.; Chouaib, S. The Effect of Hypoxia and Hypoxia-Associated Pathways in the Regulation of Antitumor Response: Friends or Foes? *Front. Immunol.* **2022**, *13*, 828875. [CrossRef] [PubMed]
23. Yamamoto, A.; Tagawa, Y.; Yoshimori, T.; Moriyama, Y.; Masaki, R.; Tashiro, Y. Bafilomycin A1 prevents maturation of autophagic vacuoles by inhibiting fusion between autophagosomes and lysosomes in rat hepatoma cell line, H-4-II-E cells. *Cell Struct. Funct.* **1998**, *23*, 33–42. [CrossRef] [PubMed]
24. Fang, Q.; Chen, H. Development of a Novel Autophagy-Related Prognostic Signature and Nomogram for Hepatocellular Carcinoma. *Front. Oncol.* **2020**, *10*, 591356. [CrossRef]
25. Titz, B.; Sewer, A.; Schneider, T.; Elamin, A.; Martin, F.; Dijon, S.; Luettich, K.; Guedj, E.; Vuillaume, G.; Ivanov, N.V.; et al. Alterations in the sputum proteome and transcriptome in smokers and early-stage COPD subjects. *J. Proteom.* **2015**, *128*, 306–320. [CrossRef]
26. Zeilinger, S.; Kuhnel, B.; Klopp, N.; Baurecht, H.; Kleinschmidt, A.; Gieger, C.; Weidinger, S.; Lattka, E.; Adamski, J.; Peters, A.; et al. Tobacco smoking leads to extensive genome-wide changes in DNA methylation. *PLoS ONE* **2013**, *8*, e63812. [CrossRef]
27. Steiling, K.; Kadar, A.Y.; Bergerat, A.; Flanigon, J.; Sridhar, S.; Shah, V.; Ahmad, Q.R.; Brody, J.S.; Lenburg, M.E.; Steffen, M.; et al. Comparison of proteomic and transcriptomic profiles in the bronchial airway epithelium of current and never smokers. *PLoS ONE* **2009**, *4*, e5043. [CrossRef]
28. Airoldi, L.; Magagnotti, C.; Iannuzzi, A.R.; Marelli, C.; Bagnati, R.; Pastorelli, R.; Colombi, A.; Santaguida, S.; Chiabrando, C.; Schiarea, S.; et al. Effects of cigarette smoking on the human urinary proteome. *Biochem. Biophys. Res. Commun.* **2009**, *381*, 397–402. [CrossRef]
29. Jessie, K.; Pang, W.W.; Haji, Z.; Rahim, A.; Hashim, O.H. Proteomic analysis of whole human saliva detects enhanced expression of interleukin-1 receptor antagonist, thioredoxin and lipocalin-1 in cigarette smokers compared to non-smokers. *Int. J. Mol. Sci.* **2010**, *11*, 4488–4505. [CrossRef]
30. Boyle, J.O.; Gumus, Z.H.; Kacker, A.; Choksi, V.L.; Bocker, J.M.; Zhou, X.K.; Yantiss, R.K.; Hughes, D.B.; Du, B.; Judson, B.L.; et al. Effects of cigarette smoke on the human oral mucosal transcriptome. *Cancer Prev. Res.* **2010**, *3*, 266–278. [CrossRef]
31. Govindan, R.; Ding, L.; Griffith, M.; Subramanian, J.; Dees, N.D.; Kanchi, K.L.; Maher, C.A.; Fulton, R.; Fulton, L.; Wallis, J.; et al. Genomic landscape of non-small cell lung cancer in smokers and never-smokers. *Cell* **2012**, *150*, 1121–1134. [CrossRef]
32. Huang, Y.T.; Lin, X.; Liu, Y.; Chirieac, L.R.; McGovern, R.; Wain, J.; Heist, R.; Skaug, V.; Zienolddiny, S.; Haugen, A.; et al. Cigarette smoking increases copy number alterations in nonsmall-cell lung cancer. *Proc. Natl. Acad. Sci. USA* **2011**, *108*, 16345–16350. [CrossRef]
33. Yu, K.; Chen, B.; Aran, D.; Charalel, J.; Yau, C.; Wolf, D.M.; van't Veer, L.J.; Butte, A.J.; Goldstein, T.; Sirota, M. Comprehensive transcriptomic analysis of cell lines as models of primary tumors across 22 tumor types. *Nat. Commun.* **2019**, *10*, 3574. [CrossRef]
34. Adcock, I.M.; Mortaz, E.; Alipoor, S.D.; Garssen, J.; Akbar Velayati, A. In Vitro effects of water-pipe smoke condensate on the endocytic activity of Type II alveolar epithelial cells (A549) with bacillus Calmette-Guerin. *Int. J. Mycobacteriol.* **2016**, *5* (Suppl. S1), S157–S158. [CrossRef]
35. Shihadeh, A.; Eissenberg, T.; Rammah, M.; Salman, R.; Jaroudi, E.; El-Sabban, M. Comparison of tobacco-containing and tobacco-free waterpipe products: Effects on human alveolar cells. *Nicotine Tob. Res.* **2014**, *16*, 496–499. [CrossRef]
36. Mortaz, E.; Alipoor, S.D.; Movassaghi, M.; Varahram, M.; Ghorbani, J.; Folkerts, G.; Garssen, J.; Adcock, I.M. Water-pipe smoke condensate increases the internalization of Mycobacterium Bovis of type II alveolar epithelial cells (A549). *BMC Pulm. Med.* **2017**, *17*, 68. [CrossRef]
37. Khalil, C.; Chahine, J.B.; Chahla, B.; Hobeika, T.; Khnayzer, R.S. Characterization and cytotoxicity assessment of nargile smoke using dynamic exposure. *Inhal. Toxicol.* **2019**, *31*, 343–356. [CrossRef]
38. Rajendran, P.; Alzahrani, A.M.; Hanieh, H.N.; Kumar, S.A.; Ben Ammar, R.; Rengarajan, T.; Alhoot, M.A. Autophagy and senescence: A new insight in selected human diseases. *J. Cell Physiol.* **2019**, *234*, 21485–21492. [CrossRef]

39. Friedberg, E.C. DNA damage and repair. *Nature* **2003**, *421*, 436–440. [CrossRef]
40. Chen, Y.S.; Song, H.X.; Lu, Y.; Li, X.; Chen, T.; Zhang, Y.; Xue, J.X.; Liu, H.; Kan, B.; Yang, G.; et al. Autophagy inhibition contributes to radiation sensitization of esophageal squamous carcinoma cells. *Dis. Esophagus* **2011**, *24*, 437–443. [CrossRef]
41. Abedin, M.J.; Wang, D.; McDonnell, M.A.; Lehmann, U.; Kelekar, A. Autophagy delays apoptotic death in breast cancer cells following DNA damage. *Cell Death Differ.* **2007**, *14*, 500–510. [CrossRef] [PubMed]
42. Ding, X.; Yue, W.; Chen, H. Effect of artesunate on apoptosis and autophagy in tamoxifen resistant breast cancer cells (TAM-R). *Transl. Cancer Res.* **2019**, *8*, 1863–1872. [CrossRef] [PubMed]
43. Khan, T.; Relitti, N.; Brindisi, M.; Magnano, S.; Zisterer, D.; Gemma, S.; Butini, S.; Campiani, G. Autophagy modulators for the treatment of oral and esophageal squamous cell carcinomas. *Med. Res. Rev.* **2020**, *40*, 1002–1060. [CrossRef] [PubMed]
44. Poillet-Perez, L.; Sharp, D.W.; Yang, Y.; Laddha, S.V.; Ibrahim, M.; Bommareddy, P.K.; Hu, Z.S.; Vieth, J.; Haas, M.; Bosenberg, M.W.; et al. Autophagy promotes growth of tumors with high mutational burden by inhibiting a T-cell immune response. *Nat. Cancer* **2020**, *1*, 923–934. [CrossRef] [PubMed]
45. Mei, P.; Freitag, C.E.; Wei, L.; Zhang, Y.; Parwani, A.V.; Li, Z. High tumor mutation burden is associated with DNA damage repair gene mutation in breast carcinomas. *Diagn. Pathol.* **2020**, *15*, 50. [CrossRef]
46. Chae, Y.K.; Davis, A.A.; Raparia, K.; Agte, S.; Pan, A.; Mohindra, N.; Villaflor, V.; Giles, F. Association of Tumor Mutational Burden with DNA Repair Mutations and Response to Anti-PD-1/PD-L1 Therapy in Non-Small-Cell Lung Cancer. *Clin. Lung Cancer* **2019**, *20*, 88–96.e86. [CrossRef]
47. Parikh, A.R.; He, Y.; Hong, T.S.; Corcoran, R.B.; Clark, J.W.; Ryan, D.P.; Zou, L.; Ting, D.T.; Catenacci, D.V.; Chao, J.; et al. Analysis of DNA Damage Response Gene Alterations and Tumor Mutational Burden Across 17,486 Tubular Gastrointestinal Carcinomas: Implications for Therapy. *Oncologist* **2019**, *24*, 1340–1347. [CrossRef]
48. Gao, L.; Chen, Y. Autophagy controls programmed death-ligand 1 expression on cancer cells (Review). *Biomed. Rep.* **2021**, *15*, 84. [CrossRef]
49. Alexandrov, L.B.; Ju, Y.S.; Haase, K.; Van Loo, P.; Martincorena, I.; Nik-Zainal, S.; Totoki, Y.; Fujimoto, A.; Nakagawa, H.; Shibata, T.; et al. Mutational signatures associated with tobacco smoking in human cancer. *Science* **2016**, *354*, 618–622. [CrossRef]
50. Yoshida, K.; Gowers, K.H.C.; Lee-Six, H.; Chandrasekharan, D.P.; Coorens, T.; Maughan, E.F.; Beal, K.; Menzies, A.; Millar, F.R.; Anderson, E.; et al. Tobacco smoking and somatic mutations in human bronchial epithelium. *Nature* **2020**, *578*, 266–272. [CrossRef]
51. Qiu, Z.; Lin, A.; Li, K.; Lin, W.; Wang, Q.; Wei, T.; Zhu, W.; Luo, P.; Zhang, J. A novel mutation panel for predicting etoposide resistance in small-cell lung cancer. *Drug Des. Devel. Ther.* **2019**, *13*, 2021–2041. [CrossRef]
52. Skaaby, T.; Husemoen, L.L.; Thyssen, J.P.; Meldgaard, M.; Thuesen, B.H.; Pisinger, C.; Jorgensen, T.; Carlsen, K.; Johansen, J.D.; Menne, T.; et al. Filaggrin loss-of-function mutations and incident cancer: A population-based study. *Br. J. Dermatol.* **2014**, *171*, 1407–1414. [CrossRef]
53. Ting, C.H.; Lee, K.Y.; Wu, S.M.; Feng, P.H.; Chan, Y.F.; Chen, Y.C.; Chen, J.Y. FOSB(-)PCDHB13 Axis Disrupts the Microtubule Network in Non-Small Cell Lung Cancer. *Cancers* **2019**, *11*, 107. [CrossRef]
54. Al-Sawalha, N.A.; Migdadi, A.M.; Alzoubi, K.H.; Khabour, O.F.; Qinna, N.A. Effect of waterpipe tobacco smoking on airway inflammation in murine model of asthma. *Inhal. Toxicol.* **2017**, *29*, 46–52. [CrossRef]
55. Nemmar, A.; Yuvaraju, P.; Beegam, S.; Ali, B.H. Short-term nose-only water-pipe (shisha) smoking exposure accelerates coagulation and causes cardiac inflammation and oxidative stress in mice. *Cell Physiol. Biochem.* **2015**, *35*, 829–840. [CrossRef]
56. Nemmar, A.; Al-Salam, S.; Yuvaraju, P.; Beegam, S.; Yasin, J.; Ali, B.H. Chronic exposure to water-pipe smoke induces cardiovascular dysfunction in mice. *Am. J. Physiol. Heart Circ. Physiol.* **2017**, *312*, H329–H339. [CrossRef]
57. Ryter, S.W.; Kim, H.P.; Hoetzel, A.; Park, J.W.; Nakahira, K.; Wang, X.; Choi, A.M. Mechanisms of cell death in oxidative stress. *Antioxid. Redox Signal.* **2007**, *9*, 49–89. [CrossRef]
58. Hasan, A.; Rizvi, S.F.; Parveen, S.; Pathak, N.; Nazir, A.; Mir, S.S. Crosstalk between ROS and Autophagy in Tumorigenesis: Understanding the Multifaceted Paradox. *Front. Oncol.* **2022**, *12*, 852424. [CrossRef]
59. Noman, M.Z.; Janji, B.; Kaminska, B.; Van Moer, K.; Pierson, S.; Przanowski, P.; Buart, S.; Berchem, G.; Romero, P.; Mami-Chouaib, F.; et al. Blocking hypoxia-induced autophagy in tumors restores cytotoxic T-cell activity and promotes regression. *Cancer Res.* **2011**, *71*, 5976–5986. [CrossRef]
60. Vijayalingam, S.; Pillai, S.G.; Rashmi, R.; Subramanian, T.; Sagartz, J.E.; Chinnadurai, G. Overexpression of BH3-Only Protein BNIP3 Leads to Enhanced Tumor Growth. *Genes Cancer* **2010**, *1*, 964–971. [CrossRef]
61. Ishihara, M.; Urushido, M.; Hamada, K.; Matsumoto, T.; Shimamura, Y.; Ogata, K.; Inoue, K.; Taniguchi, Y.; Horino, T.; Fujieda, M.; et al. Sestrin-2 and BNIP3 regulate autophagy and mitophagy in renal tubular cells in acute kidney injury. *Am. J. Physiol. Renal. Physiol.* **2013**, *305*, F495–F509. [CrossRef]
62. Pan, C.; Chen, Z.; Li, C.; Han, T.; Liu, H.; Wang, X. Sestrin2 as a gatekeeper of cellular homeostasis: Physiological effects for the regulation of hypoxia-related diseases. *J. Cell Mol. Med.* **2021**, *25*, 5341–5350. [CrossRef]
63. Chen, K.B.; Xuan, Y.; Shi, W.J.; Chi, F.; Xing, R.; Zeng, Y.C. Sestrin2 expression is a favorable prognostic factor in patients with non-small cell lung cancer. *Am. J. Transl. Res.* **2016**, *8*, 1903–1909.
64. Di Rienzo, M.; Romagnoli, A.; Antonioli, M.; Piacentini, M.; Fimia, G.M. TRIM proteins in autophagy: Selective sensors in cell damage and innate immune responses. *Cell Death Differ.* **2020**, *27*, 887–902. [CrossRef]

65. Ji, J.; Ding, K.; Luo, T.; Zhang, X.; Chen, A.; Zhang, D.; Li, G.; Thorsen, F.; Huang, B.; Li, X.; et al. TRIM22 activates NF-kappaB signaling in glioblastoma by accelerating the degradation of IkappaBalpha. *Cell Death Differ.* **2021**, *28*, 367–381. [CrossRef]
66. He, W.; Wang, Q.; Xu, J.; Xu, X.; Padilla, M.T.; Ren, G.; Gou, X.; Lin, Y. Attenuation of TNFSF10/TRAIL-induced apoptosis by an autophagic survival pathway involving TRAF2- and RIPK1/RIP1-mediated MAPK8/JNK activation. *Autophagy* **2012**, *8*, 1811–1821. [CrossRef]
67. Pecoraro, A.; Pagano, M.; Russo, G.; Russo, A. Role of Autophagy in Cancer Cell Response to Nucleolar and Endoplasmic Reticulum Stress. *Int. J. Mol. Sci.* **2020**, *21*, 7334. [CrossRef] [PubMed]
68. Mosca, L.; Pagano, M.; Borzacchiello, L.; Mele, L.; Russo, A.; Russo, G.; Cacciapuoti, G.; Porcelli, M. S-Adenosylmethionine Increases the Sensitivity of Human Colorectal Cancer Cells to 5-Fluorouracil by Inhibiting P-Glycoprotein Expression and NF-κB Activation. *Int. J. Mol. Sci.* **2021**, *22*, 9286. [CrossRef] [PubMed]
69. Mosca, L.; Pagano, M.; Pecoraro, A.; Borzacchiello, L.; Mele, L.; Cacciapuoti, G.; Porcelli, M.; Russo, G.; Russo, A. S-Adenosyl-l-Methionine Overcomes uL3-Mediated Drug Resistance in p53 Deleted Colon Cancer Cells. *Int. J. Mol. Sci.* **2020**, *22*, 103. [CrossRef] [PubMed]
70. Sun, Y.; Yang, Q.; Shen, J.; Wei, T.; Shen, W.; Zhang, N.; Luo, P.; Zhang, J. The Effect of Smoking on the Immune Microenvironment and Immunogenicity and Its Relationship with the Prognosis of Immune Checkpoint Inhibitors in Non-small Cell Lung Cancer. *Front. Cell Dev. Biol.* **2021**, *9*, 745859. [CrossRef] [PubMed]
71. Li, H. A statistical framework for SNP calling, mutation discovery, association mapping and population genetical parameter estimation from sequencing data. *Bioinformatics* **2011**, *27*, 2987–2993. [CrossRef]
72. McLaren, W.; Gil, L.; Hunt, S.E.; Riat, H.S.; Ritchie, G.R.S.; Thormann, A.; Flicek, P.; Cunningham, F. The Ensembl Variant Effect Predictor. *Genome Biol.* **2016**, *17*, 122. [CrossRef]
73. Mayakonda, A.; Lin, D.-C.; Assenov, Y.; Plass, C.; Koeffler, H.P. Maftools: Efficient and comprehensive analysis of somatic variants in cancer. *Genome Res.* **2018**, *28*, 1747–1756. [CrossRef]
74. Bergstrom, E.N.; Ni Huang, M.; Mahto, U.; Barnes, M.; Stratton, M.R.; Rozen, S.G.; Alexandrov, L.B. SigProfilerMatrixGenerator: A tool for visualizing and exploring patterns of small mutational events. *BMC Genom.* **2019**, *20*, 685. [CrossRef]
75. Newman, A.M.; Steen, C.B.; Liu, C.L.; Gentles, A.J.; Chaudhuri, A.A.; Scherer, F.; Khodadoust, M.S.; Esfahani, M.S.; Luca, B.A.; Steiner, D.; et al. Determining cell type abundance and expression from bulk tissues with digital cytometry. *Nat. Biotechnol.* **2019**, *37*, 773–782. [CrossRef]
76. Jiang, P.; Gu, S.; Pan, D.; Fu, J.; Sahu, A.; Hu, X.; Li, Z.; Traugh, N.; Bu, X.; Li, B.; et al. Signatures of T cell dysfunction and exclusion predict cancer immunotherapy response. *Nat. Med.* **2018**, *24*, 1550–1558. [CrossRef]
77. Guo, D.; Wang, M.; Shen, Z.; Zhu, J. A new immune signature for survival prediction and immune checkpoint molecules in lung adenocarcinoma. *J. Transl. Med.* **2020**, *18*, 123. [CrossRef]
78. Ling, B.; Ye, G.; Zhao, Q.; Jiang, Y.; Liang, L.; Tang, Q. Identification of an Immunologic Signature of Lung Adenocarcinomas Based on Genome-Wide Immune Expression Profiles. *Front. Mol. Biosci.* **2020**, *7*, 603701. [CrossRef]
79. Diaz-Uriarte, R. GeneSrF and varSelRF: A web-based tool and R package for gene selection and classification using random forest. *BMC Bioinform.* **2007**, *8*, 328. [CrossRef]

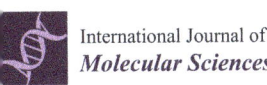

Review

Beyond Genetics: Metastasis as an Adaptive Response in Breast Cancer

Federica Ruscitto [1,†], Niccolò Roda [1,†], Chiara Priami [1], Enrica Migliaccio [1,*] and Pier Giuseppe Pelicci [1,2,*]

1. European Institute of Oncology (IEO) IRCCS, Via Ripamonti 435, 20141 Milan, Italy; federica.ruscitto@ieo.it (F.R.); niccolo.roda@ieo.it (N.R.); chiara.priami@ieo.it (C.P.)
2. Department of Oncology and Hemato-Oncology, University of Milan, Via Santa Sofia 9, 20142 Milan, Italy
* Correspondence: enrica.migliaccio@ieo.it (E.M.); piergiuseppe.pelicci@ieo.it (P.G.P.)
† These authors contributed equally to this work.

Abstract: Metastatic disease represents the primary cause of breast cancer (BC) mortality, yet it is still one of the most enigmatic processes in the biology of this tumor. Metastatic progression includes distinct phases: invasion, intravasation, hematogenous dissemination, extravasation and seeding at distant sites, micro-metastasis formation and metastatic outgrowth. Whole-genome sequencing analyses of primary BC and metastases revealed that BC metastatization is a non-genetically selected trait, rather the result of transcriptional and metabolic adaptation to the unfavorable microenvironmental conditions which cancer cells are exposed to (e.g., hypoxia, low nutrients, endoplasmic reticulum stress and chemotherapy administration). In this regard, the latest multi-omics analyses unveiled intra-tumor phenotypic heterogeneity, which determines the polyclonal nature of breast tumors and constitutes a challenge for clinicians, correlating with patient poor prognosis. The present work reviews BC classification and epidemiology, focusing on the impact of metastatic disease on patient prognosis and survival, while describing general principles and current in vitro/in vivo models of the BC metastatic cascade. The authors address here both genetic and phenotypic intrinsic heterogeneity of breast tumors, reporting the latest studies that support the role of the latter in metastatic spreading. Finally, the review illustrates the mechanisms underlying adaptive stress responses during BC metastatic progression.

Keywords: breast cancer; metastatic cascade; intra-tumor heterogeneity; mutational profile; adaptive responses

1. Breast Cancer Mortality Is Associated with Metastatic Disease

Breast cancer (BC) arises from the transformation of epithelial cells of the ductal-lobular compartment of the mammary gland [1] and it accounts for ~30% of diagnosed cancers and ~15% of cancer-related deaths in women [2]. BC incidence increases with age, being maximal between 50–70 years [3] and it is tightly linked to ethnicity, with African American women displaying the highest incidence and worst prognosis [4,5]. Several risk factors are associated with BC [6], including a family history of BC, due to inherited variants of cancer predisposing genes, such as BRCA1 and BRCA2 [7], early menarche and late menopause [8], obesity [9,10], alcohol consumption [11], physical inactivity [12] and exposure to exogenous hormones (e.g., oral contraceptives and menopausal hormone replacement therapy, [13]).

Molecular classification [14] stratifies BC patients into four major groups [15] on the basis of the expression of estrogen receptor (ESR), progesterone receptor (PR), human epidermal growth factor 2 receptor (HER2) and the proliferative marker Ki67. Tumors classified as Luminal A and B express both ESR and PR, with the A subtype displaying higher expression levels and B tumors occasionally expressing also HER2. The proliferation rate in luminal tumors is variable, but it is generally higher in the B subtype. Consistently, prognosis is usually good for the A subtype and intermediate for the B. Luminal tumors are the most frequent type of BC, with the A subtype accounting for 40%, and the B subtype for 20% of all patients. HER2 tumors account for 15–20% of patients and lack ESR and PR expression, while overexpressing HER2. They are highly proliferative tumors with intermediate prognosis. Ultimately, triple-negative breast cancer (TNBC), the least common subtype (10–20% of patients), lacks ESR, PR and HER2 expression; it is poorly differentiated and highly proliferative, leading to the worst patient prognosis [16–18].

The vast majority of BC-related deaths are not associated with primary tumor (PT) outgrowth. Rather, cancer mortality is generally (>90%) due to metastatic relapse [19,20], which rapidly results in multi-organ failure [21]. It is estimated that 20–30% of early stage BC patients will develop metastatic disease [22], while 5–10% of patients present metastases already at diagnosis [23]. The 5-year survival rate for women with metastatic BC ranges between 18% and 36% [24], compared to >90% of non-metastatic BC patients [25]. Despite the significant therapeutic progresses made in the last few years [13], metastatic BC remains mostly incurable: hence, knowledge around cellular and molecular mechanisms of metastatization and new targeted therapeutic approaches are urgently needed [26].

Traditionally, metastatic progression has been depicted as a late process in which the PT needs to grow to a certain size before releasing cells in the circulation [27]. On the contrary, recent evidence suggests that metastasis spreading can be an extremely early event [28,29], with tumor cells disseminating as early as the pre-malignant phase of tumorigenesis [30–32]. Consistently, ~1% of BC patients present metastases in the absence of a clearly identifiable PT [33].

Distant organs to which BC preferentially metastasizes are bones (~70%), lungs (~70%) and liver (~60%, [34]). Recent studies reported that commonly investigated parameters such as age at diagnosis, ethnicity and histological grade are almost never associated with sites of metastasis, whereas the subtype correlates with specific sites of colonization [35]. Indeed, bones represent the most prevalent metastatic site in Luminal A and B patients. Conversely, HER2 BC patients show metastases in both bones and liver at comparable levels, while TNBC metastases are mostly localized in bones and lungs [35,36]. The brain represents the least colonized organ across BC subtypes [34], accounting for ~20% of BC metastases, likely due to the tightness of the blood–brain barrier, which hinders extravasation of BC cells in the brain parenchyma [37]. However, patients with brain metastases generally display the worst prognosis (followed by patients with liver metastases [38]), due to the inefficient delivery of chemotherapeutic drugs to the brain [37].

Several studies investigated PT characteristics that correlate with increased metastasis risk in BC, which have been identified in larger tumor size, increased blood/lymphatic vessel and nerve fiber infiltration, ESR/PR negativity and TP53 overexpression [39–41]. However, the genetic and phenotypic determinants that specifically ignite the metastatic process within the PT mass are not yet fully understood.

2. The BC Metastatic Progression Is a Multistep Process

The BC metastatic disease can be conceptualized as a multistep process (Figure 1), characterized by a series of consecutive events: (i) epithelial-to-mesenchymal transition (EMT) and local invasion of PT cells in the surrounding tissues; (ii) intravasation and survival of tumor cells in the circulatory or lymphatic system; (iii) extravasation of circulating cells through the vascular endothelium into the parenchyma of distant organs; (iv) seeding and clonal expansion of extravasated cells which originate small colonies, henceforth referred to as "micro-metastases"; (v) micro-metastases adaptation to the foreign microenvironment and formation of clinically detectable lesions. Each of these steps will be further characterized below.

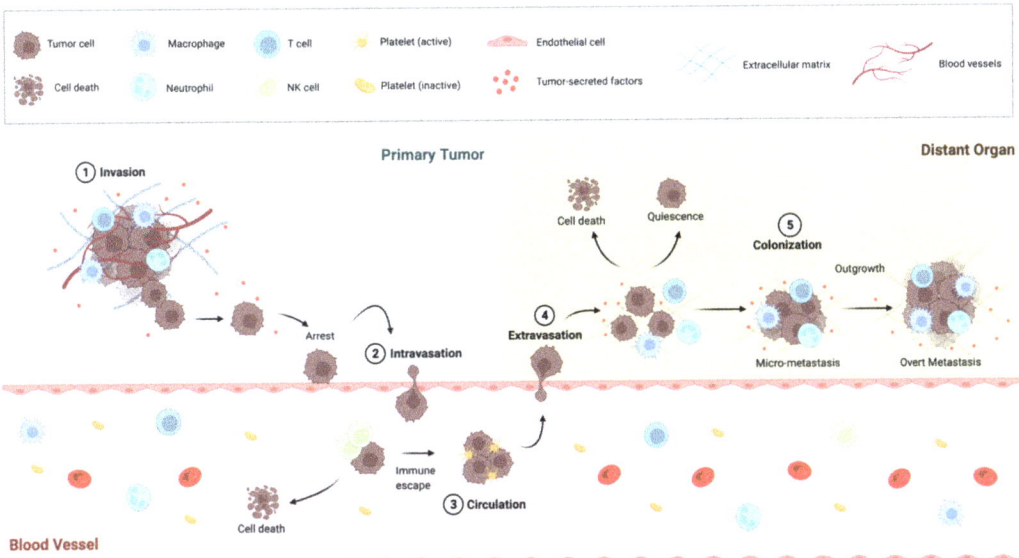

Figure 1. The BC Metastatic Progression is a Multistep Process. The metastatic process implies local invasion of the PT by cancer cells, followed by intravasation in the tumor vasculature. Once arrested in the capillary bed, cells enter the circulatory system. Cancer cells in the circulation are vulnerable to the attacks of the immune system, particularly exerted by Natural Killer cells, which proceed to tumor cell rapid clearance. Immune resistant cancer cells move along the blood vessels as single cells or clusters coated with platelets, and disseminate to secondary sites, passively following the circulatory patterns. Upon their arrival in the capillaries of a distant organ, cancer cells extravasate and start to colonize the foreign parenchyma. Colonization comprises many steps that occur in a timescale of years, during which time cells develop resistance to immunity, adapt to the novel microenvironment and settle in a pre-metastatic niche which support their survival and tumor-initiating capacity. At the metastatic site, cancer cells may be either eliminated or enter in a quiescent state as single cells or micro-metastases. Once the cancer cells break out of dormancy, they reinitiate outgrowth to form an overt metastasis in the distant organ microenvironment (figure created with BioRender.com (accessed on 26 March 2022)).

2.1. Epithelial-to-Mesenchimal Transition

To leave the PT, cancer cells must first undergo a series of transcriptional modifications that will result in a drastic phenotypical change, known as Epithelial-to-Mesenchymal Transition (EMT). EMT is the critical initial step of the metastatic cascade, which leads to loss of epithelial features, followed by acquisition of migratory and invasive capacities. EMT is a physiological program that occurs during embryo development and, in adults, in processes such as wound healing, tissue regeneration and fibrosis [42–44]. EMT induces epithelial cells to lose their polarity, to break down cell-to-cell and cell-to-basal lamina junctions, and to acquire mesenchymal phenotypes, such as a spindle-shape morphology, lack of polarization and cytoskeletal rearrangements, which enable contractility and movement [45]. In the cancer context, epithelial cancer cells undergo EMT in the growing tumor as a consequence of exogenous paracrine signals, such as the Transforming Growth Factor beta (TGFβ) and TGFβ-related cytokines, which activate multiple signaling pathways [46–51], including Wnt/β-catenin signaling [52–58], Notch signaling [59–61], interleukins [62–64] or environmental conditionings from the "reactive" tumor-associated stroma–i.e., fibroblasts, myofibroblasts, endothelial and immune cells, which activate master transcription factors such as SNAIL [65–69], SLUG [50,70–72], TWIST [73–75] and ZEB1 [76–80]. In all cases, cells undergo profound transcriptional reprogramming, which leads to the loss of epithelial markers (e.g., E-cadherin [81]), to the acquisition of mesenchymal markers (e.g., N-cadherin [82], fibronectin [83] and vimentin [84,85]), to cytoskeleton reorganization [86–88], Extracellular Matrix (ECM)-degradation [83,89,90] and, ultimately, increased migratory capacities. Notably, EMT also favors the generation of Cancer Stem Cells (CSC) [91] and prevents apoptosis and senescence via SNAIL and SLUG-mediated downregulation of p53 [92] and ZEB1-mediated downregulation of p63 and p73 [93]. Moreover, EMT increases resistance to multiple cytotoxic treatments, such as paclitaxel, docetaxel, epirubicin and doxorubicin [94,95], as well as to therapies targeting immune checkpoints (e.g., anti PDL1 and anti-CTL4 [96]). All these events are reversible, following a regulated process known as mesenchymal-to-epithelial transition (MET), which occurs when migratory mesenchymal cells have colonized distant sites and must reacquire epithelial features to infiltrate the new tissue [97].

2.2. Intravasation and Circulating Tumor Cells

During BC metastatic progression, mesenchymal-like invasive cancer cells enter the vasculature of either neighboring normal tissues or newly formed vessels within the tumor itself. Lymphatic vessels provide alternative routes for cell distribution to secondary organs. In fact, one of the earliest markers of BC metastatic disease is the presence of micro-metastases in the draining lymph nodes close to the PT site, clinically defined as "sentinel lymph nodes" [98]. Despite their early involvement, lymph nodes may represent temporary "pausing" sites but rarely end points for cancer cells [99], which most frequently seed distant regions via hematogenous dissemination. Circulating Tumor Cells (CTCs) are exposed to a variety of conditions that are potent inducers of a specific apoptotic program known as anoikis [100]. These include the flow shear stress, lack of adhesion signals and intracellular oxidative stress. CTCs are also vulnerable to immune system attacks, exerted in particular by Natural Killer (NK) cells [101]. On the other hand, the EMT phenotype is associated with anoikis resistance [102,103] and CTCs may establish interactions with several cell-types that promote their survival and extravasation. Platelets, for example, form a shield around CTCs that protects them from NK cells [104] and may prevent MET and the resulting loss of migratory/invasive traits [105]. Neutrophils also promote CTC survival via physical entrapment and, similarly to platelets, prevent CTC clearance by NK cells [106]. The balance between pro-apoptotic and pro-survival signals is, however, in favor of the first process, since CTC half-life is estimated to be between 1 and 2.4 h [107]. CTC dissemination and homing to specific organs are strongly influenced by circulatory patterns and structural differences in the capillary wall of each organ. As a consequence, metastatic tropism is considered as a passive process [108].

2.3. Extravasation

The mechanical entrapment of cancer cells in the capillary bed of a secondary organ causes CTCs to arrest. As anticipated, vessel configuration strongly contributes to determine the site of cancer cell extravasation. The fenestrated sinusoid capillaries of bone marrow and liver facilitate passive CTC extravasation, accounting for the high incidence of bone and liver BC metastases [34]. Conversely, passage through the endothelial tight junctions of lung capillaries or the blood–brain barrier necessitates to initiate specific "extravasation programs" and complex interactions with other cell types. Active extravasation requires cancer cells to pass through the endothelial wall via a process called Trans-Endothelial Migration (TEM; [109]). TEM is mediated by platelets and components of the innate immune system. Platelets interacting with CTCs trigger TEM by releasing TGFβ or enhancing vasculature wall permeability trough the secretion of adenine nucleotides [110]. Similarly, neutrophils, which are recruited by platelet-derived chemokines, adhere to the vessel wall, provide cancer cells with a physical dock and facilitate their extravasation through the secretion of metalloproteinases [106,110]. Inflammatory monocytes, which may differentiate into metastasis-associated macrophages, are recruited via cytokine CCL2 secreted by cancer cells, facilitating vascular permeability, extravasation and seeding into the host tissue parenchyma [111]. In addition to microenvironmental signals, cancer cells undergo TEM via the expression of autocrine enhancers of cell-motility and mediators of vascular permeability, including epiregulin, VEGF, MMPs, COX2 and ANGPTL4 [112,113]. In particular, Angiopoietin-like 4 (ANGPTL4) expression is induced by stromal TGFβ and it primes BC cell extravasation in the lungs via disruption of vascular integrity and TEM induction [114].

2.4. Metastatic Colonization

The development of clinically detectable metastatic lesions represents the final and most complex step in the malignant progression of a tumor. Colonization is thought to be a bottleneck of metastasis, as many cancer cells disseminate, but only 0.01% form metastases [99]. Colonization inefficiency is due to the fact that seeded cancer cells may undergo apoptosis or clearance by NK and cytotoxic T cells. Alternatively, infiltrated cancer cells may enter a quiescent state that is triggered by the intrinsically stressful condition of residing into a foreign microenvironment, which lacks all those familiar ECM constituents, stromal cells, signaling factors and mitogenic cues that had sustained their growth in the PT site [115]. As a consequence, metastatic disease may enter a phase of dormancy, which is sustained by clinical observations. A great number (20–45%) of patients who have been successfully treated for their PT never show a relapse after a long period of latency: these patients may harbor a reservoir of indolent disseminated tumor cells (DTCs) or micrometastatic clusters in distant organs and they are considered to have asymptomatic minimal residual disease, a condition that may last even for decades [116].

Despite its biological and clinical relevance, little is known about the mechanisms that promote and sustain dormancy in the metastatic context, mostly because of the difficulty to study metastatic latency in patients or experimental models (Table 1). However, it has been demonstrated that members of the TGFβ and BMP family, as well as factors present in the peri-vascular niche (i.e., the microenvironment where the vasculature harboring DTC clusters is embedded in) such as Thrombospondin-1 (TSP-1), play a role in promoting dormancy [116,117]. Successful colonization assumes that DTCs sense and respond to survival and proliferative stimuli, escape immune-surveillance, recruit the necessary supporting stroma and expand until they reach overt-metastasis formation. To do this, DTC clusters must possess at least two pre-requisites: (i) the capacity to seed and maintain a population of CSCs, responsible for initiating metastatic expansion and (ii) the ability to thrive in a hostile microenvironment through a program of organ-specific phenotypic adaptation. Adaptive responses, with regard to BC, will be covered in the following paragraphs.

3. BC Intra-Tumor Heterogeneity and Metastasis

BC evolves through the accumulation of oncogenic mutations starting from a genetically normal cell, also known as the "cell-of-origin" [1]. The "cell-of-origin" then undergoes clonal expansion, a process that is accompanied by the acquisition of further genetic and phenotypic traits, thereby generating a state of Intra-Tumor Heterogeneity (ITH; [118]). As a consequence, breast tumors, though clonal in origin, become polyclonal systems [119,120], whereby different clones (i.e., populations of cells that originate from a common ancestor) differ in terms of their genomic and phenotypic profiles [121–123].

3.1. Genetic Heterogeneity

The METABRIC (Molecular Taxonomy of Breast Cancer International Consortium) study [124,125] investigated the intra-tumor genetic heterogeneity of more than 2000 BC patients. This study reported that the mutations of several cancer-driver genes are present uniquely in a fraction of tumor cells, suggesting that populations of BC cells in the same tumor evolve distinct mutational profiles during in situ progression. Similarly, single-cell DNA analyses on patient biopsies revealed that breast tumors are composed of multiple genetic clones harboring distinct mutational profiles [126,127]. In this regard, different genetic clones are generally confined to distinct areas within the PT, although occasionally single clones can spread across multiple geographical regions in the tumor [128,129]. In line with this, a study on HER2 BC reported that the HER2 gene displays regional heterogeneity in terms of Copy Number Variations (CNVs). Notably, patients carrying highly heterogeneous HER2 amplification within the same mass poorly respond to trastuzumab, a monoclonal antibody to HER2, compared to patients with homogeneous HER2 amplification, suggesting that genetic heterogeneity represents a major challenge for BC therapy [130]. Ultimately, three studies by Aparicio and colleagues demonstrated the presence of several mutations in a small fraction of cells in the whole PT, thus suggesting that such mutations occurred at a later phase of cancer progression [131–133].

3.2. Transcriptional Heterogeneity

BC displays profound phenotypic ITH, with cells of the same PT adopting different transcriptional and metabolic profiles. Bodenmiller and colleagues investigated the expression of 35 different markers in more than 300 patient-biopsies by mass cytometry [134]. In particular, they evaluated, at single-cell spatial resolution, the expression of proteins involved in specific phenotypes, such as hypoxia response, apoptosis, EMT, proliferation and interaction with ECM. Their analyses revealed that breast PTs are organized in communities of cells, which cluster in separate regions of the tumor and display distinct phenotypes [135].

Recently, single-cell RNA sequencing technology has shed further light on phenotypic ITH. An analysis of multiple murine breast tumor models revealed that cells from the same PT can be extremely different in terms of gene expression profiles, with some cells showing activation of proliferation-related genes (e.g., Ki67), while other cells activate master regulators of EMT (e.g., TWIST1), or either basal (e.g., IGFBP5) or mesenchymal (e.g., vimentin) markers [136–138]. Single-cell analysis of the human luminal BC cell line MCF7 revealed that in vitro cultured cells could alternatively display two distinct major transcriptional programs: highly proliferative or dormant-like, with the latter showing upregulation of pathways related to stress response, hypoxia and EMT [138]. Consistently, individual PTs from TNBC patients were reported to consist of both aggressive and highly proliferating cells on one side, and slowly proliferating cells on the other [136,139].

3.3. Metabolic Heterogeneity

Single-cell transcriptional analysis of the murine BC genetic model MMTV-PyMT revealed that individual tumors may contain both glycolytic cells and cells that preferentially activate oxidative phosphorylation (OXPHOS) [140]. The switch from an oxidative to a glycolytic metabolism correlates with oxygen availability, since cells in hypoxic regions preferentially rely on glycolysis [141]. Consistently, a recent study on TNBC patient biopsies revealed that hypoxic cells hyperactivate glycolysis, while normoxic cells switch towards OXPHOS [142]. Viable cells in the necrotic core of breast tumors (where oxygen levels are extremely low as a consequence of poor vascularization) exhibit increased glucose uptake to fuel the glycolytic pathway [143]. Ultimately, it has also been reported that metabolism varies in the CSC compartment of breast tumors, with CSCs upregulating mitochondrial proteins, glycolysis and anabolic enzymes with respect to non-stem cancer cells [144,145].

3.4. Impacts of ITH on Patient Prognosis and Treatment

ITH represents a hurdle for clinicians, as it might jeopardize patient diagnosis and treatment response [146–148]. A high degree of ITH correlates with poor BC outcome and metastatic disease [149,150]. A retrospective study on 75 TNBC patients reported that the degree of heterogeneity in the CNV profile correlates with a higher risk of developing distant metastases and poor prognosis [151]. Likewise, another study quantifying the genetic intra-tumor diversity in patient-specific mutational profiles of more than 900 TCGA (The Cancer Genome Atlas) BC patients showed an inverse correlation between ITH and overall survival [152,153]. Moreover, the analysis of estrogen receptor expression across 970 different breast tumors revealed that patients with the most heterogeneous expression display an increased risk of distant metastases [154]. Thus, the co-existence of heterogeneous populations of cells within the same PT favors distant metastases, suggesting that different clones may develop cooperative interactions [155,156]. The role of clonal cooperativity in BC progression has been investigated since the late 1980s by O'Grady and colleagues, exploiting an in vitro model of rat mammary carcinoma. They showed that individual tumors are composed of both myo-epithelioid (M-cells) and epithelioid (E-cells) cells. These two populations interact through a soluble factor released by M-cells that induces collagenase secretion by E-cells, suggesting that the co-existence of two independent subpopulations is required for the expression of invasive traits [157]. Consistently, a recent study by Polyak and colleagues revealed that the metastatic behavior of certain BC clones may be actively sustained by others. Indeed, the paracrine release of IL-11 and Vascular Endothelial Growth Factor-D (VEGF-D) by a restricted clone in the PT was shown to induce microenvironmental changes (e.g., increased permeability of blood and lymphatic vessels, recruitment of pro-metastatic neutrophils), thus supporting the metastatic progression of other clones [158].

4. BC Metastatic Progression Is Not a Genetically Selected Trait

As genetic ITH positively correlates with distant metastasis spreading, it can be hypothesized that metastatic disease is indeed a genetically selected trait, which may depend on the occurrence of metastasis-driver mutations. According to this hypothesis, metastatic cells should share most somatic mutations with the whole tumor and be endowed with a separate subset of mutations capable of driving metastatic progression.

Whole Genome Sequencing (WGS) of 442 paired primary-metastasis samples [159] and Whole Exome Sequencing (WES) of 9 stage IV BC patients [160] showed increased mutational burden in metastatic lesions (i.e., single- and multiple-nucleotide variants, indels and structural variants). In both cases, however, candidate metastasis-driver genes were found at a comparable frequency in PTs and metastases (TP53, PIK3CA, ESR1, GATA3, KMT2C, and the EMT genes SMAD4, TCF7L2 and TCF4; [160]). Bioinformatic analyses of metastasis-specific genes in the former study (24% of all metastasis-associated mutations) revealed a likely "passenger-origin" for these mutations (i.e., mutations that do not confer selective advantages to cancer cells [161]). Likewise, a passenger-origin was hypothesized in the rare metastasis-specific mutations found in two independent studies on BC brain metastases [162,163] and in independent cohorts of BC patients [164–167]. Interestingly, in other cases metastasis-specific mutations have been interpreted as due to anti-cancer treatments [168]. Other reports, instead, showed that the mutational landscape of metastases and matched PTs mostly overlap [161–164]. This was also shown at a single-cell level by Navin and colleagues, who investigated the mutational profile of 10 patients affected by invasive BC and showed that invasive cancer cells harbor similar CNVs and an almost identical mutational profile [169]. In conclusion, the high genetic ITH of primary BC samples and their genomic similarity with matched metastatic lesions argue against the existence of selectable pro-metastatic genes and suggest a polyclonal origin of metastases, where clusters of genetically heterogeneous cells are shed into circulation, colonize distant organs and generate a secondary metastatic growth, with results similar to PT [165,170,171].

However, although primary and metastatic BC generally share similar genetic landscapes, several reports have shown relevant differences in mutations when metastases arise years after the PT diagnosis [2,172]. Indeed, a pivotal study by Campbell and colleagues revealed that while in the early phases of cell dissemination PT and metastatic genomic profiles were similar, metastases accumulated independent driver and passenger mutations at later phases [173]. Others reported that ~50% of genomic alterations of metachronous metastases could not be scored in the PT, thereby suggesting an independent mutational evolution of metastatic cells [174–176]. Importantly, these studies strongly suggest that the PT genomic profile may not be sufficient to assist the choice of targeting therapies for the metastatic disease.

5. Adaptive Responses in BC Metastasis

Emerging evidence suggests that the capacity to metastasize is part of an adaptive response of cancer cells to unfavorable micro-environmental conditions, including hypoxia, scarcity of nutrients, endoplasmic reticulum (ER) stress and chemotherapy (Figure 2; [177–179]).

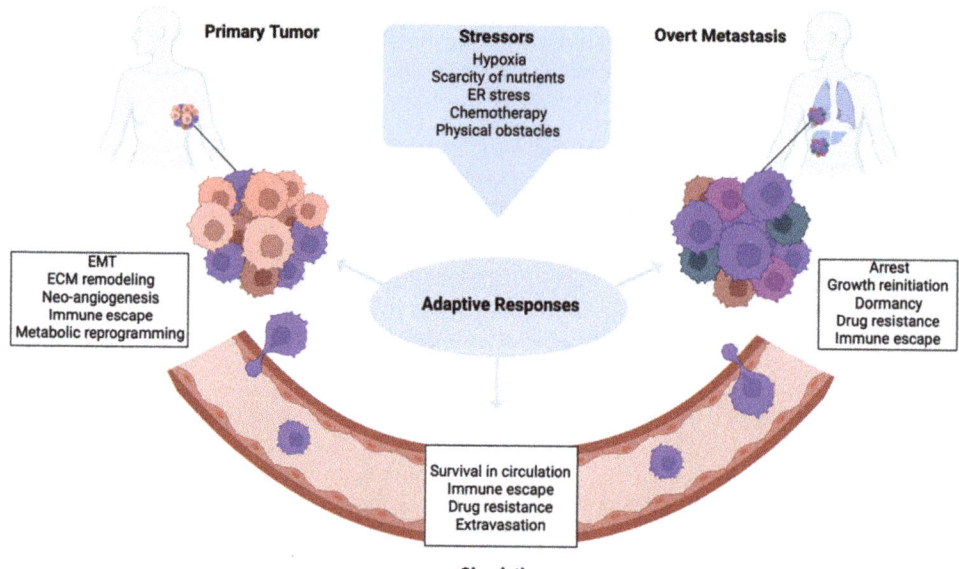

Figure 2. Adaptive Responses in BC Metastatization. During tumor progression, cancer cells encounter different kinds of microenvironmental stressors, such as hypoxia, nutrient deprivation, ER stress and physical obstacles while in transit, besides being exposed to therapeutic drugs. To increase stress tolerance and survive in a hostile environment, cells activate adaptive stress response pathways. These phenotypic adaptations are regulated in a spatial and temporal manner and foster intratumor heterogeneity, thereby endowing a subset of cancer cells with metastatic traits. Adaptive stress responses in the PT lead to EMT, immune escape, metabolic reprogramming and, through active remodeling of ECM and neo-angiogenesis events, enable cells to leave the PT site. Stress signaling also increases the capacity of cancer cells to survive in the circulation and extravasate, eluding immune surveillance and chemotherapy-induced apoptosis. Adaptive pathways at metastatic site regulate the growth dynamics of disseminated cells: once arrested in the target organ, cells can either enter dormancy to tolerate the foreign environment or reinitiate tumor growth (figure created with BioRender.com (accessed on 26 March 2022)).

5.1. Hypoxia

Hypoxia is a common feature of breast tumors and represents a major threat for cancer cell survival during tumor progression [180]. The deregulated growth of tumor masses progressively increases the distance between cancer cells and capillaries, thereby generating a hypoxic condition that hinders survival and proliferation [41]. Cancer cells respond to hypoxia with the stabilization of Hypoxia-Inducible Factor-1α (HIF-1α), which regulates transcription of several target genes, including glucose transporters, glycolysis enzymes and VEGF [181]. VEGF is secreted by BC cells and stimulates the sprouting of new vessels within the tumor mass, a process referred to as tumor neo-angiogenesis. However, these new vessels are leaky and highly permeable, thus facilitating local intravasation of cancer cells and their spreading in the circulation. Consistently, independent preclinical [182] and clinical studies [183–185] demonstrated that hypoxia and increased angiogenesis correlate with metastatic progression and poor patient prognosis.

Moreover, hypoxia was mainly shown to foster EMT in BC through upregulation of SNAIL, ZEB1 and TWIST, which in turn regulate cellular migration, loss of cell-to-cell adhesion, local invasion and stemness traits [186]. In line with this, SHARP1-mediated HIF-1α degradation reduces the expression of HIF-1α target genes, thereby severely impairing BC migration in vitro and metastatic progression in vivo [187]. Ultimately, hypoxic BC cells upregulate ANGPTL4 [181], which disrupts endothelial cell-to-cell junctions in lung capillaries, facilitating lung metastatic colonization [114].

5.2. Metabolic Stress

The deregulated growth of primary breast tumors is associated with the exhaustion of the local nutrient microenvironment, which leads to progressive nutrient deprivation, the accumulation of waste products and metabolic stress [123]. A pivotal study on transformed mammary cells revealed that glutamine deprivation strongly fosters the expression of stress-response genes (e.g., ATF4, DDIT3 and XBP1), including inflammatory mediators (e.g., KLF4, CCL2, NF-κB1 and IL20) and it increases the migratory phenotype of tumor cells [188]. In addition, a recent study using a panel of BC cell lines revealed that glutamine deficiency leads to addiction of cancer cells to asparagine and the compensatory upregulation of Asparagine Synthetase (ASNS) [189]. Notably, ASNS upregulation stimulates BC migration in vitro and metastasis spreading in vivo through EMT [190], therefore linking glutamine shortage to metastatic progression. Likewise, glucose deprivation was reported to stimulate oxidative stress in MCF7 BC cells [191], which in turn upregulate metastasis-associated genes, including VEGF and CD44 [192,193]. Ultimately, the accumulation of waste products in the tumor microenvironment leads to local acidification, which promotes metastatic progression. As an example, MCF7 chronically exposed to an acidic microenvironment were shown to acquire an invasive EMT phenotype, characterized by vimentin upregulation and E-cadherin downregulation [194]. Coherently, two studies by Lisanti and colleagues reported that BC cells exposed to the glycolytic-byproduct lactate display significantly higher metastatic potential in vivo, while PT growth remains unaffected [195]. Notably, lactate exposure increases the expression of stemness-related genes (including SP1, MAZ, SREBF1 and PAX4), which are associated with increased risk of developing metastases and poor prognosis [196].

5.3. ER Stress

Correct protein folding in the ER is fundamental to guarantee cellular homeostasis and survival. When ER protein folding capacity is hampered, unfolded proteins accumulate, threatening cellular homeostasis. The unfolded protein response (UPR) reprograms gene expression pathways in order to buffer the accumulation of aberrant peptides or to promote cellular apoptosis in case ER stress becomes irreversible [197]. ER stress is caused by several perturbations, including hypoxia, nutrient shortage, oxidative stress, chemotherapy administration and deregulated tumor growth [198–200]. ER stress is mediated by three main stress sensors: Inositol-Requiring Protein 1α (IRE1α), Protein Kinase RNA-like ER Kinase (PERK) and Activating Transcription Factor 6 (ATF6), which transduce ER-stress signals to the nucleus via three separate branches [201,202]. The upregulation of IRE1α was reported to booster the migratory phenotype of luminal BC cell lines in vitro, through degradation of several tumor suppressor miRNAs [203]. Consistently, the downregulation of the UPR stress sensor ATF6 significantly reduces BC migration and invasion in vitro [204]. In addition, an analysis of BC patient gene-expression profiles revealed that the overexpression of UPR-mediators Rhomboid Domain-Containing Protein 2 (RHBDD2) and Prion Protein (PRNP) is associated with increased metastatic spreading and poor outcome [205–207]. On top of that, the downregulation of UPR genes PERK, ATF4 and LAMP3 was shown to inhibit cellular migration and invasion of BC cells upon hypoxic conditions, linking UPR to the hypoxia-induced BC invasive phenotype [208]. Ultimately, the ER stress mediator

Endoplasmic Reticulum Oxidoreductase 1 (ERO1) is crucial for the pro-angiogenic role of HIF-1α upon hypoxia. Indeed, ERO1 deficiency significantly abrogates the secretion of pro-angiogenic factors such as VEGF, IGFBP4 and MMP1, thus inhibiting metastatic progression in vivo [209].

5.4. Chemotherapy

Despite enormous advances in BC therapy during the last few years, chemotherapy still represents one the most widely adopted therapeutic options [210–212]. However, recent evidence suggests that the administration of chemotherapeutic drugs may result in eliciting a pro-metastatic phenotype [213]. A pioneer work by Gao and colleagues revealed that, upon cyclophosphamide administration, BC cells adopt an EMT-like phenotype characterized by reduced proliferation, resistance to apoptosis, upregulation of drug-metabolizing enzymes and formation of chemoresistant metastases [214]. Ran and colleagues showed that breast tumors acquire a pro-metastatic phenotype upon Paclitaxel administration and that is mediated by Toll-like receptor 4 (TLR4), which promotes the release of inflammatory cytokines, including IL10, IL6 and IL1β, which on their turn stimulate the formation of lymphatic vessels in close proximity to the tumor; this is considered a putative path of metastasis spreading [215]. In another study, Paclitaxel was demonstrated to promote the accumulation of macrophages in the tumor microenvironment, which, in turn, induces expression in cancer cells of the invasive isoform of Mammalian-ENAbled Invasive (MENAINV) protein, an actin binding protein involved in the regulation of cell motility, leading to the intravasation and dissemination of cancer cells [216]. Likewise, Paclitaxel was reported to upregulate the mir-21/CDK5 axis, which activates the expression of EMT markers (vimentin and β-catenin), leading to increased metastasis dissemination to the lungs. Indeed, genetic or pharmacological inhibition of mir-21/CDK5 axis prevented Paclitaxel-induced lung metastases [217]. Carboplatin treatment was also shown to increase BC metastasis. It induces the overexpression of the HIF-1α target Glutathione S-Transferase Omega 1 (GSTO1), which, upon binding to type 1-Ryanodine receptor, promotes Ca^{2+} release from ER and the downstream activation of the PYK2-SRC-STAT3 axis, leading to increased expression of pluripotency genes. Intriguingly, the expression of pluripotency genes fosters the acquisition of a stem-like phenotype, which results in increased metastatic burden in the lungs [218]. Ultimately, two independent studies showed that chemotherapy elicits the release of extracellular vesicles in BC. In particular, De Palma and colleagues reported that Paclitaxel administration induces the release of Annexin A6-enriched vesicles by BC cells. These vesicles promote NF-κB-dependent endothelial cell activation, induction of monocyte-attractant chemokines and monocyte expansion in the lungs, priming the pulmonary niche for metastasis seeding [219]. Concordantly, Doxorubicin administration promotes the release of small extracellular vesicles that are enriched for the glycoprotein Pentraxin-related Protein 3 (PTX3). PTX3 binds P-selectin on the surface of vascular endothelial cells, leading to cell proliferation inhibition, increased expression of matrix metalloproteinases and endothelial cell dysfunction. Therefore, PTX3 causes vascular leakiness in the lungs, thus enhancing the pulmonary colonization of chemotherapy-treated BC cells. Indeed, the inhibition of small extracellular vesicle secretion suppresses chemotherapy-induced metastases [220]. Therefore, albeit fundamental for the treatment of BC, chemotherapy can have detrimental effects, fostering a pro-metastatic phenotype that worsens patient prognosis.

Table 1. Experimental Assays Employed to Study Metastases.

In Vitro Models	Mouse Models	Zebrafish Models

• Excellent tools to characterize migration, invasion and adhesion events at molecular level, or for drug testing.
• Cheap and rapid commercially available platforms.
• The **scratch assay** exploits a confluent monolayer cell culture in which a linear scratch generates a cell-free area that is replenished by migrating cells.
   ○ 2D cell migration can be investigated in real-time by time-lapse microscopy [221,222].
   ○ Unsuitable for non-adherent cells and for chemotaxis evaluation.
• The **trans membrane migration assay** (via modified Boyden chambers) enables to monitor cell movements between two distinct compartments separated by a microporous membrane.
   ○ Suitable for chemotaxis evaluation.
   ○ Suitable for evaluation of cancer cell-ECM interactions by coating the membrane with ECM proteins [223].
   ○ Migrating cells can be selectively recovered for further studies.
• These systems lack a faithful recapitulation of tumor-associated micro-environment and the three-dimensional architecture provided by ECM.
	• Most appropriate model organisms to investigate human cancer in all its complexity.
	• Genetic engineered mouse models (GEMMs) allow to study the de novo formation of tumors and metastases.
	   ○ They allow for a complete recapitulation of tumor-associated microenvironment.
	   ○ Their drawbacks are inter-individual variability in penetrance and time lagging before metastasis onset [224].
	   ○ The MMTV-PyMT mouse, obtained through the transgenic expression of Polyomavirus Middle T Antigen, is prone to multifocal mammary carcinomas with 100% penetrance and develop pulmonary metastases in 85% of cases, with a latency of 3 months [225].
	• Transplantable models can be syngeneic or xenografts.
	• Syngeneic models are obtained by the transplantation of murine cancer cells in mice with matching genetic background.
	   ○ They allow for a complete conservation of the host tumor-associated micro-environment.
	   ○ They may not fully recapitulate human breast cancers.
	• Xenograft models are obtained by the transplantation of human cancer cells into immunocompromised animals.
	   ○ They allow for the recapitulation of human breast cancer features.
	   ○ They do not permit to study interactions with the immune system.
	• Both models can be generated applying two opposite approaches.
	• The experimental metastasis approach is the direct transplantation of cancer cells in the circulation.
	   ○ It ensures rapidity and high reproducibility, by-passing the early steps of the metastatic cascade.
	   ○ It negatively selects dormant pro-metastatic cells.
	• The spontaneous metastasis approach is based on the subcutaneous or orthotopic transplantation of cancer cells in the host.
	   ○ The emergence of distant metastases may be less frequent and highly variable among individuals.
	   ○ It more closely resembles human cancer features, including early steps of the metastatic cascade [224,226].
	• Imaging metastases in mice often requires euthanasia and post-mortem organ examination.
	• Approaches for live imaging are generally laborious: magnetic resonance imaging, positron enhanced tomography scan and intravital microscopy.
	• Bioluminescence is the simplest live-imaging technique.
	   ○ It relies on detection of photons emitted by genetically-engineered transplanted cancer cells, upon the enzymatic reaction catalyzed by luciferase.
	   ○ Although non-invasive, it has a poor anatomical resolution [227].
	• Intravital microscopy provides high-resolution and single-cell level visualization of dynamic metastatic events.
	   ○ It exploits surgical optical windows exposed at specific anatomic regions.
	   ○ It provides both spatial and temporal information about cancer cell behavior and enables to follow individual cells over time.
	   ○ It remains experimentally challenging and limited to few specialized laboratories [228].
		• The use of non-mammalian hosts, as zebrafish, has emerged as an alternative or complementary system to mouse models of cancer metastases [229].
		• The transparency and small dimensions of zebrafish larvae, together with fluorescently labeled cancer cells, enables high-resolution real-time visualization of:
		   ○ Proliferation,
		   ○ Intravasation,
		   ○ Extravasation,
		   ○ Distant organ colonization by live imaging [230–233].
		• The lack of adaptive immune system eliminates the need for immunosuppression.
		• Several transgenic reporter lines with fluorescently labeled components of the host micro-environment (e.g. the vasculature, macrophages and neutrophils) allows for the visualization of complex phenotypes:
		   ○ Neo-angiogenesis,
		   ○ Interaction of human cancer cells with the host innate immune system [234–237].
		• Large numbers of animals are attainable, with significantly reduced costs and increased statistical power [238].
		• These characteristics make the zebrafish xenograft assay an appealing tool which allows to recapitulate and dissect each step of the metastatic cascade in real-time, with an unprecedented rapidity and optical resolution for an in vivo model.

6. Concluding Remarks

Metastasis spreading accounts for the vast majority of patient deaths and it represents therefore the deadliest outcome of BC. However, the molecular mechanisms that force cells to abandon the tumor microenvironment and to colonize distant organs are not yet fully understood. In particular, it is not completely clear whether the metastatic phenotype depends on the acquisition of specific metastasis-driver mutations that endow cells with a selective advantage over all the others. In this case, metastasis spreading should represent a genetically selected trait that improves the fitness of specific subpopulations in the PT, by conferring them the capacity to migrate towards distant organs. However, this hypothesis does not properly fit the basic principles of natural selection [239], as metastasizing cells do not display a higher fitness as compared to non-metastasizing ones. Rather, metastasis spreading often represents an inefficient process, in which tumor cells die long before reaching distant organs. On top of that, the outgrowth of BC cells in a different microenvironment may require, even decades after colonization, a period during which PT cells could hugely expand, while the metastatic ones linger in dormancy. Therefore, the hypothesis that metastasis represents a genetically selected trait does not easily fit the Darwinian concepts of selection. In line with this, recent literature largely failed in identifying metastasis-driver mutations (i.e., mutations that characterize the total of metastatic cells and are nearly absent in the PT). This failure can be largely due to the difficulty in having cohorts of patients where PT and metastases are synchronous, as the time-window between PT and metastasis diagnosis comes along with a significant alteration in the mutational profile of metastatic BC cells. This aspect should be carefully considered when studying the mechanisms that underlie metastatization. However, when synchronous primary and distant diseases have been investigated [169,173], results clearly showed that the mutational profile of the two significantly overlap, hence excluding the major role for metastasis-driver mutations in this process. In this review, we focused on this concept, reporting recent evidence that interpret metastatic spreading as an adaptive response to stress conditions (namely, hypoxia, unfolded proteins accumulation, metabolic stress and chemotherapy). Indeed, the important phenotypic determinants of metastatization were identified within BC stress response pathways, whose inactivation turned out to significantly decrease the metastatic progression in preclinical settings. However, the nature and the key players of these adaptive responses are still largely unknown and should be, in our opinion, the major focus of BC metastasis studies in the future (Table 2). In this regard, the use of both *in vitro* and *in vivo* appropriate preclinical models (summarized in Table 1) is of capital importance to dissect the role of specific genes in metastatization and to aggressively determine their exploitability, in order to identify possible drugs which can improve BC patient prognosis in the future.

Table 2. Questions to be addressed in future studies on BC metastatization.

1.	Despite metastasis is not a genetically selected trait, are there mutational backgrounds that are more prone than others to activate metastasis as an adaptive response to stress?
2.	Is the high mutational overlap between primary tumors and metastases due to ecological reasons (i.e., to the necessity of maintaining specific subpopulations at specific frequencies)?
3.	Which are the molecular triggers that ignite the passage from micro- to overt metastases?
4.	Are mouse models of patient-derived xenografts truly reliable in recapitulating patient's metastatic progression, since only cancer stem cells survive and form a new tumor upon transplantation?
5.	Given the early nature of metastatization, could be worth not to lose more differentiated ("progenitor-like") cells when modeling the metastatic cascade? In this scenario, could zebrafish be more suitable than mouse in finding "metastasis-prone (differentiated) cells"?

Author Contributions: Conceptualization, F.R., N.R., P.G.P.; writing—original draft preparation, F.R., N.R. and C.P.; writing—review and editing, E.M. and P.G.P.; supervision, E.M. and P.G.P. All authors have read and agreed to the published version of the manuscript.

Funding: AIRC (Associazione Italiana per la Ricerca sul Cancro): AIRC-IG-2017-20162. MIUR (Italian Ministry of University and Research): PRIN 2017L8FWY8. N.R was recipient of Fondazione IEO-CCM fellowship.

Conflicts of Interest: The authors declare no conflict of interest.

References

1. Sims, A.H.; Howell, A.; Howell, S.J.; Clarke, R.B. Origins of breast cancer subtypes and therapeutic implications. *Nat. Clin. Pract. Oncol.* **2007**, *4*, 516–525. [CrossRef] [PubMed]
2. Siegel, R.L.; Miller, K.D.; Jemal, A. Cancer statistics, 2020. *CA Cancer J. Clin.* **2020**, *70*, 7–30. [CrossRef] [PubMed]
3. McGuire, A.; Brown, J.A.; Malone, C.; McLaughlin, R.; Kerin, M.J. Effects of age on the detection and management of breast cancer. *Cancers* **2015**, *7*, 908–929. [CrossRef] [PubMed]
4. Chlebowski, R.T.; Chen, Z.; Anderson, G.L.; Rohan, T.; Aragaki, A.; Lane, D.; Dolan, N.C.; Paskett, E.D.; McTiernan, A.; Hubbell, F.A.; et al. Ethnicity and breast cancer: Factors influencing differences in incidence and outcome. *J. Natl. Cancer Inst.* **2005**, *97*, 439–448. [CrossRef]
5. DeSantis, C.E.; Ma, J.; Goding Sauer, A.; Newman, L.A.; Jemal, A. Breast cancer statistics, 2017, racial Dis.parity in mortality by state. *CA Cancer J. Clin.* **2017**, *67*, 439–448. [CrossRef]
6. Kaminska, M.; Ciszewski, T.; Lopacka-Szatan, K.; Miotla, P.; Staroslawska, E. Breast cancer risk factors. *Prz. Menopauzalny* **2015**, *14*, 196–202. [CrossRef]
7. Ford, D.; Easton, D.F.; Stratton, M.; Narod, S.; Goldgar, D.; Devilee, P.; Bishop, D.T.; Weber, B.; Lenoir, G.; Chang-Claude, J.; et al. Genetic heterogeneity and penetrance analysis of the BRCA1 and BRCA2 genes in breast cancer families. The Breast Cancer Linkage Consortium. *Am. J. Hum. Genet.* **1998**, *62*, 676–689. [CrossRef]
8. Collaborative Group on Hormonal Factors in Breast, C. Menarche, menopause, and breast cancer risk: Individual participant meta-analysis, including 118 964 women with breast cancer from 117 epidemiological studies. *Lancet Oncol.* **2012**, *13*, 1141–1151. [CrossRef]
9. James, F.R.; Wootton, S.; Jackson, A.; Wiseman, M.; Copson, E.R.; Cutress, R.I. Obesity in breast cancer–what is the risk factor? *Eur. J. Cancer* **2015**, *51*, 705–720. [CrossRef]
10. Mohanty, S.S.; Mohanty, P.K. Obesity as potential breast cancer risk factor for postmenopausal women. *Genes Dis.* **2021**, *8*, 117–123. [CrossRef]
11. Chen, W.Y.; Rosner, B.; Hankinson, S.E.; Colditz, G.A.; Willett, W.C. Moderate alcohol consumption during adult life, drinking patterns, and breast cancer risk. *JAMA* **2011**, *306*, 1884–1890. [CrossRef]
12. Danaei, G.; Vander Hoorn, S.; Lopez, A.D.; Murray, C.J.; Ezzati, M.; Comparative Risk Assessment collaborating, g. Causes of cancer in the world: Comparative risk assessment of nine behavioural and environmental risk factors. *Lancet* **2005**, *366*, 1784–1793. [CrossRef]
13. Torre, L.A.; Islami, F.; Siegel, R.L.; Ward, E.M.; Jemal, A. Global Cancer in Women: Burden and Trends. *Cancer Epidemiol. Biomark. Prev.* **2017**, *26*, 444–457. [CrossRef]
14. Malhotra, G.K.; Zhao, X.; Band, H.; Band, V. Histological, molecular and functional subtypes of breast cancers. *Cancer Biol.* **2010**, *10*, 955–960. [CrossRef]
15. Eliyatkin, N.; Yalcin, E.; Zengel, B.; Aktas, S.; Vardar, E. Molecular Classification of Breast Carcinoma: From Traditional, Old-Fashioned Way to A New Age, and A New Way. *J. Breast Health* **2015**, *11*, 59–66. [CrossRef]
16. Prat, A.; Pineda, E.; Adamo, B.; Galvan, P.; Fernandez, A.; Gaba, L.; Diez, M.; Viladot, M.; Arance, A.; Munoz, M. Clinical implications of the intrinsic molecular subtypes of breast cancer. *Breast* **2015**, *24* (Suppl. S2), S26–S35. [CrossRef]
17. Li, X.; Yang, J.; Peng, L.; Sahin, A.A.; Huo, L.; Ward, K.C.; O'Regan, R.; Torres, M.A.; Meisel, J.L. Triple-negative breast cancer has worse overall survival and cause-specific survival than non-triple-negative breast cancer. *Breast. Cancer Res. Treat.* **2017**, *161*, 279–287. [CrossRef]
18. Harbeck, N.; Penault-Llorca, F.; Cortes, J.; Gnant, M.; Houssami, N.; Poortmans, P.; Ruddy, K.; Tsang, J.; Cardoso, F. Breast cancer. *Nat. Rev. Dis. Primers* **2019**, *5*, 66. [CrossRef]
19. Foulkes, W.D.; Smith, I.E.; Reis-Filho, J.S. Triple-negative breast cancer. *N. Engl. J. Med.* **2010**, *363*, 1938–1948. [CrossRef]
20. Dillekas, H.; Rogers, M.S.; Straume, O. Are 90% of deaths from cancer caused by metastases? *Cancer Med.* **2019**, *8*, 5574–5576. [CrossRef]
21. Kaskel, P.; Orth, M.; Arndt, E.; Leiter, U.; Peter, R.U.; Krahn, G. Fulminating multi-organ failure in a young woman caused by rapidly progressing melanoma metastases. *Dermatology* **2000**, *201*, 79–80. [CrossRef]
22. Riggio, A.I.; Varley, K.E.; Welm, A.L. The lingering mysteries of metastatic recurrence in breast cancer. *Br. J. Cancer* **2021**, *124*, 13–26. [CrossRef]
23. Lim, B.; Hortobagyi, G.N. Current challenges of metastatic breast cancer. *Cancer Metastasis. Rev.* **2016**, *35*, 495–514. [CrossRef]

24. Mariotto, A.B.; Etzioni, R.; Hurlbert, M.; Penberthy, L.; Mayer, M. Estimation of the Number of Women Living with Metastatic Breast Cancer in the United States. *Cancer Epidemiol. Biomark. Prev.* **2017**, *26*, 809–815. [CrossRef]
25. Lucci, A.; Hall, C.S.; Lodhi, A.K.; Bhattacharyya, A.; Anderson, A.E.; Xiao, L.; Bedrosian, I.; Kuerer, H.M.; Krishnamurthy, S. Circulating tumour Cells in non-metastatic breast cancer: A prospective study. *Lancet Oncol.* **2012**, *13*, 688–695. [CrossRef]
26. Caswell-Jin, J.L.; Plevritis, S.K.; Tian, L.; Cadham, C.J.; Xu, C.; Stout, N.K.; Sledge, G.W.; Mandelblatt, J.S.; Kurian, A.W. Change in Survival in Metastatic Breast Cancer with Treatment Advances: Meta-Analysis and Systematic Review. *JNCI Cancer Spectr.* **2018**, *2*, pky062. [CrossRef]
27. Yachida, S.; Jones, S.; Bozic, I.; Antal, T.; Leary, R.; Fu, B.; Kamiyama, M.; Hruban, R.H.; Eshleman, J.R.; Nowak, M.A.; et al. Distant metastasis occurs late during the genetic evolution of pancreatic cancer. *Nature* **2010**, *467*, 1114–1117. [CrossRef]
28. Kang, Y.; Pantel, K. Tumor Cell Dissemination: Emerging Biological insights from animal models and cancer patients. *Cancer Cell* **2013**, *23*, 573–581. [CrossRef] [PubMed]
29. Klein, C.A. Selection and adaptation during metastatic cancer progression. *Nature* **2013**, *501*, 365–372. [CrossRef] [PubMed]
30. Husemann, Y.; Geigl, J.B.; Schubert, F.; Musiani, P.; Meyer, M.; Burghart, E.; Forni, G.; Eils, R.; Fehm, T.; Riethmuller, G.; et al. Systemic spread is an early step in breast cancer. *Cancer Cell* **2008**, *13*, 58–68. [CrossRef] [PubMed]
31. Hosseini, H.; Obradovic, M.M.S.; Hoffmann, M.; Harper, K.L.; Sosa, M.S.; Werner-Klein, M.; Nanduri, L.K.; Werno, C.; Ehrl, C.; Maneck, M.; et al. Early Dis.semination seeds metastasis in breast cancer. *Nature* **2016**, *540*, 552–558. [CrossRef]
32. Harper, K.L.; Sosa, M.S.; Entenberg, D.; Hosseini, H.; Cheung, J.F.; Nobre, R.; Avivar-Valderas, A.; Nagi, C.; Girnius, N.; Davis, R.J.; et al. Mechanism of early Dis.semination and metastasis in Her2(+) mammary cancer. *Nature* **2016**, *540*, 588–592. [CrossRef]
33. Ofri, A.; Moore, K. Occult breast cancer: Where are we at? *Breast* **2020**, *54*, 211–215. [CrossRef]
34. Weigelt, B.; Peterse, J.L.; Van 't Veer, L.J. Breast cancer metastasis: Markers and models. *Nat. Rev. Cancer* **2005**, *5*, 591–602. [CrossRef]
35. Soni, A.; Ren, Z.; Hameed, O.; Chanda, D.; Morgan, C.J.; Siegal, G.P.; Wei, S. Breast cancer subtypes predispose the site of distant metastases. *Am. J. Clin. Pathol.* **2015**, *143*, 471–478. [CrossRef]
36. Press, D.J.; Miller, M.E.; Liederbach, E.; Yao, K.; Huo, D. De novo metastasis in breast cancer: Occurrence and overall survival stratified by molecular subtype. *Clin. Exp. Metastasis* **2017**, *34*, 457–465. [CrossRef]
37. Arshad, F.; Wang, L.; Sy, C.; Avraham, S.; Avraham, H.K. Blood-brain barrier Int.egrity and breast cancer metastasis to the brain. *Pathol. Res. Int.* **2010**, *2011*, 920509. [CrossRef]
38. Chen, S.; Yang, J.; Liu, Y.; You, H.; Dong, Y.; Lyu, J. Prognostic factors and survival outcomes according to tumor subtype in patients with breast cancer lung metastases. *PeerJ* **2019**, *7*, e8298. [CrossRef]
39. Gasparini, G.; Weidner, N.; Bevilacqua, P.; Maluta, S.; Dalla Palma, P.; Caffo, O.; Barbareschi, M.; Boracchi, P.; Marubini, E.; Pozza, F. Tumor microvessel density, p53 expression, tumor size, and peritumoral lymphatic vessel invasion are relevant prognostic markers in node-negative breast carcinoma. *J. Clin. Oncol.* **1994**, *12*, 454–466. [CrossRef]
40. Fitzpatrick, D.J.; Lai, C.S.; Parkyn, R.F.; Walters, D.; Humeniuk, V.; Walsh, D.C. Time to breast cancer relapse predicted by primary tumour characteristics, not lymph node involvement. *World J. Surg.* **2014**, *38*, 1668–1675. [CrossRef]
41. Roda, N.; Blandano, G.; Pelicci, P.G. Blood Vessels and Peripheral Nerves as Key Players in Cancer Progression and Therapy Resistance. *Cancers* **2021**, *13*, 4471. [CrossRef] [PubMed]
42. Fazilaty, H.; Rago, L.; Kass Youssef, K.; Ocana, O.H.; Garcia-Asencio, F.; Arcas, A.; Galceran, J.; Nieto, M.A. A gene regulatory network to control EMT programs in development and Disease. *Nat. Commun.* **2019**, *10*, 5115. [CrossRef] [PubMed]
43. Aharonov, A.; Shakked, A.; Umansky, K.B.; Savidor, A.; Genzelinakh, A.; Kain, D.; Lendengolts, D.; Revach, O.Y.; Morikawa, Y.; Dong, J.; et al. ERBB2 drives YAP activation and EMT-like processes during cardiac regeneration. *Nat. Cell Biol.* **2020**, *22*, 1346–1356. [CrossRef] [PubMed]
44. Sheng, G. Defining epithelial-mesenchymal transitions in animal development. *Development* **2021**, *148*, 198036. [CrossRef] [PubMed]
45. Kalluri, R.; Weinberg, R.A. The basics of epithelial-mesenchymal transition. *J. Clin. Invest* **2009**, *119*, 1420–1428. [CrossRef]
46. Zhang, H.; Meng, F.; Liu, G.; Zhang, B.; Zhu, J.; Wu, F.; Ethier, S.P.; Miller, F.; Wu, G. Forkhead transcription factor foxq1 promotes epithelial-mesenchymal transition and breast cancer metastasis. *Cancer Res.* **2011**, *71*, 1292–1301. [CrossRef]
47. Horiguchi, K.; Sakamoto, K.; Koinuma, D.; Semba, K.; Inoue, A.; Inoue, S.; Fujii, H.; Yamaguchi, A.; Miyazawa, K.; Miyazono, K.; et al. TGF-beta drives epithelial-mesenchymal transition through deltaEF1-mediated downregulation of ESRP. *Oncogene* **2012**, *31*, 3190–3201. [CrossRef]
48. Stankic, M.; Pavlovic, S.; Chin, Y.; Brogi, E.; Padua, D.; Norton, L.; Massague, J.; Benezra, R. TGF-beta-Id1 signaling opposes Twist1 and promotes metastatic colonization via a mesenchymal-to-epithelial transition. *Cell Rep.* **2013**, *5*, 1228–1242. [CrossRef]
49. Yu, Y.; Xiao, C.H.; Tan, L.D.; Wang, Q.S.; Li, X.Q.; Feng, Y.M. Cancer-associated fibroblasts induce epithelial-mesenchymal transition of breast cancer Cells through paracrine TGF-beta signalling. *Br. J. Cancer* **2014**, *110*, 724–732. [CrossRef]
50. Lee, Y.J.; Park, J.H.; Oh, S.M. Activation of NF-kappaB by TOPK upregulates Snail/Slug expression in TGF-beta1 signaling to induce epithelial-mesenchymal transition and invasion of breast cancer Cells. *Biochem. Biophys. Res. Commun.* **2020**, *530*, 122–129. [CrossRef]
51. Han, D.; Wang, L.; Chen, B.; Zhao, W.; Liang, Y.; Li, Y.; Zhang, H.; Liu, Y.; Wang, X.; Chen, T.; et al. USP1-WDR48 deubiquitinase complex enhances TGF-beta induced epithelial-mesenchymal transition of TNBC Cells via stabilizing TAK1. *Cell Cycle* **2021**, *20*, 320–331. [CrossRef]

52. Incassati, A.; Pinderhughes, A.; Eelkema, R.; Cowin, P. Links between transforming growth factor-beta and canonical Wnt signaling yield new insights into breast cancer susceptibility, suppression and tumor heterogeneity. *Breast. Cancer Res.* 2009, *11*, 103. [CrossRef]
53. Serra, R.; Easter, S.L.; Jiang, W.; Baxley, S.E. Wnt5a as an effector of TGFbeta in mammary development and cancer. *J. Mammary Gland. Biol. Neoplasia* 2011, *16*, 157–167. [CrossRef]
54. Johnson, R.W.; Merkel, A.R.; Page, J.M.; Ruppender, N.S.; Guelcher, S.A.; Sterling, J.A. Wnt signaling induces gene expression of factors associated with bone destruction in lung and breast cancer. *Clin. Exp. Metastasis* 2014, *31*, 945–959. [CrossRef]
55. Ma, F.; Li, W.; Liu, C.; Li, W.; Yu, H.; Lei, B.; Ren, Y.; Li, Z.; Pang, D.; Qian, C. MiR-23a promotes TGF-beta1-induced EMT and tumor metastasis in breast cancer Cells by directly targeting CDH1 and activating Wnt/beta-catenin signaling. *Oncotarget* 2017, *8*, 69538–69550. [CrossRef]
56. Zhuang, X.; Zhang, H.; Li, X.; Li, X.; Cong, M.; Peng, F.; Yu, J.; Zhang, X.; Yang, Q.; Hu, G. Differential effects on lung and bone metastasis of breast cancer by Wnt signalling inhibitor DKK1. *Nat. Cell Biol.* 2017, *19*, 1274–1285. [CrossRef]
57. Buechel, D.; Sugiyama, N.; Rubinstein, N.; Saxena, M.; Kalathur, R.K.R.; Luond, F.; Vafaizadeh, V.; Valenta, T.; Hausmann, G.; Cantu, C.; et al. Parsing beta-catenin's cell adhesion and Wnt signaling functions in malignant mammary tumor progression. *Proc. Natl. Acad. Sci. USA* 2021, *118*, e2020227118. [CrossRef]
58. Esposito, M.; Fang, C.; Cook, K.C.; Park, N.; Wei, Y.; Spadazzi, C.; Bracha, D.; Gunaratna, R.T.; Laevsky, G.; DeCoste, C.J.; et al. TGF-beta-induced DACT1 biomolecular condensates repress Wnt signalling to promote bone metastasis. *Nat. Cell Biol.* 2021, *23*, 257–267. [CrossRef]
59. Sun, Y.; Lowther, W.; Kato, K.; Bianco, C.; Kenney, N.; Strizzi, L.; Raafat, D.; Hirota, M.; Khan, N.I.; Bargo, S.; et al. Notch4 intracellular domain binding to Smad3 and inhibition of the TGF-beta signaling. *Oncogene* 2005, *24*, 5365–5374. [CrossRef]
60. Leong, K.G.; Niessen, K.; Kulic, I.; Raouf, A.; Eaves, C.; Pollet, I.; Karsan, A. Jagged1-mediated Notch activation induces epithelial-to-mesenchymal transition through Slug-induced repression of E-cadherin. *J. Exp. Med.* 2007, *204*, 2935–2948. [CrossRef]
61. Sethi, N.; Dai, X.; Winter, C.G.; Kang, Y. Tumor-derived JAGGED1 promotes osteolytic bone metastasis of breast cancer by engaging notch signaling in bone Cells. *Cancer Cell* 2011, *19*, 192–205. [CrossRef]
62. Bendre, M.S.; Gaddy-Kurten, D.; Mon-Foote, T.; Akel, N.S.; Skinner, R.A.; Nicholas, R.W.; Suva, L.J. Expression of interleukin 8 and not parathyroid hormone-related protein by human breast cancer Cells correlates with bone metastasis in vivo. *Cancer Res.* 2002, *62*, 5571–5579.
63. Studebaker, A.W.; Storci, G.; Werbeck, J.L.; Sansone, P.; Sasser, A.K.; Tavolari, S.; Huang, T.; Chan, M.W.; Marini, F.C.; Rosol, T.J.; et al. Fibroblasts isolated from common sites of breast cancer metastasis enhance cancer cell growth rates and invasiveness in an interleukin-6-dependent manner. *Cancer Res.* 2008, *68*, 9087–9095. [CrossRef]
64. Oh, K.; Ko, E.; Kim, H.S.; Park, A.K.; Moon, H.G.; Noh, D.Y.; Lee, D.S. Transglutaminase 2 facilitates the distant hematogenous metastasis of breast cancer by modulating interleukin-6 in cancer Cells. *Breast. Cancer Res.* 2011, *13*, R96. [CrossRef] [PubMed]
65. Cheng, L.; Zha, Z.; Lang, B.; Liu, J.; Yao, X. Heregulin-beta1 promotes metastasis of breast cancer cell line SKBR3 through upregulation of Snail and induction of epithelial-mesenchymal transition. *Cancer Lett.* 2009, *280*, 50–60. [CrossRef] [PubMed]
66. Vincent, T.; Neve, E.P.; Johnson, J.R.; Kukalev, A.; Rojo, F.; Albanell, J.; Pietras, K.; Virtanen, I.; Philipson, L.; Leopold, P.L.; et al. A SNAIL1-SMAD3/4 transcriptional repressor complex promotes TGF-beta mediated epithelial-mesenchymal transition. *Nat. Cell Biol.* 2009, *11*, 943–950. [CrossRef]
67. Yuen, H.F.; Chan, Y.K.; Grills, C.; McCrudden, C.M.; Gunasekharan, V.; Shi, Z.; Wong, A.S.; Lappin, T.R.; Chan, K.W.; Fennell, D.A.; et al. Polyomavirus enhancer activator 3 protein promotes breast cancer metastatic progression through Snail-induced epithelial-mesenchymal transition. *J. Pathol.* 2011, *224*, 78–89. [CrossRef] [PubMed]
68. Chimge, N.O.; Baniwal, S.K.; Little, G.H.; Chen, Y.B.; Kahn, M.; Tripathy, D.; Borok, Z.; Frenkel, B. Regulation of breast cancer metastasis by Runx2 and estrogen signaling: The role of SNAI2. *Breast. Cancer Res.* 2011, *13*, R127. [CrossRef]
69. Gupta, P.; Srivastava, S.K. HER2 mediated de novo production of TGFbeta leads to SNAIL driven epithelial-to-mesenchymal transition and metastasis of breast cancer. *Mol. Oncol.* 2014, *8*, 1532–1547. [CrossRef]
70. Wu, Z.Q.; Li, X.Y.; Hu, C.Y.; Ford, M.; Kleer, C.G.; Weiss, S.J. Canonical Wnt signaling regulates Slug activity and links epithelial-mesenchymal transition with epigenetic Breast Cancer 1, Early Onset (BRCA1) repression. *Proc. Natl. Acad. Sci. USA* 2012, *109*, 16654–16659. [CrossRef] [PubMed]
71. Jiang, Y.; Zhao, X.; Xiao, Q.; Liu, Q.; Ding, K.; Yu, F.; Zhang, R.; Zhu, T.; Ge, G. Snail and Slug mediate tamoxifen resistance in breast cancer cells through activation of EGFR-ERK independent of epithelial-mesenchymal transition. *J. Mol. Cell Biol.* 2014, *6*, 352–354. [CrossRef]
72. Shao, S.; Zhao, X.; Zhang, X.; Luo, M.; Zuo, X.; Huang, S.; Wang, Y.; Gu, S.; Zhao, X. Notch1 signaling regulates the epithelial-mesenchymal transition and invasion of breast cancer in a Slug-dependent manner. *Mol. Cancer* 2015, *14*, 28. [CrossRef]
73. Li, N.Y.; Weber, C.E.; Wai, P.Y.; Cuevas, B.D.; Zhang, J.; Kuo, P.C.; Mi, Z. An MAPK-dependent pathway induces epithelial-mesenchymal transition via Twist activation in human breast cancer cell lines. *Surgery* 2013, *154*, 404–410. [CrossRef]
74. Lim, J.C.; Koh, V.C.; Tan, J.S.; Tan, W.J.; Thike, A.A.; Tan, P.H. Prognostic significance of epithelial-mesenchymal transition proteins Twist and Foxc2 in phyllodes tumours of the breast. *Breast. Cancer Res. Treat.* 2015, *150*, 19–29. [CrossRef]
75. Yang, J.; Hou, Y.; Zhou, M.; Wen, S.; Zhou, J.; Xu, L.; Tang, X.; Du, Y.E.; Hu, P.; Liu, M. Twist induces epithelial-mesenchymal transition and cell motility in breast cancer via ITGB1-FAK/ILK signaling axis and its associated downstream network. *Int. J. Biochem. Cell Biol.* 2016, *71*, 62–71. [CrossRef]

76. Cieply, B.; Farris, J.; Denvir, J.; Ford, H.L.; Frisch, S.M. Epithelial-mesenchymal transition and tumor suppression are controlled by a reciprocal feedback loop between ZEB1 and Grainyhead-like-2. *Cancer Res.* **2013**, *73*, 6299–6309. [CrossRef]
77. Hugo, H.J.; Pereira, L.; Suryadinata, R.; Drabsch, Y.; Gonda, T.J.; Gunasinghe, N.P.; PInto, C.; Soo, E.T.; Van Denderen, B.J.; Hill, P.; et al. Direct repression of MYB by ZEB1 suppresses proliferation and epithelial gene expression during epithelial-to-mesenchymal transition of breast cancer cells. *Breast Cancer Res.* **2013**, *15*, R113. [CrossRef]
78. Avtanski, D.B.; Nagalingam, A.; Bonner, M.Y.; Arbiser, J.L.; Saxena, N.K.; Sharma, D. Honokiol inhibits epithelial-mesenchymal transition in breast cancer cells by targeting signal transducer and activator of transcription 3/Zeb1/E-cadherin axis. *Mol. Oncol.* **2014**, *8*, 565–580. [CrossRef]
79. Lee, J.Y.; Park, M.K.; Park, J.H.; Lee, H.J.; Shin, D.H.; Kang, Y.; Lee, C.H.; Kong, G. Loss of the polycomb protein Mel-18 enhances the epithelial-mesenchymal transition by ZEB1 and ZEB2 expression through the downregulation of miR-205 in breast cancer. *Oncogene* **2014**, *33*, 1325–1335. [CrossRef]
80. Liang, W.; Song, S.; Xu, Y.; Li, H.; Liu, H. Knockdown of ZEB1 suppressed the formation of vasculogenic mimicry and epithelial-mesenchymal transition in the human breast cancer cell line MDA-MB-231. *Mol. Med. Rep.* **2018**, *17*, 6711–6716. [CrossRef]
81. Onder, T.T.; Gupta, P.B.; Mani, S.A.; Yang, J.; Lander, E.S.; Weinberg, R.A. Loss of E-cadherin promotes metastasis via multiple downstream transcriptional pathways. *Cancer Res.* **2008**, *68*, 3645–3654. [CrossRef]
82. Nieman, M.T.; Prudoff, R.S.; Johnson, K.R.; Wheelock, M.J. N-cadherin promotes motility in human breast cancer cells regardless of their E-cadherin expression. *J. Cell Biol.* **1999**, *147*, 631–644. [CrossRef]
83. Fernandez-Garcia, B.; Eiro, N.; Marin, L.; Gonzalez-Reyes, S.; Gonzalez, L.O.; Lamelas, M.L.; Vizoso, F.J. Expression and prognostic significance of fibronectin and matrix metalloproteases in breast cancer metastasis. *HistoPathology* **2014**, *64*, 512–522. [CrossRef]
84. Korsching, E.; Packeisen, J.; Liedtke, C.; Hungermann, D.; Wulfing, P.; Van Diest, P.J.; Brandt, B.; Boecker, W.; Buerger, H. The origin of vimentin expression in invasive breast cancer: Epithelial-mesenchymal transition, myoepithelial histogenesis or histogenesis from progenitor cells with bilinear differentiation potential? *J. Pathol.* **2005**, *206*, 451–457. [CrossRef]
85. Vuoriluoto, K.; Haugen, H.; Kiviluoto, S.; Mpindi, J.P.; Nevo, J.; Gjerdrum, C.; Tiron, C.; Lorens, J.B.; Ivaska, J. Vimentin regulates EMT induction by Slug and oncogenic H-Ras and migration by governing Axl expression in breast cancer. *Oncogene* **2011**, *30*, 1436–1448. [CrossRef]
86. Whipple, R.A.; Matrone, M.A.; Cho, E.H.; Balzer, E.M.; Vitolo, M.I.; Yoon, J.R.; Ioffe, O.B.; Tuttle, K.C.; Yang, J.; Martin, S.S. Epithelial-to-mesenchymal transition promotes tubulin detyrosination and microtentacles that enhance endothelial engagement. *Cancer Res.* **2010**, *70*, 8127–8137. [CrossRef]
87. Zhang, Z.; Yang, M.; Chen, R.; Su, W.; Li, P.; Chen, S.; Chen, Z.; Chen, A.; Li, S.; Hu, C. IBP regulates epithelial-to-mesenchymal transition and the motility of breast cancer cells via Rac1, RhoA and Cdc42 signaling pathways. *Oncogene* **2014**, *33*, 3374–3382. [CrossRef]
88. Pereira De Carvalho, B.; Chern, Y.J.; He, J.; Chan, C.H. The ubiquitin ligase RNF8 regulates Rho GTPases and promotes cytoskeletal changes and motility in triple-negative breast cancer cells. *FEBS Lett.* **2021**, *595*, 241–252. [CrossRef]
89. Wang, X.; Lu, H.; Urvalek, A.M.; Li, T.; Yu, L.; Lamar, J.; DiPersio, C.M.; Feustel, P.J.; Zhao, J. KLF8 promotes human breast cancer cell invasion and metastasis by transcriptional activation of MMP9. *Oncogene* **2011**, *30*, 1901–1911. [CrossRef]
90. Eckert, M.A.; Santiago-Medina, M.; Lwin, T.M.; Kim, J.; Courtneidge, S.A.; Yang, J. ADAM12 induction by Twist1 promotes tumor invasion and metastasis via regulation of invadopodia and focal adhesions. *J. Cell Sci.* **2017**, *130*, 2036–2048. [CrossRef]
91. Mani, S.A.; Guo, W.; Liao, M.J.; Eaton, E.N.; Ayyanan, A.; Zhou, A.Y.; Brooks, M.; Reinhard, F.; Zhang, C.C.; Shipitsin, M.; et al. The epithelial-mesenchymal transition generates cells with properties of stem cells. *Cell* **2008**, *133*, 704–715. [CrossRef] [PubMed]
92. Kurrey, N.K.; Jalgaonkar, S.P.; Joglekar, A.V.; Ghanate, A.D.; Chaskar, P.D.; Doiphode, R.Y.; Bapat, S.A. Snail and slug mediate radioresistance and chemoresistance by antagonizing p53-mediated apoptosis and acquiring a stem-like phenotype in ovarian cancer cells. *Stem Cells* **2009**, *27*, 2059–2068. [CrossRef] [PubMed]
93. Fontemaggi, G.; Gurtner, A.; Strano, S.; Higashi, Y.; Sacchi, A.; Piaggio, G.; Blandino, G. The transcriptional repressor ZEB regulates p73 expression at the crossroad between proliferation and differentiation. *Mol. Cell. Biol.* **2001**, *21*, 8461–8470. [CrossRef] [PubMed]
94. Iseri, O.D.; Kars, M.D.; Arpaci, F.; Atalay, C.; Pak, I.; Gunduz, U. Drug resistant MCF-7 Cells exhibit epithelial-mesenchymal transition gene expression pattern. *Biomed. Pharm.* **2011**, *65*, 40–45. [CrossRef]
95. Xu, X.; Zhang, L.; He, X.; Zhang, P.; Sun, C.; Xu, X.; Lu, Y.; Li, F. TGF-beta plays a vital role in triple-negative breast cancer (TNBC) drug-resistance through regulating stemness, EMT and apoptosis. *Biochem. Biophys. Res. Commun.* **2018**, *502*, 160–165. [CrossRef]
96. Soundararajan, R.; Fradette, J.J.; Konen, J.M.; Moulder, S.; Zhang, X.; Gibbons, D.L.; Varadarajan, N.; Wistuba, I.I.; Tripathy, D.; Bernatchez, C.; et al. Targeting the Interplay between Epithelial-to-Mesenchymal-Transition and the Immune System for Effective Immunotherapy. *Cancers* **2019**, *11*, 714. [CrossRef]
97. Gunasinghe, N.P.; Wells, A.; Thompson, E.W.; Hugo, H.J. Mesenchymal-epithelial transition (MET) as a mechanism for metastatic colonisation in breast cancer. *Cancer Metastasis. Rev.* **2012**, *31*, 469–478. [CrossRef]
98. Maguire, A.; Brogi, E. Sentinel lymph nodes for breast carcinoma: An update on current practice. *HistoPathology* **2016**, *68*, 152–167. [CrossRef]
99. Chambers, A.F.; Groom, A.C.; MacDonald, I.C. Dissemination and growth of cancer cells in metastatic sites. *Nat. Rev. Cancer* **2002**, *2*, 563–572. [CrossRef]

100. Paoli, P.; Giannoni, E.; Chiarugi, P. Anoikis molecular pathways and its role in cancer progression. *Biochim. Biophys. Acta* **2013**, *1833*, 3481–3498. [CrossRef]
101. Hanna, N.; Fidler, I.J. Role of natural killer cells in the destruction of circulating tumor emboli. *J. Natl. Cancer Inst.* **1980**, *65*, 801–809. [CrossRef]
102. Adorno, M.; Cordenonsi, M.; Montagner, M.; Dupont, S.; Wong, C.; Hann, B.; Solari, A.; Bobisse, S.; Rondina, M.B.; Guzzardo, V.; et al. A Mutant-p53/Smad complex opposes p63 to empower TGFbeta-induced metastasis. *Cell* **2009**, *137*, 87–98. [CrossRef]
103. Smit, M.A.; Geiger, T.R.; Song, J.Y.; Gitelman, I.; Peeper, D.S. A Twist-Snail axis critical for TrkB-induced epithelial-mesenchymal transition-like transformation, anoikis resistance, and metastasis. *Mol. Cell. Biol.* **2009**, *29*, 3722–3737. [CrossRef]
104. Palumbo, J.S.; Talmage, K.E.; Massari, J.V.; La Jeunesse, C.M.; Flick, M.J.; Kombrinck, K.W.; Hu, Z.; Barney, K.A.; Degen, J.L. Tumor cell-associated tissue factor and circulating hemostatic factors cooperate to increase metastatic potential through natural killer cell-dependent and-independent mechanisms. *Blood* **2007**, *110*, 133–141. [CrossRef]
105. Labelle, M.; Begum, S.; Hynes, R.O. Direct signaling between platelets and cancer cells induces an epithelial-mesenchymal-like transition and promotes metastasis. *Cancer Cell* **2011**, *20*, 576–590. [CrossRef]
106. Spiegel, A.; Brooks, M.W.; Houshyar, S.; Reinhardt, F.; Ardolino, M.; Fessler, E.; Chen, M.B.; Krall, J.A.; DeCock, J.; Zervantonakis, I.K.; et al. Neutrophils Suppress Intraluminal NK Cell.-Mediated Tumor Cell Clearance and Enhance Extravasation of disseminated Carcinoma cells. *Cancer Discov.* **2016**, *6*, 630–649. [CrossRef]
107. Alix-Panabieres, C.; Pantel, K. Challenges in circulating tumour cell research. *Nat. Rev. Cancer* **2014**, *14*, 623–631. [CrossRef]
108. Chaffer, C.L.; Weinberg, R.A. A perspective on cancer cell metastasis. *Science* **2011**, *331*, 1559–1564. [CrossRef]
109. Reymond, N.; D'Agua, B.B.; Ridley, A.J. Crossing the endothelial barrier during metastasis. *Nat. Rev. Cancer* **2013**, *13*, 858–870. [CrossRef]
110. Schumacher, D.; Strilic, B.; Sivaraj, K.K.; Wettschureck, N.; Offermanns, S. Platelet-derived nucleotides promote tumor-cell transendothelial migration and metastasis via P2Y2 receptor. *Cancer Cell* **2013**, *24*, 130–137. [CrossRef]
111. Qian, B.Z.; Li, J.; Zhang, H.; Kitamura, T.; Zhang, J.; Campion, L.R.; Kaiser, E.A.; Snyder, L.A.; Pollard, J.W. CCL2 recruits inflammatory monocytes to facilitate breast-tumour metastasis. *Nature* **2011**, *475*, 222–225. [CrossRef]
112. Weis, S.; Cui, J.; Barnes, L.; Cheresh, D. Endothelial barrier Disruption by VEGF-mediated Src activity potentiates tumor cell extravasation and metastasis. *J. Cell Biol.* **2004**, *167*, 223–229. [CrossRef]
113. Gupta, G.P.; Nguyen, D.X.; Chiang, A.C.; Bos, P.D.; Kim, J.Y.; Nadal, C.; Gomis, R.R.; Manova-Todorova, K.; Massague, J. Mediators of vascular remodelling co-opted for sequential steps in lung metastasis. *Nature* **2007**, *446*, 765–770. [CrossRef]
114. Padua, D.; Zhang, X.H.; Wang, Q.; Nadal, C.; Gerald, W.L.; Gomis, R.R.; Massague, J. TGFbeta primes breast tumors for lung metastasis seeding through angiopoietin-like 4. *Cell* **2008**, *133*, 66–77. [CrossRef]
115. Luzzi, K.J.; MacDonald, I.C.; Schmidt, E.E.; Kerkvliet, N.; Morris, V.L.; Chambers, A.F.; Groom, A.C. Multistep nature of metastatic inefficiency: Dormancy of solitary cells after successful extravasation and limited survival of early micrometastases. *Am. J. Pathol.* **1998**, *153*, 865–873. [CrossRef]
116. Ghajar, C.M.; Peinado, H.; Mori, H.; Matei, I.R.; Evason, K.J.; Brazier, H.; Almeida, D.; Koller, A.; Hajjar, K.A.; Stainier, D.Y.; et al. The perivascular niche regulates breast tumour dormancy. *Nat. Cell Biol.* **2013**, *15*, 807–817. [CrossRef]
117. Gao, H.; Chakraborty, G.; Lee-Lim, A.P.; Mo, Q.; Decker, M.; Vonica, A.; Shen, R.; Brogi, E.; Brivanlou, A.H.; Giancotti, F.G. The BMP inhibitor Coco reactivates breast cancer cells at lung metastatic sites. *Cell* **2012**, *150*, 764–779. [CrossRef]
118. Skibinski, A.; Kuperwasser, C. The origin of breast tumor heterogeneity. *Oncogene* **2015**, *34*, 5309–5316. [CrossRef]
119. Symmans, W.F.; Liu, J.; Knowles, D.M.; Inghirami, G. Breast cancer heterogeneity: Evaluation of clonality in primary and metastatic lesions. *Hum. Pathol.* **1995**, *26*, 210–216. [CrossRef]
120. Teixeira, M.R.; Tsarouha, H.; Kraggerud, S.M.; Pandis, N.; Dimitriadis, E.; Andersen, J.A.; Lothe, R.A.; Heim, S. Evaluation of breast cancer polyclonality by combined chromosome banding and comparative genomic hybridization analysis. *Neoplasia* **2001**, *3*, 204–214. [CrossRef]
121. Zhang, M.; Lee, A.V.; Rosen, J.M. The Cellular Origin and Evolution of Breast Cancer. *Cold. Spring Harb. Perspect. Med.* **2017**, *7*, a027128. [CrossRef] [PubMed]
122. Jewer, M.; Lee, L.; Leibovitch, M.; Zhang, G.; Liu, J.; Findlay, S.D.; Vincent, K.M.; Tandoc, K.; Dieters-Castator, D.; Quail, D.F.; et al. Translational control of breast cancer plasticity. *Nat. Commun.* **2020**, *11*, 2498. [CrossRef] [PubMed]
123. Roda, N.; Gambino, V.; Giorgio, M. Metabolic Constrains Rule Metastasis Progression. *Cells* **2020**, *9*, 2081. [CrossRef] [PubMed]
124. Curtis, C.; Shah, S.P.; Chin, S.F.; Turashvili, G.; Rueda, O.M.; Dunning, M.J.; Speed, D.; Lynch, A.G.; Samarajiwa, S.; Yuan, Y.; et al. The genomic and transcriptomic architecture of 2000 breast tumours reveals novel subgroups. *Nature* **2012**, *486*, 346–352. [CrossRef] [PubMed]
125. Pereira, B.; Chin, S.F.; Rueda, O.M.; Vollan, H.K.; Provenzano, E.; Bardwell, H.A.; Pugh, M.; Jones, L.; Russell, R.; Sammut, S.J.; et al. The somatic mutation profiles of 2433 breast cancers refines their genomic and transcriptomic landscapes. *Nat. Commun.* **2016**, *7*, 11479. [CrossRef] [PubMed]
126. Navin, N.; Kendall, J.; Troge, J.; Andrews, P.; Rodgers, L.; McIndoo, J.; Cook, K.; Stepansky, A.; Levy, D.; Esposito, D.; et al. Tumour evolution inferred by single-cell sequencing. *Nature* **2011**, *472*, 90–94. [CrossRef]
127. Yates, L.R.; Gerstung, M.; Knappskog, S.; Desmedt, C.; Gundem, G.; Van Loo, P.; Aas, T.; Alexandrov, L.B.; Larsimont, D.; Davies, H.; et al. Subclonal diversification of primary breast cancer revealed by multiregion sequencing. *Nat. Med.* **2015**, *21*, 751–759. [CrossRef]

128. Geyer, F.C.; Weigelt, B.; Natrajan, R.; Lambros, M.B.; De Biase, D.; Vatcheva, R.; Savage, K.; Mackay, A.; Ashworth, A.; Reis-Filho, J.S. Molecular analysis reveals a genetic basis for the phenotypic diversity of metaplastic breast carcinomas. *J. Pathol.* **2010**, *220*, 562–573. [CrossRef]
129. Patani, N.; Barbashina, V.; Lambros, M.B.; Gauthier, A.; Mansour, M.; Mackay, A.; Reis-Filho, J.S. Direct evidence for concurrent morphological and genetic heterogeneity in an invasive ductal carcinoma of triple-negative phenotype. *J. Clin. Pathol.* **2011**, *64*, 822–828. [CrossRef]
130. Lee, H.J.; Seo, A.N.; Kim, E.J.; Jang, M.H.; Suh, K.J.; Ryu, H.S.; Kim, Y.J.; Kim, J.H.; Im, S.A.; Gong, G.; et al. HER2 heterogeneity affects trastuzumab responses and survival in patients with HER2-positive metastatic breast cancer. *Am. J. Clin. Pathol.* **2014**, *142*, 755–766. [CrossRef]
131. Shah, S.P.; Morin, R.D.; Khattra, J.; Prentice, L.; Pugh, T.; Burleigh, A.; Delaney, A.; Gelmon, K.; Guliany, R.; Senz, J.; et al. Mutational evolution in a lobular breast tumour profiled at single nucleotide resolution. *Nature* **2009**, *461*, 809–813. [CrossRef]
132. Shah, S.P.; Roth, A.; Goya, R.; Oloumi, A.; Ha, G.; Zhao, Y.; Turashvili, G.; Ding, J.; Tse, K.; Haffari, G.; et al. The clonal and mutational evolution spectrum of primary triple-negative breast cancers. *Nature* **2012**, *486*, 395–399. [CrossRef]
133. Eirew, P.; Steif, A.; Khattra, J.; Ha, G.; Yap, D.; Farahani, H.; Gelmon, K.; Chia, S.; Mar, C.; Wan, A.; et al. Dynamics of genomic clones in breast cancer patient xenografts at single-cell resolution. *Nature* **2015**, *518*, 422–426. [CrossRef]
134. Giesen, C.; Wang, H.A.; Schapiro, D.; Zivanovic, N.; Jacobs, A.; Hattendorf, B.; Schuffler, P.J.; Grolimund, D.; Buhmann, J.M.; Brandt, S.; et al. Highly multiplexed imaging of tumor tissues with subcellular resolution by mass cytometry. *Nat. Methods* **2014**, *11*, 417–422. [CrossRef]
135. Jackson, H.W.; Fischer, J.R.; Zanotelli, V.R.T.; Ali, H.R.; Mechera, R.; Soysal, S.D.; Moch, H.; Muenst, S.; Varga, Z.; Weber, W.P.; et al. The single-cell Pathology landscape of breast cancer. *Nature* **2020**, *578*, 615–620. [CrossRef]
136. Karaayvaz, M.; Cristea, S.; Gillespie, S.M.; Patel, A.P.; Mylvaganam, R.; Luo, C.C.; Specht, M.C.; Bernstein, B.E.; Michor, F.; Ellisen, L.W. Unravelling subclonal heterogeneity and aggressive Disease states in TNBC through single-cell RNA-seq. *Nat. Commun.* **2018**, *9*, 3588. [CrossRef]
137. Rios, A.C.; Capaldo, B.D.; Vaillant, F.; Pal, B.; Van Ineveld, R.; Dawson, C.A.; Chen, Y.; Nolan, E.; Fu, N.Y.; Group, D.; et al. Intraclonal Plasticity in Mammary Tumors Revealed through Large-Scale Single-Cell Resolution 3D Imaging. *Cancer Cell* **2019**, *35*, 618–632.e616. [CrossRef]
138. Chen, F.; Ding, K.; Priedigkeit, N.; Elangovan, A.; Levine, K.M.; Carleton, N.; Savariau, L.; Atkinson, J.M.; Oesterreich, S.; Lee, A.V. Single-Cell Transcriptomic Heterogeneity in Invasive Ductal and Lobular Breast Cancer Cells. *Cancer Res.* **2021**, *81*, 268–281. [CrossRef]
139. Wu, S.Z.; Al-Eryani, G.; Roden, D.L.; Junankar, S.; Harvey, K.; Andersson, A.; Thennavan, A.; Wang, C.; Torpy, J.R.; Bartonicek, N.; et al. A single-cell and spatially resolved atlas of human breast cancers. *Nat. Genet.* **2021**, *53*, 1334–1347. [CrossRef]
140. Yeo, S.K.; Zhu, X.; Okamoto, T.; Hao, M.; Wang, C.; Lu, P.; Lu, L.J.; Guan, J.L. Single-Cell RNA-sequencing reveals Dis.tinct patterns of cell state heterogeneity in mouse models of breast cancer. *Elife* **2020**, *9*, e58810. [CrossRef]
141. Jose, C.; Bellance, N.; Rossignol, R. Choosing between glycolysis and oxidative phosphorylation: A tumor's dilemma? *Biochim. Biophys. Acta* **2011**, *1807*, 552–561. [CrossRef]
142. Jia, D.; Lu, M.; Jung, K.H.; Park, J.H.; Yu, L.; Onuchic, J.N.; Kaipparettu, B.A.; Levine, H. Elucidating cancer metabolic plasticity by coupling gene regulation with metabolic pathways. *Proc. Natl. Acad. Sci. USA* **2019**, *116*, 3909–3918. [CrossRef]
143. Xu, H.N.; Zheng, G.; Tchou, J.; Nioka, S.; Li, L.Z. Characterizing the metabolic heterogeneity in human breast cancer xenografts by 3D high resolution fluorescence imaging. *Springerplus* **2013**, *2*, 73. [CrossRef]
144. Farnie, G.; Sotgia, F.; Lisanti, M.P. High mitochondrial mass identifies a sub-population of stem-like cancer cells that are chemo-resistant. *Oncotarget* **2015**, *6*, 30472–30486. [CrossRef]
145. Lamb, R.; Ozsvari, B.; Bonuccelli, G.; Smith, D.L.; Pestell, R.G.; Martinez-Outschoorn, U.E.; Clarke, R.B.; Sotgia, F.; Lisanti, M.P. Dissecting tumor metabolic heterogeneity: Telomerase and large cell size metabolically define a sub-population of stem-like, mitochondrial-rich, cancer cells. *Oncotarget* **2015**, *6*, 21892–21905. [CrossRef]
146. Komaki, K.; Sano, N.; Tangoku, A. Problems in histological grading of malignancy and its clinical significance in patients with operable breast cancer. *Breast. Cancer* **2006**, *13*, 249–253. [CrossRef]
147. Bhang, H.E.; Ruddy, D.A.; Krishnamurthy Radhakrishna, V.; Caushi, J.X.; Zhao, R.; Hims, M.M.; Singh, A.P.; Kao, I.; Rakiec, D.; Shaw, P.; et al. Studying clonal dynamics in response to cancer therapy using high-complexity barcoding. *Nat. Med.* **2015**, *21*, 440–448. [CrossRef] [PubMed]
148. Koren, S.; Bentires-Alj, M. Breast Tumor Heterogeneity: Source of Fitness, Hurdle for Therapy. *Mol. Cell* **2015**, *60*, 537–546. [CrossRef] [PubMed]
149. Turashvili, G.; Brogi, E. Tumor Heterogeneity in Breast Cancer. *Front. Med.* **2017**, *4*, 227. [CrossRef] [PubMed]
150. Ramon, Y.C.S.; Sese, M.; Capdevila, C.; Aasen, T.; De Mattos-Arruda, L.; Diaz-Cano, S.J.; Hernandez-Losa, J.; Castellvi, J. Clinical implications of intratumor heterogeneity: Challenges and opportunities. *J. Mol. Med.* **2020**, *98*, 161–177. [CrossRef] [PubMed]
151. Yang, F.; Wang, Y.; Li, Q.; Cao, L.; Sun, Z.; Jin, J.; Fang, H.; Zhu, A.; Li, Y.; Zhang, W.; et al. Intratumor heterogeneity predicts metastasis of triple-negative breast cancer. *Carcinogenesis* **2017**, *38*, 900–909. [CrossRef]
152. Mroz, E.A.; Tward, A.D.; Hammon, R.J.; Ren, Y.; Rocco, J.W. Int.ra-tumor genetic heterogeneity and mortality in head and neck cancer: Analysis of data from the Cancer Genome Atlas. *PLoS Med.* **2015**, *12*, e1001786. [CrossRef]

153. Ma, D.; Jiang, Y.Z.; Liu, X.Y.; Liu, Y.R.; Shao, Z.M. Clinical and molecular relevance of mutant-allele tumor heterogeneity in breast cancer. *Breast. Cancer Res. Treat.* **2017**, *162*, 39–48. [CrossRef]
154. Saha, A.; Harowicz, M.R.; Cain, E.H.; Hall, A.H.; Hwang, E.S.; Marks, J.R.; Marcom, P.K.; Mazurowski, M.A. Intra-tumor molecular heterogeneity in breast cancer: Definitions of measures and association with distant recurrence-free survival. *Breast. Cancer Res. Treat.* **2018**, *172*, 123–132. [CrossRef]
155. McGranahan, N.; Swanton, C. Clonal Heterogeneity and Tumor Evolution: Past, Present, and the Future. *Cell* **2017**, *168*, 613–628. [CrossRef]
156. Zhou, H.; Neelakantan, D.; Ford, H.L. Clonal cooperativity in heterogenous cancers. *Semin. Cell Dev. Biol.* **2017**, *64*, 79–89. [CrossRef]
157. Lyons, J.G.; Siew, K.; O'Grady, R.L. Cellular Int.eractions determining the production of collagenase by a rat mammary carcinoma cell line. *Int. J. Cancer* **1989**, *43*, 119–125. [CrossRef]
158. Janiszewska, M.; Tabassum, D.P.; Castano, Z.; Cristea, S.; Yamamoto, K.N.; Kingston, N.L.; Murphy, K.C.; Shu, S.; Harper, N.W.; Del Alcazar, C.G.; et al. Subclonal cooperation drives metastasis by modulating local and systemic immune microenvironments. *Nat. Cell Biol.* **2019**, *21*, 879–888. [CrossRef]
159. Angus, L.; Smid, M.; Wilting, S.M.; Van Riet, J.; Van Hoeck, A.; Nguyen, L.; Nik-Zainal, S.; Steenbruggen, T.G.; Tjan-Heijnen, V.C.G.; Labots, M.; et al. The genomic landscape of metastatic breast cancer highlights changes in mutation and signature frequencies. *Nat. Genet.* **2019**, *51*, 1450–1458. [CrossRef]
160. Ng, C.K.Y.; Bidard, F.C.; Piscuoglio, S.; Geyer, F.C.; Lim, R.S.; De Bruijn, I.; Shen, R.; Pareja, F.; Berman, S.H.; Wang, L.; et al. Genetic Heterogeneity in Therapy-Naive Synchronous Primary Breast Cancers and Their Metastases. *Clin. Cancer Res.* **2017**, *23*, 4402–4415. [CrossRef]
161. Stratton, M.R.; Campbell, P.J.; Futreal, P.A. The cancer genome. *Nature* **2009**, *458*, 719–724. [CrossRef]
162. Ding, L.; Ellis, M.J.; Li, S.; Larson, D.E.; Chen, K.; Wallis, J.W.; Harris, C.C.; McLellan, M.D.; Fulton, R.S.; Fulton, L.L.; et al. Genome remodelling in a basal-like breast cancer metastasis and xenograft. *Nature* **2010**, *464*, 999–1005. [CrossRef]
163. Lee, J.Y.; Park, K.; Lim, S.H.; Kim, H.S.; Yoo, K.H.; Jung, K.S.; Song, H.N.; Hong, M.; Do, I.G.; Ahn, T.; et al. Mutational profiling of brain metastasis from breast cancer: Matched pair analysis of targeted sequencing between brain metastasis and primary breast cancer. *Oncotarget* **2015**, *6*, 43731–43742. [CrossRef]
164. Moelans, C.B.; Van der Groep, P.; Hoefnagel, L.D.C.; Van de Vijver, M.J.; Wesseling, P.; Wesseling, J.; Van der Wall, E.; Van Diest, P.J. Genomic evolution from primary breast carcinoma to Distant metastasis: Few copy number changes of breast cancer related genes. *Cancer Lett.* **2014**, *344*, 138–146. [CrossRef]
165. Hoadley, K.A.; Siegel, M.B.; Kanchi, K.L.; Miller, C.A.; Ding, L.; Zhao, W.; He, X.; Parker, J.S.; Wendl, M.C.; Fulton, R.S.; et al. Tumor Evolution in Two Patients with Basal-like Breast Cancer: A Retrospective Genomics Study of Multiple Metastases. *PLoS Med.* **2016**, *13*, e1002174. [CrossRef]
166. Bertucci, F.; Finetti, P.; Guille, A.; Adelaide, J.; Garnier, S.; Carbuccia, N.; Monneur, A.; Charafe-Jauffret, E.; Goncalves, A.; Viens, P.; et al. Comparative genomic analysis of primary tumors and metastases in breast cancer. *Oncotarget* **2016**, *7*, 27208–27219. [CrossRef] [PubMed]
167. Aftimos, P.; Oliveira, M.; Irrthum, A.; Fumagalli, D.; Sotiriou, C.; Gal-Yam, E.N.; Robson, M.E.; Ndozeng, J.; Di Leo, A.; Ciruelos, E.M.; et al. Genomic and Transcriptomic Analyses of Breast Cancer Primaries and Matched Metastases in AURORA, the Breast International Group (BIG) Molecular Screening Initiative. *Cancer Discov.* **2021**, *11*, 2796–2811. [CrossRef] [PubMed]
168. Hu, Z.; Li, Z.; Ma, Z.; Curtis, C. Multi-cancer analysis of clonality and the timing of systemic spread in paired primary tumors and metastases. *Nat. Genet.* **2020**, *52*, 701–708. [CrossRef] [PubMed]
169. Casasent, A.K.; Schalck, A.; Gao, R.; Sei, E.; Long, A.; Pangburn, W.; Casasent, T.; Meric-Bernstam, F.; Edgerton, M.E.; Navin, N.E. Multiclonal Invasion in Breast Tumors Identified by Topographic Single Cell Sequencing. *Cell* **2018**, *172*, 205–217 e212. [CrossRef]
170. Cheung, K.J.; Padmanaban, V.; Silvestri, V.; Schipper, K.; Cohen, J.D.; Fairchild, A.N.; Gorin, M.A.; Verdone, J.E.; Pienta, K.J.; Bader, J.S.; et al. Polyclonal breast cancer metastases arise from collective Dis.semination of keratin 14-expressing tumor cell clusters. *Proc. Natl. Acad. Sci. USA* **2016**, *113*, E854–E863. [CrossRef]
171. Tiede, S.; Kalathur, R.K.R.; Luond, F.; Von Allmen, L.; Szczerba, B.M.; Hess, M.; Vlajnic, T.; Muller, B.; Canales Murillo, J.; Aceto, N.; et al. Multi-color clonal tracking reveals intra-stage proliferative heterogeneity during mammary tumor progression. *Oncogene* **2021**, *40*, 12–27. [CrossRef]
172. Paul, M.R.; Pan, T.C.; Pant, D.K.; Shih, N.N.; Chen, Y.; Harvey, K.L.; Solomon, A.; Lieberman, D.; Morrissette, J.J.; Soucier-Ernst, D.; et al. Genomic landscape of metastatic breast cancer identifies preferentially dysregulated pathways and targets. *J. Clin. Invest* **2020**, *130*, 4252–4265. [CrossRef]
173. Yates, L.R.; Knappskog, S.; Wedge, D.; Farmery, J.H.R.; Gonzalez, S.; Martincorena, I.; Alexandrov, L.B.; Van Loo, P.; Haugland, H.K.; Lilleng, P.K.; et al. Genomic Evolution of Breast Cancer Metastasis and Relapse. *Cancer Cell* **2017**, *32*, 169–184 e167. [CrossRef]
174. Brastianos, P.K.; Carter, S.L.; Santagata, S.; Cahill, D.P.; Taylor-Weiner, A.; Jones, R.T.; Van Allen, E.M.; Lawrence, M.S.; Horowitz, P.M.; Cibulskis, K.; et al. Genomic Characterization of Brain Metastases Reveals Branched Evolution and Potential Therapeutic Targets. *Cancer Discov.* **2015**, *5*, 1164–1177. [CrossRef]

175. Diossy, M.; Reiniger, L.; Sztupinszki, Z.; Krzystanek, M.; Timms, K.M.; Neff, C.; Solimeno, C.; Pruss, D.; Eklund, A.C.; Toth, E.; et al. Breast cancer brain metastases show increased levels of genomic aberration-based homologous recombination deficiency scores relative to their corresponding primary tumors. *Ann. Oncol.* **2018**, *29*, 1948–1954. [CrossRef]
176. Schrijver, W.; Selenica, P.; Lee, J.Y.; Ng, C.K.Y.; Burke, K.A.; Piscuoglio, S.; Berman, S.H.; Reis-Filho, J.S.; Weigelt, B.; Van Diest, P.J.; et al. Mutation Profiling of Key Cancer Genes in Primary Breast Cancers and Their Distant Metastases. *Cancer Res.* **2018**, *78*, 3112–3121. [CrossRef]
177. Marjon, P.L.; Bobrovnikova-Marjon, E.V.; Abcouwer, S.F. Expression of the pro-angiogenic factors vascular endothelial growth factor and interleukin-8/CXCL8 by human breast carcinomas is responsive to nutrient deprivation and endoplasmic reticulum stress. *Mol. Cancer* **2004**, *3*, 4. [CrossRef]
178. Quintavalle, M.; Elia, L.; Price, J.H.; Heynen-Genel, S.; Courtneidge, S.A. A cell-based high-content screening assay reveals activators and inhibitors of cancer cell invasion. *Sci Signal.* **2011**, *4*, ra49. [CrossRef]
179. Shen, X.; Xue, Y.; Si, Y.; Wang, Q.; Wang, Z.; Yuan, J.; Zhang, X. The unfolded protein response potentiates epithelial-to-mesenchymal transition (EMT) of gastric cancer cells under severe hypoxic conditions. *Med. Oncol.* **2015**, *32*, 447. [CrossRef]
180. Semenza, G.L. The hypoxic tumor microenvironment: A driving force for breast cancer progression. *Biochim. Biophys. Acta* **2016**, *1863*, 382–391. [CrossRef]
181. Semenza, G.L. Molecular mechanisms mediating metastasis of hypoxic breast cancer cells. *Trends Mol. Med.* **2012**, *18*, 534–543. [CrossRef]
182. Chen, A.; Sceneay, J.; Godde, N.; Kinwel, T.; Ham, S.; Thompson, E.W.; Humbert, P.O.; Moller, A. Intermittent hypoxia induces a metastatic phenotype in breast cancer. *Oncogene* **2018**, *37*, 4214–4225. [CrossRef]
183. Weidner, N.; Semple, J.P.; Welch, W.R.; Folkman, J. Tumor angiogenesis and metastasis–correlation in invasive breast carcinoma. *N. Engl. J. Med.* **1991**, *324*, 1–8. [CrossRef]
184. Horak, E.R.; Leek, R.; Klenk, N.; LeJeune, S.; Smith, K.; Stuart, N.; Greenall, M.; Stepniewska, K.; Harris, A.L. Angiogenesis, assessed by platelet/endothelial Cell. adhesion molecule antibodies, as indicator of node metastases and survival in breast cancer. *Lancet* **1992**, *340*, 1120–1124. [CrossRef]
185. Vaupel, P.; Hockel, M.; Mayer, A. Detection and characterization of tumor hypoxia using pO2 histography. *Antioxid. Redox. Signal.* **2007**, *9*, 1221–1235. [CrossRef]
186. Gao, T.; Li, J.Z.; Lu, Y.; Zhang, C.Y.; Li, Q.; Mao, J.; Li, L.H. The mechanism between epithelial mesenchymal transition in breast cancer and hypoxia microenvironment. *Biomed. Pharm.* **2016**, *80*, 393–405. [CrossRef]
187. Montagner, M.; Enzo, E.; Forcato, M.; Zanconato, F.; Parenti, A.; Rampazzo, E.; Basso, G.; Leo, G.; Rosato, A.; Bicciato, S.; et al. SHARP1 suppresses breast cancer metastasis by promoting degradation of hypoxia-inducible factors. *Nature* **2012**, *487*, 380–384. [CrossRef]
188. Gameiro, P.A.; Struhl, K. Nutrient Deprivation Elicits a Transcriptional and Translational Inflammatory Response Coupled to Decreased Protein Synthesis. *Cell Rep.* **2018**, *24*, 1415–1424. [CrossRef]
189. Pavlova, N.N.; Hui, S.; Ghergurovich, J.M.; Fan, J.; Intlekofer, A.M.; White, R.M.; Rabinowitz, J.D.; Thompson, C.B.; Zhang, J. As Extracellular Glutamine Levels Decline, Asparagine Becomes an Essential Amino Acid. *Cell. Metab.* **2018**, *27*, 428–438 e425. [CrossRef]
190. Knott, S.R.V.; Wagenblast, E.; Khan, S.; Kim, S.Y.; Soto, M.; Wagner, M.; Turgeon, M.O.; Fish, L.; Erard, N.; Gable, A.L.; et al. Asparagine bioavailability governs metastasis in a model of breast cancer. *Nature* **2018**, *554*, 378–381. [CrossRef]
191. Lee, Y.J.; Galoforo, S.S.; Berns, C.M.; Chen, J.C.; Davis, B.H.; Sim, J.E.; Corry, P.M.; Spitz, D.R. Glucose deprivation-induced cytotoxicity and alterations in mitogen-activated protein kinase activation are mediated by oxidative stress in multidrug-resistant human breast carcinoma Cells. *J. Biol. Chem.* **1998**, *273*, 5294–5299. [CrossRef] [PubMed]
192. Brown, N.S.; Bicknell, R. Hypoxia and oxidative stress in breast cancer. Oxidative stress: Its effects on the growth, metastatic potential and response to therapy of breast cancer. *Breast Cancer Res.* **2001**, *3*, 323–327. [CrossRef] [PubMed]
193. Mahalingaiah, P.K.; Singh, K.P. Chronic oxidative stress increases growth and tumorigenic potential of MCF-7 breast cancer cells. *PLoS ONE* **2014**, *9*, e87371. [CrossRef] [PubMed]
194. Sadeghi, M.; Ordway, B.; Rafiei, I.; Borad, P.; Fang, B.; Koomen, J.L.; Zhang, C.; Yoder, S.; Johnson, J.; Damaghi, M. Int.egrative Analysis of Breast Cancer Cells Reveals an Epithelial-Mesenchymal Transition Role in Adaptation to Acidic Microenvironment. *Front. Oncol.* **2020**, *10*, 304. [CrossRef]
195. Bonuccelli, G.; Tsirigos, A.; Whitaker-Menezes, D.; Pavlides, S.; Pestell, R.G.; Chiavarina, B.; Frank, P.G.; Flomenberg, N.; Howell, A.; Martinez-Outschoorn, U.E.; et al. Ketones and lactate "fuel" tumor growth and metastasis: Evidence that epithelial cancer cells use oxidative mitochondrial metabolism. *Cell Cycle* **2010**, *9*, 3506–3514. [CrossRef]
196. Martinez-Outschoorn, U.E.; Prisco, M.; Ertel, A.; Tsirigos, A.; Lin, Z.; Pavlides, S.; Wang, C.; Flomenberg, N.; Knudsen, E.S.; Howell, A.; et al. Ketones and lactate increase cancer cell "stemness," driving recurrence, metastasis and poor clinical outcome in breast cancer: Achieving personalized medicine via Metabolo-Genomics. *Cell Cycle* **2011**, *10*, 1271–1286. [CrossRef]
197. Hetz, C. The unfolded protein response: Controlling cell fate decisions under ER stress and beyond. *Nat. Rev. Mol. Cell Biol.* **2012**, *13*, 89–102. [CrossRef]
198. Ma, Y.; Hendershot, L.M. The role of the unfolded protein response in tumour development: Friend or foe? *Nat. Rev. Cancer* **2004**, *4*, 966–977. [CrossRef]

199. Avril, T.; Vauleon, E.; Chevet, E. Endoplasmic reticulum stress signaling and chemotherapy resistance in solid cancers. *Oncogenesis* **2017**, *6*, e373. [CrossRef]
200. Tsai, Y.C.; Weissman, A.M. The Unfolded Protein Response, Degradation from Endoplasmic Reticulum and Cancer. *Genes Cancer* **2010**, *1*, 764–778. [CrossRef]
201. Wang, M.; Wey, S.; Zhang, Y.; Ye, R.; Lee, A.S. Role of the unfolded protein response regulator GRP78/BiP in development, cancer and neurological disorders. *Antioxid. Redox. Signal.* **2009**, *11*, 2307–2316. [CrossRef]
202. McGrath, E.P.; Logue, S.E.; Mnich, K.; Deegan, S.; Jager, R.; Gorman, A.M.; Samali, A. The Unfolded Protein Response in Breast Cancer. *Cancers* **2018**, *10*, 344. [CrossRef]
203. Zhang, K.; Liu, H.; Song, Z.; Jiang, Y.; Kim, H.; Samavati, L.; Nguyen, H.M.; Yang, Z.Q. The UPR Transducer IRE1 Promotes Breast Cancer Malignancy by Degrading Tumor Suppressor microRNAs. *iScience* **2020**, *23*, 101503. [CrossRef]
204. Sicari, D.; Fantuz, M.; Bellazzo, A.; Valentino, E.; Apollonio, M.; Pontisso, I.; Di Cristino, F.; Dal Ferro, M.; Bicciato, S.; Del Sal, G.; et al. Mutant p53 improves cancer Cells' resistance to endoplasmic reticulum stress by sustaining activation of the UPR regulator ATF6. *Oncogene* **2019**, *38*, 6184–6195. [CrossRef]
205. Abba, M.C.; Lacunza, E.; Nunez, M.I.; Colussi, A.; Isla-Larrain, M.; Segal-Eiras, A.; Croce, M.V.; Aldaz, C.M. Rhomboid domain containing 2 (RHBDD2): A novel cancer-related gene over-expressed in breast cancer. *Biochim. Biophys. Acta* **2009**, *1792*, 988–997. [CrossRef]
206. Dery, M.A.; Jodoin, J.; Ursini-Siegel, J.; Aleynikova, O.; Ferrario, C.; Hassan, S.; Basik, M.; LeBlanc, A.C. Endoplasmic reticulum stress induces PRNP prion protein gene expression in breast cancer. *Breast Cancer Res.* **2013**, *15*, R22. [CrossRef]
207. Lacunza, E.; Rabassa, M.E.; Canzoneri, R.; Pellon-Maison, M.; Croce, M.V.; Aldaz, C.M.; Abba, M.C. Identification of signaling pathways modulated by RHBDD2 in breast cancer Cells: A link to the unfolded protein response. *Cell. Stress Chaperones* **2014**, *19*, 379–388. [CrossRef]
208. Nagelkerke, A.; Bussink, J.; Mujcic, H.; Wouters, B.G.; Lehmann, S.; Sweep, F.C.; Span, P.N. Hypoxia stimulates migration of breast cancer cells via the PERK/ATF4/LAMP3-arm of the unfolded protein response. *Breast. Cancer Res.* **2013**, *15*, R2. [CrossRef]
209. Varone, E.; Decio, A.; Chernorudskiy, A.; Minoli, L.; Brunelli, L.; Ioli, F.; Piotti, A.; Pastorelli, R.; Fratelli, M.; Gobbi, M.; et al. The ER stress response mediator ERO1 triggers cancer metastasis by favoring the angiogenic switch in hypoxic conditions. *Oncogene* **2021**, *40*, 1721–1736. [CrossRef]
210. Piccart-Gebhart, M.J.; Procter, M.; Leyland-Jones, B.; Goldhirsch, A.; Untch, M.; Smith, I.; Gianni, L.; Baselga, J.; Bell, R.; Jackisch, C.; et al. Trastuzumab after adjuvant chemotherapy in HER2-positive breast cancer. *N. Engl. J. Med.* **2005**, *353*, 1659–1672. [CrossRef]
211. O'Shaughnessy, J.; Osborne, C.; Pippen, J.E.; Yoffe, M.; Patt, D.; Rocha, C.; Koo, I.C.; Sherman, B.M.; Bradley, C. Iniparib plus chemotherapy in metastatic triple-negative breast cancer. *N. Engl. J. Med.* **2011**, *364*, 205–214. [CrossRef]
212. Burstein, H.J. Systemic Therapy for Estrogen Receptor-Positive, HER2-Negative Breast Cancer. *N. Engl. J. Med.* **2020**, *383*, 2557–2570. [CrossRef]
213. Middleton, J.D.; Stover, D.G.; Hai, T. Chemotherapy-Exacerbated Breast Cancer Metastasis: A Paradox Explainable by Dysregulated Adaptive-Response. *Int. J. Mol. Sci* **2018**, *19*, 3333. [CrossRef]
214. Fischer, K.R.; Durrans, A.; Lee, S.; Sheng, J.; Li, F.; Wong, S.T.; Choi, H.; El Rayes, T.; Ryu, S.; Troeger, J.; et al. Epithelial-to-mesenchymal transition is not required for lung metastasis but contributes to chemoresistance. *Nature* **2015**, *527*, 472–476. [CrossRef]
215. Volk-Draper, L.; Hall, K.; Griggs, C.; Rajput, S.; Kohio, P.; DeNardo, D.; Ran, S. Paclitaxel therapy promotes breast cancer metastasis in a TLR4-dependent manner. *Cancer Res.* **2014**, *74*, 5421–5434. [CrossRef]
216. Karagiannis, G.S.; Pastoriza, J.M.; Wang, Y.; Harney, A.S.; Entenberg, D.; Pignatelli, J.; Sharma, V.P.; Xue, E.A.; Cheng, E.; D'Alfonso, T.M.; et al. Neoadjuvant chemotherapy induces breast cancer metastasis through a TMEM-mediated mechanism. *Sci. Transl. Med.* **2017**, *9*, eaan0026. [CrossRef]
217. Ren, Y.; Zhou, X.; Yang, J.J.; Liu, X.; Zhao, X.H.; Wang, Q.X.; Han, L.; Song, X.; Zhu, Z.Y.; Tian, W.P.; et al. AC1MMYR2 impairs high dose paclitaxel-induced tumor metastasis by targeting miR-21/CDK5 axis. *Cancer Lett.* **2015**, *362*, 174–182. [CrossRef] [PubMed]
218. Lu, H.; Chen, I.; Shimoda, L.A.; Park, Y.; Zhang, C.; Tran, L.; Zhang, H.; Semenza, G.L. Chemotherapy-Induced Ca(2+) Release Stimulates Breast Cancer Stem Cell Enrichment. *Cell Rep.* **2017**, *18*, 1946–1957. [CrossRef]
219. Keklikoglou, I.; Cianciaruso, C.; Guc, E.; Squadrito, M.L.; Spring, L.M.; Tazzyman, S.; Lambein, L.; Poissonnier, A.; Ferraro, G.B.; Baer, C.; et al. Chemotherapy elicits pro-metastatic extracellular vesicles in breast cancer models. *Nat. Cell Biol.* **2019**, *21*, 190–202. [CrossRef] [PubMed]
220. Wills, C.A.; Liu, X.; Chen, L.; Zhao, Y.; Dower, C.M.; Sundstrom, J.; Wang, H.G. Chemotherapy-Induced Upregulation of Small Extracellular Vesicle-Associated PTX3 Accelerates Breast Cancer Metastasis. *Cancer Res.* **2021**, *81*, 452–463. [CrossRef] [PubMed]
221. Liang, C.C.; Park, A.Y.; Guan, J.L. In vitro scratch assay: A convenient and inexpensive method for analysis of cell migration in vitro. *Nat. Protoc.* **2007**, *2*, 329–333. [CrossRef]
222. Cory, G. Scratch-wound assay. *Methods Mol. Biol.* **2011**, *769*, 25–30. [CrossRef]
223. Hulkower, K.I.; Herber, R.L. Cell migration and invasion assays as tools for drug discovery. *Pharmaceutics* **2011**, *3*, 107–124. [CrossRef]
224. Khanna, C.; Hunter, K. Modeling metastasis in vivo. *Carcinogenesis* **2005**, *26*, 513–523. [CrossRef]

225. Guy, C.T.; Cardiff, R.D.; Muller, W.J. Induction of mammary tumors by expression of polyomavirus middle T oncogene: A transgenic mouse model for metastatic Disease. *Mol. Cell. Biol.* **1992**, *12*, 954–961. [CrossRef]
226. Bibby, M.C. Orthotopic models of cancer for preclinical drug evaluation: Advantages and disadvantages. *Eur. J. Cancer* **2004**, *40*, 852–857. [CrossRef]
227. Kim, J.B.; Urban, K.; Cochran, E.; Lee, S.; Ang, A.; Rice, B.; Bata, A.; Campbell, K.; Coffee, R.; Gorodinsky, A.; et al. Non-invasive detection of a small number of Bioluminescent cancer Cells in vivo. *PLoS ONE* **2010**, *5*, e9364. [CrossRef]
228. Ritsma, L.; Steller, E.J.; Beerling, E.; Loomans, C.J.; Zomer, A.; Gerlach, C.; Vrisekoop, N.; Seinstra, D.; Van Gurp, L.; Schafer, R.; et al. Intravital microscopy through an abdominal imaging window reveals a pre-micrometastasis stage during liver metastasis. *Sci. Transl. Med.* **2012**, *4*, 158ra145. [CrossRef]
229. Hason, M.; Bartunek, P. Zebrafish Models of Cancer-New Insights on Modeling Human Cancer in a Non-Mammalian Vertebrate. *Genes* **2019**, *10*, 935. [CrossRef]
230. Fior, R.; Povoa, V.; Mendes, R.V.; Carvalho, T.; Gomes, A.; Figueiredo, N.; Ferreira, M.G. Single-Cell. functional and chemosensitive profiling of combinatorial colorectal therapy in zebrafish xenografts. *Proc. Natl. Acad. Sci. USA* **2017**, *114*, E8234–E8243. [CrossRef]
231. Follain, G.; Osmani, N.; Fuchs, C.; Allio, G.; Harlepp, S.; Goetz, J.G. Using the Zebrafish Embryo to Dissect the Early Steps of the Metastasis Cascade. *Methods Mol. Biol.* **2018**, *1749*, 195–211. [CrossRef] [PubMed]
232. Follain, G.; Osmani, N.; Azevedo, A.S.; Allio, G.; Mercier, L.; Karreman, M.A.; Solecki, G.; Garcia Leon, M.J.; Lefebvre, O.; Fekonja, N.; et al. Hemodynamic Forces Tune the Arrest, Adhesion, and Extravasation of Circulating Tumor Cells. *Dev. Cell.* **2018**, *45*, 33–52.e12. [CrossRef] [PubMed]
233. Asokan, N.; Daetwyler, S.; Bernas, S.N.; Schmied, C.; Vogler, S.; Lambert, K.; Wobus, M.; Wermke, M.; Kempermann, G.; Huisken, J.; et al. Long-term in vivo imaging reveals tumor-specific Dissemination and captures host tumor Interaction in zebrafish xenografts. *Sci. Rep.* **2020**, *10*, 13254. [CrossRef] [PubMed]
234. Nicoli, S.; Ribatti, D.; Cotelli, F.; Presta, M. Mammalian tumor xenografts induce neovascularization in zebrafish embryos. *Cancer Res.* **2007**, *67*, 2927–2931. [CrossRef]
235. Roh-Johnson, M.; Shah, A.N.; Stonick, J.A.; Poudel, K.R.; Kargl, J.; Yang, G.H.; Di Martino, J.; Hernandez, R.E.; Gast, C.E.; Zarour, L.R.; et al. Macrophage-Dependent Cytoplasmic Transfer during Melanoma Invasion In Vivo. *Dev. Cell.* **2017**, *43*, 549–562.e546. [CrossRef]
236. Britto, D.D.; Wyroba, B.; Chen, W.; Lockwood, R.A.; Tran, K.B.; Shepherd, P.R.; Hall, C.J.; Crosier, K.E.; Crosier, P.S.; Astin, J.W. Macrophages enhance Vegfa-driven angiogenesis in an embryonic zebrafish tumour xenograft model. *Dis. Model. Mech.* **2018**, *11*, dmm.035998. [CrossRef]
237. Povoa, V.; Rebelo de Almeida, C.; Maia-Gil, M.; Sobral, D.; Domingues, M.; Martinez-Lopez, M.; De Almeida Fuzeta, M.; Silva, C.; Grosso, A.R.; Fior, R. Innate immune evasion revealed in a colorectal zebrafish xenograft model. *Nat. Commun.* **2021**, *12*, 1156. [CrossRef]
238. Costa, B.; Estrada, M.F.; Mendes, R.V.; Fior, R. Zebrafish Avatars towards Personalized Medicine-A Comparative Review between Avatar Models. *Cells* **2020**, *9*, 293. [CrossRef]
239. Gregory, T.R. Understanding Natural Selection: Essential Concepts and Common Misconceptions. *Evo. Edu. Outreach* **2009**, *2*, 156–175. [CrossRef]

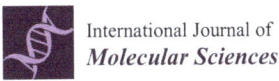

International Journal of Molecular Sciences

Article

CD146+ Pericytes Subset Isolated from Human Micro-Fragmented Fat Tissue Display a Strong Interaction with Endothelial Cells: A Potential Cell Target for Therapeutic Angiogenesis

Ekta Manocha [1,*], Alessandra Consonni [2], Fulvio Baggi [2], Emilio Ciusani [3], Valentina Cocce [4], Francesca Paino [4], Carlo Tremolada [5], Arnaldo Caruso [1] and Giulio Alessandri [1,5]

1. Section of Microbiology, Department of Molecular and Translational Medicine, University of Brescia Medical School, 25123 Brescia, Italy; arnaldo.caruso@unibs.it (A.C.); cisiamo2@yahoo.com (G.A.)
2. Neurology IV—Neuroimmunology and Neuromuscular Diseases Unit, Fondazione IRCCS Istituto Neurologico Carlo Besta, 20133 Milan, Italy; alessandra.consonni@istituto-besta.it (A.C.); fulvio.baggi@istituto-besta.it (F.B.)
3. Laboratory of Neurological Biochemistry and Neuropharmacology, Fondazione IRCCS Istituto Neurologico Carlo Besta, 20133 Milan, Italy; emilio.ciusani@istituto-besta.it
4. CRC StaMeTec, Department of Biomedical, Surgical and Dental Sciences, University of Milan, 20122 Milan, Italy; valentina.cocce@unimi.it (V.C.); francesca.paino@unimi.it (F.P.)
5. Department of Stem Cells and Regenerative Medicine, Image Institute, 20122 Milan, Italy; carlo.tremolada@gmail.com
* Correspondence: e.manocha@unibs.it

Citation: Manocha, E.; Consonni, A.; Baggi, F.; Ciusani, E.; Cocce, V.; Paino, F.; Tremolada, C.; Caruso, A.; Alessandri, G. CD146+ Pericytes Subset Isolated from Human Micro-Fragmented Fat Tissue Display a Strong Interaction with Endothelial Cells: A Potential Cell Target for Therapeutic Angiogenesis. *Int. J. Mol. Sci.* **2022**, *23*, 5806. https://doi.org/10.3390/ijms23105806

Academic Editors: Bozena Smolkova, Julie Earl and Agapi Kataki

Received: 29 April 2022
Accepted: 19 May 2022
Published: 22 May 2022

Publisher's Note: MDPI stays neutral with regard to jurisdictional claims in published maps and institutional affiliations.

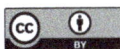

Copyright: © 2022 by the authors. Licensee MDPI, Basel, Switzerland. This article is an open access article distributed under the terms and conditions of the Creative Commons Attribution (CC BY) license (https://creativecommons.org/licenses/by/4.0/).

Abstract: Pericytes (PCs) are mesenchymal stromal cells (MSCs) that function as support cells and play a role in tissue regeneration and, in particular, vascular homeostasis. PCs promote endothelial cells (ECs) survival which is critical for vessel stabilization, maturation, and remodeling. In this study, PCs were isolated from human micro-fragmented adipose tissue (MFAT) obtained from fat lipoaspirate and were characterized as $NG2^+/PDGFR\beta^+/CD105^+$ cells. Here, we tested the fat-derived PCs for the dispensability of the CD146 marker with the aim of better understanding the role of these PC subpopulations on angiogenesis. Cells from both CD146-positive ($CD146^+$) and negative ($CD146^-$) populations were observed to interact with human umbilical vein ECs (HUVECs). In addition, fat-derived PCs were able to induce angiogenesis of ECs in spheroids assay; and conditioned medium (CM) from both PCs and fat tissue itself led to the proliferation of ECs, thereby marking their role in angiogenesis stimulation. However, we found that $CD146^+$ cells were more responsive to PDGF-BB-stimulated migration, adhesion, and angiogenic interaction with ECs, possibly owing to their higher expression of NCAM/CD56 than the corresponding $CD146^-$ subpopulation. We conclude that in fat tissue, CD146-expressing cells may represent a more mature pericyte subpopulation that may have higher efficacy in controlling and stimulating vascular regeneration and stabilization than their CD146-negative counterpart.

Keywords: angiogenesis; pericytes; adipose tissue; cell adhesion; endothelial cells

1. Introduction

Mesenchymal Stromal Cells (MSCs) are medicinal signaling cells involved in tissue regeneration but are not stem cells [1]. This cell population, which can be isolated from many tissues, such as bone marrow, placenta, adipose tissue (AT), and umbilical cord blood, has been shown to be identical to the vascular associated cell phenotype, namely pericytes (PCs) [2]. Indeed, both MSCs and PCs express similar markers and, most importantly, display very similar functional activity. They both are considered safe for allogenic transplantation due to the lack of expression of membrane-bound molecules involved in immune rejection [3]. MSCs have the potential to turn out as drug stores and be involved in immune modulation, tissue regeneration, and secretion of angiogenic molecules [4,5]. They prevent inflammatory cascades by secreting cytokines and paracrine factors to interact directly with different immune cells to suppress the over-activation of the immune system [6–8]. Overall, they appeared as a quite heterogeneous cell population that includes stromal cells at different levels of maturation and differentiation [7,8]. More specifically, PCs are vascular mural cells that interact with the abluminal surface of endothelial cells (ECs) from capillaries, arterioles, and venules and share a common basement membrane with ECs. They can be found around blood capillaries, precapillary arterioles, postcapillary venules, and collecting venules and are morphologically distinct in different organs [9]. Moreover, PCs have been found to regulate capillary diameter, blood flow, vessel permeability, and stabilization of ECs [10].

The synergism between the ECs and PCs in maintaining a functional vasculature is well studied in terms of regulation of different stages of vessel maturity as PCs may regulate both destabilization of nascent vessels and stabilization of mature vasculature [11,12]. Endothelial-free PC assemblies were observed to regulate sprouting in retinal neovascularization, adult mouse cornea, and mouse tumor models, by recruiting ECs from the parental vessel, signifying the guidance exerted by PCs for invading ECs [13]. Genetic or acquired deficiencies in pericyte coverage of EC-lined capillaries can lead to the instability of micro-vessels [14].

Little is known about the "maturity stage" of PCs involved in ECs migration or its role in mediating angiogenesis. The primary reason for this lack of knowledge is probably related to the fact that PCs are a heterogeneous cell population, difficult to characterize due to the absence of specific markers. Usually, PCs are characterized by many molecular markers [15], among them, NG2, PDGF-β receptor, and Endoglin (CD105) are indicated as the most common ones. In addition, CD146 which was originally identified as an endothelial marker involved in the angiogenesis process was also found significantly expressed in PCs [2,16]. Interestingly, it has been known that $CD146^+$ stem cells appear to have a greater therapeutic potential than $CD146^-$ stem cells in inflammatory diseases [17], as well as CD146 expression on MSCs was associated with their vascular smooth muscle commitment [18]. However, the role of these two PC populations on angiogenesis is poorly investigated.

Therefore, in this study, we investigated PCs distinguished by the presence of CD146 in regulating interaction with ECs and their efficacy on the angiogenesis process in vitro. PCs were isolated from AT upon a process of mechanical micro-fragmentation which allows obtaining a significant number of mesenchymal cells/pericytes [19,20]. Briefly, we found that $CD146^+$ PCs were highly effective in interacting with ECs compared to their CD146-negative counterpart and consequently were more efficient in stimulating angiogenesis. We also postulated that the variable expression of CD56/NCAM by $CD146^+$ PCs was related to their capacity to adhere to endothelium.

2. Results

2.1. Characterization of Pericytes (PCs)/Mesenchymal Stromal Cells (MSCs) from Adipose Tissue (AT)

The common pericyte-specific markers that correspond to MSCs are often used for the unambiguous identification of the cells from the stromal vascular fraction (SVF) of AT along with a meticulous analysis of morphological criteria. Magnetic-activated cell sorting (MACS)-based CD31 selection was performed on the stromal cell population extracted from collagenase-treated micro-fragmented adipose tissue (MFAT). The $CD31^-$ subset cells (that were around $0.62 \pm 0.08 \times 10^6$/mL of MFAT) were investigated for typical MSC markers. Immunostaining results identified the extracted CD31-negative cells to be mostly $NG2^+$, $PDGFR\beta^+$, $CD105^+$, and slightly positive for αSMA (Figure 1A). Furthermore, the $CD31^-$ cells were investigated for other common markers using flow cytometric analysis and were observed to be $CD34^-/CD105^+/CD73^+/CD90^+/CD44^+$; thus, expressing the typical markers of MSCs derived from adipose tissue (Figure 1B) thereby demonstrating their PC origin. The same cells were also majorly positive for adhesion molecules such as intracellular adhesion molecule 1 (ICAM1) (Figure 1B) and Vascular Endothelial Cadherin (VECAD) (Figure S1). As flow cytometric analysis showed the majority of the CD31$^-$ cells as negative for CD146 (Figure S1), to separate this cell population we performed a second cell sorting (MACS)-based CD146 selection. The isolated CD146$^+$ cells showed no morphological difference from the CD146$^-$ cell populations. Nonetheless, it is important to have both CD146 subpopulations phenotypically different from CD31$^+$ cells (Figure 1C) since the CD146 marker has also been shown to be expressed by ECs [21]. Consequently, both CD146$^-$ and CD146$^+$ subpopulations were screened for typical MSC markers by flow cytometry (Figure S2A–C). CD146$^+$ cells showed higher expression levels of ICAM1, CD44, CD105, and CD90 while CD146$^-$ cells expressed a slightly higher proportion of CD73 surface marker (Figure 2A). In this regard, CD31 initial selection was crucial for removing all the ECs present in the MFAT tissue preparations; thus, excluding the possible presence of residual ECs contaminating the isolated PCs population. This was also confirmed by the negative expression of von Willebrand factor (data not shown), while both of the CD146-sorted populations do express characteristic MSC markers.

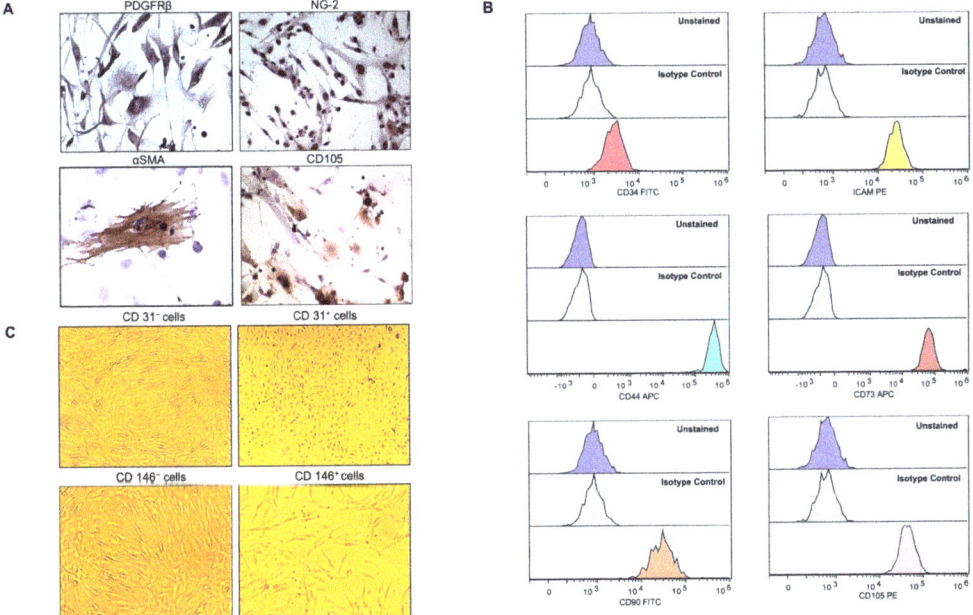

Figure 1. Expression of mesenchymal cell markers (MSCs) on cultured pericytes (PCs). (**A**) Immunohistochemistry staining with CD31$^-$ PCs were strongly positive for PDGFRβ, NG-2, and most of the cells were positive for CD105 but slightly for αSMA. Pictures were taken at magnification 40× after avidin-biotin peroxide staining. (**B**) Flow cytometry demonstrated CD31$^-$ PCs to be mostly negative for CD34, and positive for ICAM1, CD44, CD73, CD90, and CD105. Histograms in the lowest panels (multicolor) represent the staining for specific antibodies as compared to the unstained and unrelated isotype-matched antibodies in blue and light grey histograms, respectively. (**C**) Bright-field microscopy depicting the morphology of CD31$^-$ PCs versus CD31$^+$ cells as the latter were distinguished by the endothelial-cell-like cobblestone morphology from the elongated and slender shape of the former. CD31$^-$ cells, selected for CD146-based MACS (CD146$^-$ and CD146$^+$), were similar in shape and morphology. Pictures were taken at a magnification of 10×.

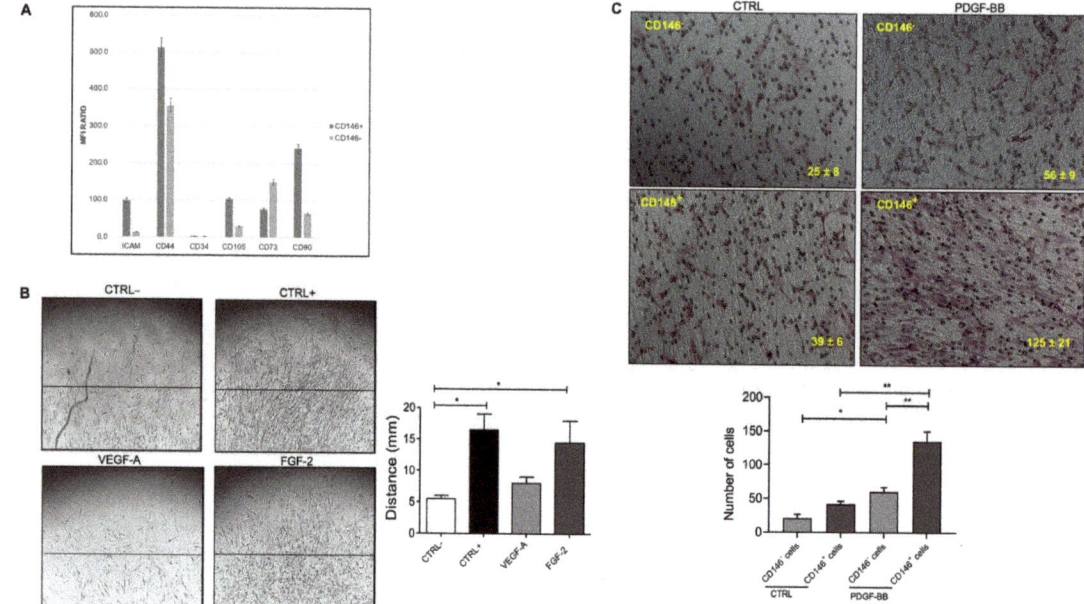

Figure 2. (**A**) The bar graph represents the mean fluorescence intensity (MFI) ratio of each specific antibody and the relative isotype control by flow cytometric analysis of CD146$^+$ and CD146$^-$ cell populations. Values greater than 1 indicate the expression of the specific marker. (**B**) PDGF-BB induced pericyte migration. The presence of FGF-2 promoted CD31$^-$ PCs migration but not VEGF-A as compared to the negative control (EBM-2 + 0.5% FBS). PCs stimulated with complete medium (EGM-2 + 10% FBS) were used as a positive control. The bar chart represents the relative distance migrated outwards from the collagen layer towards the edge of the wells upon stimulation with VEGF-A and FGF-2. At least 3 different fields/well were counted at 10× magnification in triplicates. Scale bar = 100 µM. (**C**) PDGF-BB promoted PCs migration for CD146$^+$ cells higher than CD146$^-$ cells in the basal medium in a transwell assay. The bar chart represents the number of cells that migrated across the membrane and were counted by microscopically examining the lower surface of the transwell chamber. Reported data represent the means ± standard deviation (SD) of the number of cells found in each field. At least 5 different fields for each membrane were counted at 10× magnification. Scale bar = 100 µM. Images are representative of at least three independent experiments with similar results performed in triplicates. Statistical analysis was performed by one way ANOVA and Bonferroni's post-test; * $p < 0.05$, ** $p < 0.01$. CTRL$^+$—positive control; CTRL$^-$—negative control; VEGF-A—vascular endothelial growth factor-A; FGF-2—fibroblast growth factor-2; PDGF-BB—platelet-derived growth factor-BB.

Under our experimental conditions, we found that the number of the isolated CD31$^-$CD146$^-$ cells was around $0.51 \pm 0.09 \times 10^6$ (per 5 mL of MFAT) and was almost 4–5-fold that of CD31$^-$CD146$^+$ cells ($0.13 \pm 0.02 \times 10^6$ per 5 mL of MFAT).

2.2. Fat Pericytes Respond to Platelet Derived Growth Factor (PDGF-BB) Signaling

Pericytes have been identified as important regulators of ECs signaling and vascular patterning as the release of platelet derived growth factor (PDGF-BB) by ECs activates PDGFR on PCs which, in turn, controls angiogenesis by regulating vascular endothelial growth factor (VEGF-A)/VEGFR-2 signaling [12,22]. Fibroblast growth factor (FGF-2) binds to FGFR2 to stimulate pericyte proliferation and orchestrates the PDGFRβ signaling, directly and indirectly, for vascular recruitment. In angiogenic vessels, ECs produce PDGF-BB to recruit PDGFRβ⁺ pericytes onto the nascent vasculature [23,24].

To this aim, we asked whether CD31⁻ PCs can sustain differential migratory potential toward common growth factors. Cultured CD31⁻PCs from fat tissue exhibited strong chemotaxis towards FGF-2 stimulation (Figure 2B). However, they were not found to be stimulated with VEGF-A signals, therefore, speculating towards basic FGF mediated downstream signaling in a collagen-containing medium. The migration response to FGF-2 was comparable to the positive control, stimulated with endothelial growth medium (EGM) in the presence of serum and other growth factors. The negative control, on the other hand, basal medium without the presence of any growth factors, appeared to be quite slow to respond to the migratory stimuli.

PDGF is released from angiogenic ECs and the binding of PDGF-BB to PDGFRβ on the pericytes induces their migration by activating the Ras/Rho/Rac and protein kinase C pathway [9]. Since FGF-2 activates downstream PDGF signaling and owing to the same origin of CD146-sorted PCs, we attempted to test the different migratory properties of CD146⁺ and CD146⁻ subpopulation upon stimulation with PDGF-BB. CD146⁺ PCs were found to migrate and proliferate much higher in number than CD146⁻ cells in response to PDGF-BB in the basal medium (Figure 2C). To our surprise, CD146⁺ PCs migrated much slower than their CD146⁻ counterparts upon collagen embedding in a complete medium in the absence of PDGF-BB which was evident starting from day 4 until day 7 post-stimulation (Figure S3A,B).

2.3. Pericytes from Fat Tissue Interact with Human Umbilical Vein ECs (HUVECs)

The interaction of PCs with ECs is crucial in maintaining the mechanical stability of micro-vessels and can be studied with the help of adhesion assays. For this reason, we determined the adhesion of CD31⁻ PCs to the surface of quiescent ECs monolayer at 15, 30, and 60 min of incubation where 30 min was chosen as the optimum time point for the identification of round-shaped PCs attached to the resting elliptical-shaped ECs (Figure S4). At the mentioned time point, a reasonable number of PCs among both subpopulations were observed to be in the vicinity of ECs. As a negative control, only HUVECs, without the presence of PCs, were used (Figure 3A). Interestingly, the adhesion of CD146⁻ PCs to the HUVECs monolayer was significantly lower than that of CD146⁺ PCs (Figure 3A) suggesting that CD146⁺ PCs may have much more efficacy than their CD146⁻ counterpart in the angiogenesis process, particularly in remodeling and stabilization of ECs during micro-vessels neoformation.

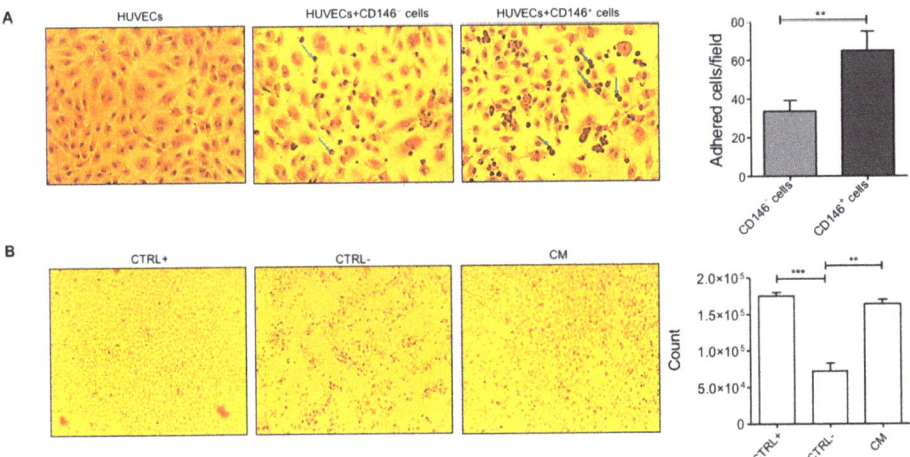

Figure 3. ECs-PCs interaction (**A**) Adhesion assay. PCs detached from tissue culture flasks were seeded on

a cultured ECs monolayer. In the figure, adherent PCs appear as darker round cells (for example, indicated by blue arrows) adhered to the elliptical-shaped HUVECs monolayer. CD146$^+$ cells were relatively more adherent than CD146$^-$ cells to ECs. Images are representative of three different experiments performed in triplicates. The left corner image represents the HUVECs monolayer as a negative control in the absence of adhered pericytes. The bar graph displays the number of adhered cells per frame (counted for three different frames/well) performed in triplicates at 10× magnification. (**B**) Cell proliferation assay. Cells cultured under starvation conditions proliferated in the presence of CM from MFAT (diluted 2-fold in RPMI medium). Images were taken after 16 h of treatment at 4× magnification. ECs cultured in the complete medium (EGM + 10% FBS) were used as a positive control. ECs cultured under starvation conditions (EBM + 0.5% FBS; NC) were used as a negative control. The bar graph shows the cell count after overnight treatment with CM. Images are representative of one out of three independent experiments with similar results performed in triplicates. Statistical analysis was performed by Student's t-test and one way ANOVA following Bonferroni's post-test; ** $p < 0.01$, *** $p < 0.001$. CM—conditioned medium.

2.4. Micro Fragmented Adipose Tissue (MFAT)-Derived CD146$^+$ PCs Subset Promotes Vascular Stability

We initially investigated if the conditioned medium (CM), obtained by incubation of the whole PCs population derived from MFAT tissue and cultured at very low serum concentration in basal medium, was able to preserve ECs vascular monolayer integrity. Thus PCs-CM was added (2-fold diluted) to the HUVECs monolayer and then cultured under starvation for 24 h. PCs-CM demonstrated potent efficacy in preserving ECs monolayer integrity. The effect of CM was equal to that of the complete growth medium (EGM + 10% FBS). In contrast, the EC monolayer cultured under starved conditions (medium consisting of only EBM + 0.5% FBS) and in the absence of PCs-CM was significantly damaged: cells were non-viable and almost completely detached as observed by the presence of floating cells in the culture (Figure 3B). Furthermore, ECs stimulated with PCs-CM up to a dilution of 64-fold were able to survive under starved conditions (Figure S5).

Once the efficacy of PCs on vascular monolayer integrity was established, we next performed a 3-D spheroids assay by mixing CD31$^-$ PCs and ECs in a ratio of 1:5. As shown in Figure 4A, the presence of PCs not only perturbated the angiogenesis process but also aggravated the same as observed by a higher number of sprouts formed by HUVECs. This strong effect was also confirmed by CD31$^+$ endothelial cells derived from the fat tissue itself. Then, we asked if the two subpopulations of PCs, CD146$^-$ and CD146$^+$, could modulate vascular sprouting and stabilization differently. We found that the induction of sprouting by ECs combined with the CD146$^+$ cell population was, in general, higher than that induced by CD146$^-$, but not statistically different (Figure 4B). However, CD146$^+$ cells induced a significantly higher sprout length than CD146$^-$ cells (Figure 4C) suggesting that CD146$^+$ cells may have been more tightly integrated with ECs as observed by longer cytoplasmic extensions to the spheroid core and therefore higher capacity to support ECs stability. This was confirmed by an investigation of capillary-like structures via tube formation assay. In this case, we tested the effect of CM derived from cultured CD146$^+$ and CD146$^-$ fat PCs on HUVECs seeded on polymerized plugs of growth factor reduced (GFR)-basement membrane extract (BME). The addition of CD146$^+$ PCs-derived CM was more effective as compared to CD146$^-$-CM to induce the significant production of cord-like formation by ECs when seeded on the Matrigel. Indeed, the effect of CD146$^+$-CM was most effective after 24 h of incubation. At this time of observation, while cord formation persisted in CD146$^+$-CM-treated wells, the cords were completely regressed in the control medium and CD146$^-$-CM (1:2 dilution) treated wells (Figure 4D). Interestingly, under these experimental conditions, the addition of CM derived from CD146$^+$ PCs was much more effective than the CM of the CD146$^-$ PC subset in stimulating EC sprouting number in a 3-D spheroids assay (Figure 4E).

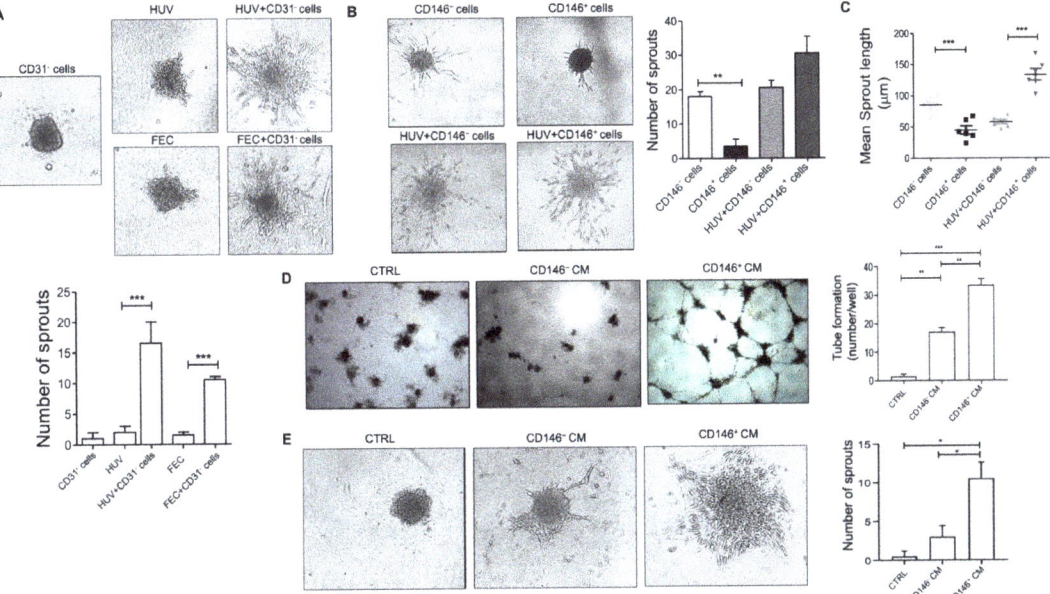

Figure 4. Sprout formation from ECs and PCs co-culture spheroids. (**A**) Representative images of sprout formation from ECs-only (HUVECs or CD31$^+$ Fat ECs), and CD31$^-$ PCs:ECs (1:5) co-culture spheroids embedded in type I collagen gel at 24 h (magnification, 20×). The quantitative graph shows sprout numbers formed from CD31$^-$ PCs- or ECs-only (HUVECs or CD31$^+$ fat ECs), compared to co-culture spheroids (mean ± SD, $n = 3$). (**B**) Sprout formation from CD146$^-$ and CD146$^+$ PCs-only, and PCs + ECs (HUVECs) co-culture spheroids in collagen after 24 h of embedding (magnification, 20×). The quantitative graph displays the number of sprouts at 24 h from PCs-only and PCs:ECs (1:5) co-culture spheroids (mean ± SD, $n = 3$). (**C**) The scatter plot displays the mean sprout length (in μm) per spheroid at 24 h (mean ± SD, $n \leq 6$). Images are representative of one out of three independent experiments with similar results performed in triplicates. (**D**) HUVECs were seeded on BME-coated plates and stimulated with CM from CD146$^-$ and CD146$^+$ pericytes in culture. Images were taken after 24 h of plating the assay (original magnification, 10×). HUVECs treated with EGM complete medium were used as a control. The number of cords was counted as a parameter for the quantification of tube formation. (**E**) The 3-D spheroids assay of HUVECs in the presence of CM from CD146$^-$ and CD146$^+$ cells. HUVECs treated with EGM complete medium were used as a control. Images were taken after 24 h at 10× magnification. Images are representative of one out of two independent experiments with similar results performed in triplicates. Statistical analysis was performed by one way ANOVA and Bonferroni's post-test; * $p \leq 0.05$, ** $p < 0.01$, *** $p < 0.001$. HUV—human umbilical vein endothelial cells; FEC—endothelial cells from fat tissue.

2.5. Upregulation of CD56 (NCAM) Expression by CD146$^+$ PCs

Pericyte–endothelial cell interaction is crucial in tissue regeneration which is related to the activation of signals that regulate endothelial cell function. Among the presence of other adhesion molecules such as ICAM1, VECAD, and TGFβ signaling as previously reported, we attempted to investigate if NCAM (CD56), another marker known to mediate endothelial cell–pericyte interactions [25] is also differentially expressed among CD146-sorted pericyte population. As shown in Figure 5A, CD146$^+$ PCs relatively expressed NCAM as punctate staining in the cytoplasm. On the contrary, CD146$^-$ PCs do not show a marked expression of NCAM. However, both the populations did exhibit PDGFRβ expression but CD146$^+$ cells showed a relatively higher expression of the same in the cytoplasm and plasma membrane than their counterpart. Labeling studies demonstrated that CD146$^+$ cells were strongly positive for CD44, CD56, and negative for αSMA, whereas the CD146$^-$ cells stained strongly for CD44 but significantly less intense for CD56, and negative for αSMA (Figure 5B). Under our experimental conditions, we identified the higher expression of CD105 by CD146$^+$ cells (also confirmed by flow cytometry) while a dim expression by CD146$^-$ cells was observed whereas the two subpopulations that stained positive for NG-2 with CD146$^+$ cells displayed a relatively stronger expression in both nucleus and cytoplasm (Figure 5C). Since a higher level of PDGFRβ receptor upregulates cell adhesion molecules in vitro and in vivo, we examined the NCAM expression of PCs upon adhesion to ECs. We found that CD146$^+$ PCs, which adhere to a greater extent than CD146$^-$ PCs, also appeared to express NCAM at a higher level (Figure 6B,C). The negative control IgG and IgG1 isotype stained negatively for anti-PDGFRβ and anti-NCAM antibodies, respectively (Figure 6A). Therefore, these experiments seem to confirm that NCAM may play a role in the interaction of PCs with endothelial cells and the CD146$^+$ PCs subset may have an important role in mediating vascular stability.

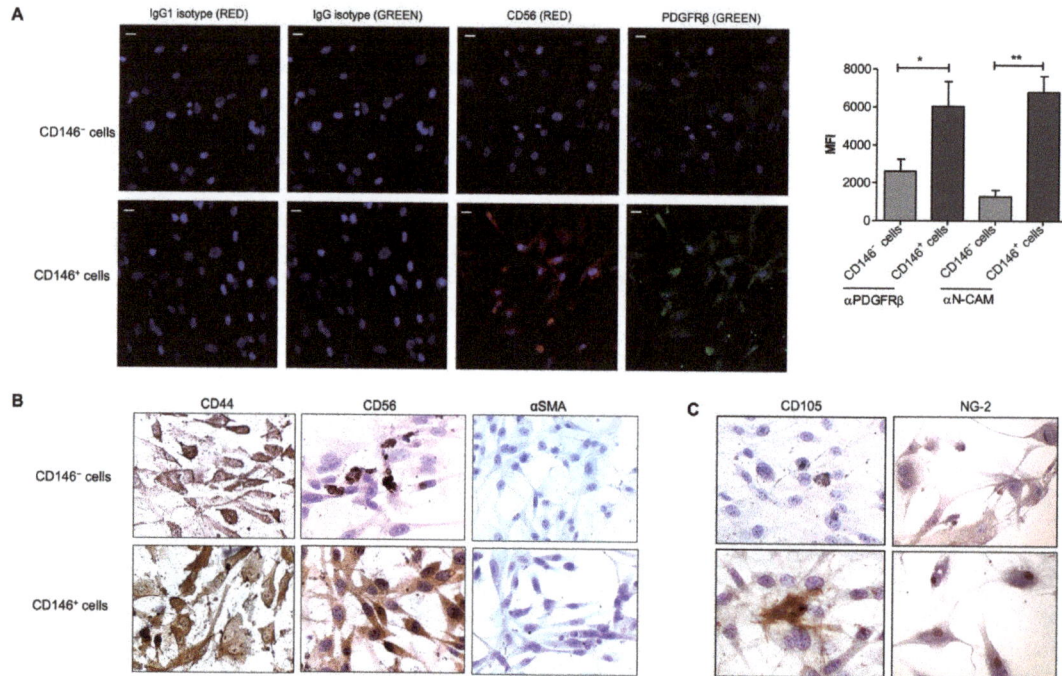

Figure 5. Expression of CD56 (NCAM). (**A**) Representative confocal images of CD146$^-$ cells (upper side) and CD146$^+$ (lower side). Immunofluorescence was performed to identify PDGFRβ and CD56 expression by both the cell subpopulations. Images display PDGFRβ in green, CD56 in red, and cell nuclei in blue; magnification, 40×. Scale bar = 25 μM. The corresponding IgG- (green) or IgG1-isotype (red) was used as a negative control. The bar graph was generated using the mean fluorescence intensity of two different experiments performed in triplicates. One-way ANOVA and Bonferroni's post-test were used to compare the data; * $p \leq 0.05$, ** $p < 0.01$. (**B**) CD146$^-$ (upper) and CD146$^+$ (lower) cells were stained for peculiar mesenchymal markers CD44, CD56 (NCAM), and αSMA. Images were taken at 60× magnification. (**C**) Immunostaining images represent CD146$^-$ (upper) and CD146$^+$ cells (lower) for the expression of common mesenchymal markers, CD105 and NG-2 at 40× and 20× magnification, respectively. Images are representative of one out of three experiments performed in duplicates. NCAM—neural cell adhesion molecule (CD56).

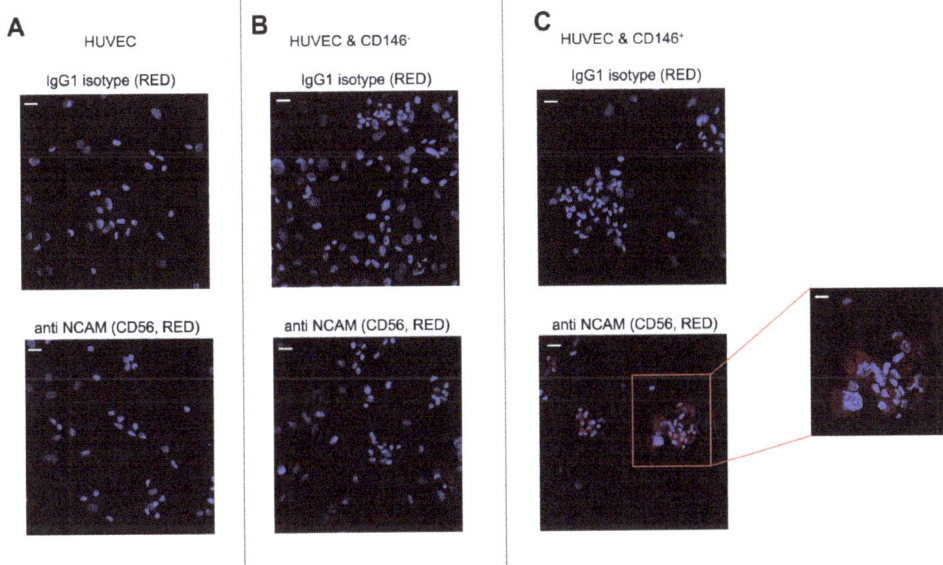

Figure 6. Differential expression of CD56 by CD146⁻ and CD146⁺ pericytes adhered to HUVECs. (**A**) The upper image represents HUVECs stained with an anti-IgG1 isotype. The bottom image represents the HUVECs monolayer stained with antibody to CD56 (NCAM) as a negative control. (**B,C**) PCs detached from culture flasks were seeded on the cultured ECs monolayer. The two different morphologies in the figure represent adherent PCs as round cells adjacent to relatively long-shaped HUVECs. The upper images represent ECs-PCs co-culture stained with the negative control IgG1 isotype. The bottom images represent ECs-PCs co-culture stained with CD56 (NCAM). Images are representative of two different experiments performed in triplicates; magnification, 40×. Scale bar = 25 µM. The extreme right image displays the higher magnification image; magnification, 100×. Scale bar = 10 µM. Images display pericytes in red, adhered to HUVECs, and nuclei in blue.

3. Discussion

PCs are involved in various stages of angiogenesis including EC migration, proliferation, and subsequent endothelial tubulogenesis and vessel stabilization [26]. This implies that the interaction of ECs–PCs may influence the parenchymal–stromal cell cross-talk and may provide insights into specific treatment therapy [27]. In this study, we investigated two distinct subpopulations of PCs, isolated from human MFAT which represent a very rich tissue source for stromal cells [28,29], and, based on CD146 segregation, we analyzed their angiogenic activity along with their interaction with human vascular endothelial cells.

Owing to the heterogeneity of pericytes, a number of molecular markers have been used to identify this cell population. Crisan et al. validated that $CD146^+$ $NG2^+$ $PDGFR\beta^+$ ALP^+ $CD34^-$ $CD45^-$ vWF^- $CD144^-$ phenotype is an indicator of pericytes or perivascular cells throughout human fetal and adult organs mostly associated with capillaries and micro-vessels. Particularly, the presence of NG2 and CD146 mark myogenic progenitors at the periphery of larger veins and arteries or blood vessels [2]. We here identified MFAT-derived pericytes by the expression of $CD146^+$, $NG2^+$, $PDGFR\beta^+$, $CD105^+$, $CD73^+$, $CD90^+$, $CD44^+$, $CD34$, and mostly αSMA^-. Alongside, we found another phenotypically similar population which is devoid of CD146. Comparing the two PC populations, we found that CD146-positive ($CD146^+$) PCs were more adherent to the ECs monolayer than CD146-negative ($CD146^-$) PCs and also expressed higher levels of molecules such as ICAM1 and CD105. This leads to the speculation that the distinction between the two populations of PCs from human AT may aid in elucidating the critical molecules involved in the adhesion or eventually vascularization process of ECs. Thus, supporting the idea that clarifying the mechanisms by which PCs may adhere to endothelial cells' surfaces may better define their role in vascular remodeling and formation. However, the expression of MSC markers among the two subpopulations may vary in culture depending on the passage number, culture conditions, and differentiation potential.

PCs release VEGF that binds VEGFR2 on ECs, thereby recruiting them to mediate angiogenesis whereas Ang-1 and PDGF-BB regulate PC coverage of ECs differently in normal and pathological conditions [13,30]. Additionally, placental PCs are known to secrete significant quantities of HGF (hepatocyte growth factor) that can be a potent paracrine angiogenic stimulus for EC sprouting where PCs were recruited to the sprouts by PDGF-BB [14,31,32]. Interestingly, we here observed that CD146$^+$ PCs respond very consistently and rigorously to PDGF-BB-stimulated migration in a concerted way, whereas they do not respond at the same pace to migration in the presence of multiple growth factors containing complete media. On the contrary, CD146$^-$ PCs responded highly to different growth factors containing complete media but not enough to PDGF-BB stimulation. This observation corresponds to a low expression of PDGFβ-receptors on the surface of CD146-negative cells and possibly the variable expression of other growth factor receptors similar to microvascular cells. Furthermore, FGF-2 synchronizes with the PDGF-BB–PDGFRβ signaling pathway by modulating their expression and activation [24]. This was postulated in our results as MFAT-derived pericytes, in particular, respond positively to both FGF-2- and PDGF-BB-mediated migration but not the stimuli meant for ECs. Since CD146-expressing cells are known to lose their expression on expansion in vitro [21], we observed the same effect in our studies at higher passage (data not shown) while the differential migratory activity between both the subpopulations remained intact.

PCs have been long known to regulate angiogenesis either by direct contact or paracrine effect. In a previous study, the Diptheria toxin-mediated ablation of PCs led to morphological changes in endothelial sprouts at the leading edge of the vascular plexus with thicker and blunt-ended sprouts compared to slender morphology of sprouts in the presence of PCs [12]. Our study reports the difference between both populations of pericyte-driven angiogenesis where the mix of EC-CD146$^-$ PCs is not able to carry out integrated sprouting of ECs, mimicking the pericyte ablation condition. Opposite to the former, EC-CD146$^+$ PCs direct a sustained and robust sprouting pattern, thereby making CD146 an indispensable marker for pericyte-driven vessel stabilization. Of note, the destabilizing effect of low pericyte coverage can lead to inappropriate extensive angiogenesis [33] which may be the case for CD146$^-$ PCs.

In another finding, human muscle PCs were shown to inhibit cord formation by dermal microvascular cells through CXCR3-induced ECs involution [10]. On the other hand, CD146$^+$ PCs have been reported to induce remodeling of vessels under circumstances such as tumor growth and invasion of hypoxia-induced angiogenesis [13,34,35]. Comparably, we identified MFAT-derived PCs to aggravate sprout formation by macrovascular endothelial cells. MFAT- and MSCs-secretome has already been identified to release factors such as β-FGF, HGF, IL-8, IL-16, and VEGF, SCGF-β, IL-6, and MCP-1, respectively [19]. Similarly, CM derived from CD146$^+$ PCs facilitated higher tube formation as well as sprouting by endothelial cells than CD146$^-$ PCs-CM, emphasizing that CD146$^+$ PCs provide paracrine survival support for ECs.

Finally, NCAM (CD56) expression modulation has been implicated in the progression of different human cancers. TGF-β1 was shown to reduce the interaction between stromal cells and liver ECs through its capacity to down-modulate NCAM expression, thereby attesting to the important role of NCAM in pericyte–EC interaction and thus in vascular stability [25]. Since CD146$^+$ PCs were observed to upregulate NCAM expression but not CD146$^-$ cells, this information provides us with a rationale to support the importance of the stromal cells–EC interaction in mediating angiogenesis. To our knowledge, this is the first report which highlights the fat PCs as composed of CD146$^-$/CD56$^-$ and CD146$^+$/CD56$^+$ subpopulations in displaying a differential angiogenic activity. NCAM expression was evident in both resting and adhered states of CD146$^+$ PCs, confirming the postulation that NCAM expression has a role in the interaction and/or adhesion of PCs with endothelial cells [36]. Since CD146 seems important for PDGFRβ-induced PCs recruitment [37], whether the expression of NCAM also has a potential role in driving PCs to upregulate the expression of PDGFRβ remains to be elucidated. Understanding the mechanism by which the pericyte population interacts with the endothelial cells to induce vascular stability represents a fundamental stem for the development of both pro- and anti-angiogenic therapies [24,38]. This study highlights the importance of the PCs subpopulation expressing CD146$^+$/NCAM markers to represent a step forward in this direction.

4. Materials and Methods

4.1. Lipoaspiration

Samples of human MFAT were obtained by liposuction of subcutaneous tissue as previously described elsewhere by using disposable cannulas provided with the Lipogems® kit [39,40]. Tissue samples were collected from plastic surgery operations after signed informed consent by the patient, in accordance with the Declaration of Helsinki. Written informed consent, specifying that residual material destined to be disposed of could be used for research, was signed by each participant before the biological materials were removed, in agreement with Rec (2006)4 of the Committee of Ministers Council of Europe on research on biological materials of human origin. The approval for their use was obtained from the Institutional Ethical Committee of Milan University (n.59/15, C.E. UNIMI, 09.1115).

For all the in vitro experiments performed in this study, the fat tissue was obtained from five different human donors (4 females and 1 male, age median 54 ± 7) that underwent plastic surgery. The fat tissue was harvested from the abdominal site. Each experiment was performed with the material obtained from a single donor and similar results were acquired with the material from other donors. The cell confluence rate was variable for different donors.

4.2. Cells and Media

PCs were maintained in EGM-2 MV media (Lonza, Basel, Switzerland) containing 10% FBS and growth factors (EGM-MV2 Bullet Kit, Lonza). PCs were passaged every 2 days. Cells were cultured until 70–80% confluence for all the experiments until passages 3-4. HUVECs were maintained in complete EGM MV media (Promo cell, Heidelberg, Germany) containing growth factors with 10% FBS. HUVECs were cultured until 70-80% confluence for all the experiments until passage 6. Wherever mentioned, ECs and PCs were starved in EBM (Promo cell) or EBM-2 (Lonza) basal medium containing 0.5% FBS.

4.3. Isolation and Cell Cultures of Pericytes from Fat Tissue

To discriminate the AT-derived MSCs (CD31$^-$) from ECs (CD31$^+$), 3–5 mL of fat samples (fresh MFAT specimens) were used. The MFAT was collected in 15 mL conical tubes and washed twice with RPMI-1640 media (Sigma, St. Louis, MO, USA) containing 0.2% BSA. The fat specimens were digested with collagenase (0.25% w/v, Sigma) to evaluate the total cells and MSC content. After collagenase digestion for 1 h at 37 °C, DMEM/F-12 medium (Gibco, Life Technologies, Monza, Italy) + 10% FBS was added to the tube to stop the enzymatic reaction followed by centrifugation for 5 min, 1200 rpm. The obtained cell pellets were processed for selection with CD31-magnetic microbeads (BD biosciences, Italy) as previously described [19] followed by culturing of cells in EGM-2 + 10% FBS for 5 days or until confluence. Once the cells reached confluence, they were further processed for selection with CD146-magnetic beads (Miltenyi Biotec, Germany) to distinguish CD146$^+$ from the CD146$^-$ population. Both CD146$^+$ and CD146$^-$ populations were maintained in culture and passaged every 2–3 days.

4.4. Immunophenotyping by Flow Cytometry

Phenotypical characterization of donor PCs was performed by multicolor flow cytometry. PCs were harvested after CD31-based selection followed by CD146 selection (as mentioned above), washed with EGM-2 complete medium followed by PBS, and incubated with PE- or FITC- or APC-conjugated antibodies for 1 h at 4 °C according to the manufacturer's recommendation and then analyzed. CD31$^-$ PCs were characterized with the following antibodies: anti-CD34-FITC, anti-CD44-APC, anti-CD73-APC, anti-CD90-FITC, anti-CD146-FITC (all from BD Pharmingen Franklin Lakes, NJ, USA); anti-CD105-PE (Immuno tools, Friesoythe, Germany); anti-ICAM1-PE and anti-VECAD-FITC (both from Biolegend, San Diego, CA, USA).

For CD146-selected PCs, CD34-FITC/CD105-PE/CD73-APC and CD146-FITC/ICAM1-PE/CD44-APC were detected as triple stains, while CD90-FITC was detected as a single stain. Isotype-matched nonreactive fluorochrome-conjugated antibodies were used as controls and quantitative analysis was performed using a Navios EX flow cytometer (Beckman Coulter, Brea, CA, USA) with software Navios (Beckman Coulter, Brea, CA, USA). In this study, at least 10,000 events were analyzed for each sample excluding non-viable cells based on forward scatter and side scatter parameters. The data are expressed as the ratio of mean fluorescence intensity (MFI) of each specific antibody and the relative isotype control. Values greater than 1 indicate the expression of the specific marker.

4.5. Immunohistochemical Staining for Pericyte Markers

In total, 50,000 cells were plated on 8-well chamber slides (Labtek, Thermofisher Scientific, Waltham, MA, USA) and fixed with 4% paraformaldehyde. Immunohistochemical analysis was performed as mentioned previously [24]. The antibodies used for this assay were anti-CD105 (1:50, Histo-line Laboratories, Italy), anti-NG2 (1:50, Santa Cruz Biotechnology, Dallas, TX, USA), anti-CD44 (1:50, Agilent Technologies, Santa Clara, CA, USA), anti-PDGFRβ (1:200, Santa Cruz Biotechnology), and anti-αSMA (1:1000, Biocare Medical, Italy). Digital photographs were obtained using the Olympus DP73 digital camera (Olympus Corporation, Milan, Italy).

4.6. Spheroids Assay

Spheroids were generated by mixing 0.2×10^5 PCs and 1×10^5 HUVECs in a 1:5 ratio in 10 mL of complete EGM with methylcellulose (Sigma) and incubated at 37 °C in 96-well (100 µL/well) non-adherent plates (Greiner Bio-one, Kremsmünster, Austria). The collagen solution was formed with Rat tail collagen I (Corning, NY, USA), 1X PBS, 1X NaOH, and final pH 7.4 after neutralization with 0.1 N NaOH. The next day, spheroids were collected, centrifuged at $2000 \times g$ for 10 s, resuspended in neutralized collagen solution, and plated on neutralized collagen-coated chamber slides. After 1 h of incubation, the cells were treated with complete EGM-2 medium or CM from PCs for overnight incubation at 37 °C. Wherever mentioned, CD31$^+$ cells from fat tissue were used to generate spheroids. Sprouting was observed from the spheroid core, and the sprout length (mean ± SD) was measured using the Image-J software for at least five spheroids with similar sizes and sprout numbers from three wells/conditions.

4.7. Adhesion Assay

All cells were washed with RPMI media containing 0.2% BSA. In total, 6000 PCs were counted using a hemocytometer (Sigma), added in the same number for each condition to the HUVECs monolayer (30,000 cells) seeded in a 96-well plate, and incubated for 30 min at 37 °C, 5% CO_2 in a humidified incubator. Afterward, cells were fixed and stained with a Diff-Quik staining kit (Medion Diagnostics, Düdingen, Switzerland) and the number of round-shaped PCs adhered to the elliptical-shaped HUVECs layer was analyzed and counted manually based on the phenotypic distinction in 3 different frames/well for at least 3 wells per condition. For the cytostaining, the HUVECs monolayer was seeded in 8-well chamber slides (Labtek, Thermofisher Scientific) for performing the adhesion assay.

4.8. Collagen Migration Assay

A total of 25,000 PCs were detached from the flasks and resuspended in a mixture of collagen I, 1X DMEM/F-12 medium, and 1X sodium bicarbonate solution. Gel drops were then created in a 4-well plate (Nunc., Thermofisher Scientific) and incubated at 37 °C for 1 h. After incubation, cell-loaded collagen drops were bathed in a medium containing FGF-2 (50 ng/mL) (Santa Cruz Biotechnology) or VEGF-A (50 ng/mL) (Miltenyi Biotec). Collagen drops bathed in EBM-2 media with 0.5% serum or EGM-2 media with 10% FBS were used as a negative and positive control, respectively. PCs migration outside collagen drops was quantified as the distance covered at least after 72 h obtained with a DM-IRB microscope system (Leica, Wetzlar, Germany) and photographed with a Hitachi KP-D50 camera. The distance was measured manually as a parameter of length from the edge of the collagen drops to the leading edge of the cells.

4.9. Transwell Assay

Corning Costar Transwell supports were used to test spontaneous and PDGF-BB-stimulated pericytes migration. The 6.5 mm Transwell with 5 µm pore size polycarbonate membrane inserts was coated with Coll-1 as previously described [41]. For each test, 1×10^5 CD146$^+$ and CD146$^-$ PCs in 200 mL of EBM + 0.2% BSA were routinely placed on the top of the membrane insert (the upper compartment of the well). To evaluate spontaneous migration, 500 mL of control EBM medium was added to the lower compartment of the wells. To evaluate PDGF-BB-induced CD146$^+$ and CD146$^-$ PCs migration, 10 ng/mL of PDGF-BB (ReliaTech, Wolfenbüttel, Germany) was added to the lower compartment of each well. A substance placed in the lower compartment of the well acts as a chemoattractant, and the cells move from the surface through the membrane against a concentration gradient. The migration assay was carried out for 8 h at 37 °C in 5% CO_2. Then, the membrane inserts were removed, fixed in 10% formalin, and stained with Wright's solution. Cells attached to the upper surface of the filter were removed with a swab, and the cells that migrated across the membrane were counted by microscopically examining the lower surface. Reported data represent the means ± standard deviation (SD) of the number of cells found in each field. At least 5 different fields for each membrane were counted at 10× magnification.

4.10. Cell Proliferation Assay

The specimens of fat tissue (MFAT), freshly obtained from patients, were washed in PBS at 1200 rpm for 5 min. Then, 3 mL of washed tissue was seeded in almost 6 mL of serum-free RPMI-1640 medium in a T25 flask and incubated for 3–4 days at 37 °C in a humidified incubator. At the end of incubation, the CM was collected and an equal volume of fresh serum-free RPMI-1640 medium was added. Separately, 25,000 HUVECs were seeded for overnight incubation in a 24-well plate. The next day, cells were washed with RPMI + 0.2% BSA and treated with the CM in a serum-free RPMI medium. Cells treated with endothelial basal medium (EBM) + 0.5% FBS and diluted two-fold with serum-free RPMI medium were used as a negative control. Cells treated with complete medium (EGM + 10% FBS) were used as a positive control. Following overnight incubation, cells were photographed, trypsinized, and counted using trypan blue exclusion. Images were recorded using an inverted Hitachi KP-D50 camera (Hitachi Ltd., Tokyo, Japan) at 4× magnification.

4.11. Tube Formation Assay

The CM from cultured pericytes in EGM-2 complete medium was collected post 3 days of incubation at 37 °C, clarified at 1200 rpm, 5min, and stored at −20 °C. A tube formation assay was used to test the effect of CM from pericytes on vascular morphogenesis of ECs. Briefly, around 50 µL of GFR matrigel (Sigma) was placed into cold wells of a 96-multiwell plate (Corning, NY, USA) at 37 °C for 30 min until jellification. HUVECs were then seeded on Matrigel at a concentration of 10^4 cells/well in 50 µL of EGM basal medium diluted two times with CM from the corresponding PCs subpopulation. ECs treated with EGM complete medium were used as a control. The number of cords was analyzed, photographed, and counted after 24 h as a parameter of tube formation with an inverted microscope at 10× magnification.

4.12. Immunofluorescence Staining for CD56 (NCAM)

Cultures of PCs were seeded on 8-well chamber slides at a confluence of 70% and maintained overnight in culture. For immunofluorescence analysis, cells were fixed with 4% paraformaldehyde in PBS, pH 7.0, permeabilized with 0.5% Triton-X100 in PBS, at RT, and blocked with PBS-BSA5%-NGS2%. Then, cells were stained with a mouse monoclonal antibody anti-CD56 (NCAM/ERIC 1:250; Santa Cruz Biotechnology), and a rabbit polyclonal antibody against PDGFRβ (1:100; Invitrogen), followed by Alexa Fluor-555 donkey anti-mouse and Alexa Fluor-488 goat anti-rabbit secondary antibodies (Thermofisher Scientific). Nuclei were stained with 4′,6-diamidino-2-phenylindole (DAPI) (Thermofisher Scientific). Maximum projection images were acquired via confocal microscopy (C1/TE2000-E microscope; Nikon) using 40× or 100× objectives for evaluation of NCAM and PDGFRβ staining on at least 5 adjacent image fields. Parameters for image acquisition were defined and not modified to allow the comparison of fluorescence intensity as a measure of relative quantification. Image analysis was performed with Image J and FIJI software [42] (NIH, USA).

4.13. Statistical Analysis

Results are expressed as mean ± standard deviation (s.d.). Statistical significance was evaluated by one-way analysis of variance following the Bonferroni post-test and Student's t-test. Statistical significance of differences was set at p-value < 0.05. Statistical tests were performed using Prism8 software (GraphPad, San Diego, CA, USA).

5. Conclusions

MSCs produce and recruit different growth factors to promote tissue regeneration and improve the microenvironment while their ablation or insufficient coverage can lead to abnormal vasculature and leaky cancers. The two immunophenotypically different subpopulations of MSCs were derived from fat tissue also known as pericytes (CD31−CD146+) and supra-adventitial adipose stromal cells (SA-ASC; CD31−CD146−) [29], respectively. Both the populations may tend to develop similar immunophenotypes under similar culture conditions [2,43]. We found that the one expressing the CD146 marker was able to interact better with ECs via higher expression of the NCAM/CD56 adhesion molecule when compared with their CD146 negative counterpart. Consequently, we propose that CD146-expressing pericytes that promote the interaction with endothelial cells can therefore be utilized as a therapeutic target for both repairing unstable vessels as well as newly formed damaged vessels.

Supplementary Materials: The following supporting information can be downloaded at: https://www.mdpi.com/article/10.3390/ijms23105806/s1.

Author Contributions: Conceptualization, E.M., A.C. (Arnaldo Caruso) and G.A.; methodology, E.M., A.C. (Alessandra Consonni), F.B., E.C., C.T., V.C. and F.P.; formal analysis, E.M., A.C. (Alessandra Consonni), E.C. and G.A.; investigation, E.M., A.C. (Alessandra Consonni), F.B., E.C., V.C. and F.P.; resources, C.T., A.C. (Arnaldo Caruso) and G.A.; data curation, E.M., A.C. (Alessandra Consonni) and E.C.; writing—original draft preparation, E.M.; writing—review and editing, G.A.; visualization, E.M. and A.C. (Alessandra Consonni); supervision, F.B., A.C. (Arnaldo Caruso) and G.A.; project administration, A.C. (Arnaldo Caruso) and G.A. All authors have read and agreed to the published version of the manuscript.

Funding: This research received no external funding.

Institutional Review Board Statement: Tissue samples were collected from plastic surgery operations after signed informed consent by the patient, in accordance with the Declaration of Helsinki. All procedures in this study were conducted in accordance with the Rec (2006)4 of the Committee of Ministers Council of Europe on research on biological materials of human origin. The approval for their use was obtained from the Institutional Ethical Committee of Milan University (n.59/15, C.E. UNIMI, 09.1115).

Informed Consent Statement: Informed consent was obtained from all subjects involved in the study.

Data Availability Statement: The data presented in this study are available in this paper and supplementary file.

Acknowledgments: The authors are thankful to Moris Cadei (Pathological Anatomy, University of Brescia) and Tiziana Gulotta (Pathological Anatomy Unit, Ospedali Civili di Brescia) for their technical assistance.

Conflicts of Interest: The authors declare no conflict of interest.

References

1. Caplan, A.I. Mesenchymal stem cells: Time to change the name! *Stem Cells Transl. Med.* **2017**, *6*, 1445–1451. [CrossRef] [PubMed]
2. Crisan, M.; Yap, S.; Casteilla, L.; Chen, C.W.; Corselli, M.; Park, T.S.; Andriolo, G.; Sun, B.; Zheng, B.; Zhang, L.; et al. A Perivascular Origin for Mesenchymal Stem Cells in Multiple Human Organs. *Cell Stem Cell* **2008**, *3*, 301–313. [CrossRef] [PubMed]
3. Meng, F.; Xu, R.; Wang, S.; Xu, Z.; Zhang, C.; Li, Y.; Yang, T.; Shi, L.; Fu, J.; Jiang, T.; et al. Human umbilical cord-derived mesenchymal stem cell therapy in patients with COVID-19: A phase 1 clinical trial. *Signal Transduct. Target Ther.* **2020**, *5*, 172. [CrossRef] [PubMed]
4. Gao, F.; Chiu, S.M.; Motan, D.A.L.; Zhang, Z.; Chen, L.; Ji, H.L.; Tse, H.F.; Fu, Q.L.; Lian, Q. Mesenchymal stem cells and immunomodulation: Current status and future prospects. *Cell Death Dis.* **2016**, *7*, e2062. [CrossRef] [PubMed]
5. Thompson, M.; Mei, S.H.J.; Wolfe, D.; Champagne, J.; Fergusson, D.; Stewart, D.J.; Sullivan, K.J.; Doxtator, E.; Lalu, M.; English, S.W.; et al. Cell therapy with intravascular administration of mesenchymal stromal cells continues to appear safe: An updated systematic review and meta-analysis. *EClinicalMedicine* **2020**, *19*, 100249. [CrossRef] [PubMed]
6. Atluri, S.; Manchikanti, L.; Hirsch, J.A. Expanded umbilical cord mesenchymal stem cells (UC-MSCs) as a therapeutic strategy in managing critically ILL COVID-19 patients: The case for compassionate use. *Pain Physician* **2020**, *23*, E71–E83.
7. Dominici, M.; Le Blanc, K.; Mueller, I.; Slaper-Cortenbach, I.; Marini, F.C.; Krause, D.S.; Deans, R.J.; Keating, A.; Prockop, D.J.; Horwitz, E.M. Minimal Criteria for Defining Multipotent Mesenchymal Stromal Cells. The International Society for Cellular Therapy Position Statement. *Cytotherapy* **2006**, *8*, 315–317. [CrossRef]
8. Galderisi, U.; Giordano, A. The Gap between the Physiological and Therapeutic Roles of Mesenchymal Stem Cells. *Med. Res. Rev.* **2014**, *34*, 1100–1126. [CrossRef]
9. Aguilera, K.Y.; Brekken, R.A. Recruitment and retention: Factors that affect pericyte migration. *Cell Mol. Life Sci.* **2014**, *71*, 299–309. [CrossRef]
10. Bodnar, R.J.; Rodgers, M.E.; Chen, W.C.W.; Wells, A. Pericyte regulation of vascular remodeling through the CXC receptor 3, 2013. *Arter. Thromb Vasc. Biol.* **2013**, *33*, 2818–2829. [CrossRef]
11. Teichert, M.; Milde, L.; Holm, A.; Stanicek, L.; Gengenbacher, N.; Savant, S.; Ruckdeschel, T.; Hasanov, Z.; Srivastava, K.; Hu, J.; et al. Pericyte-expressed Tie2 controls angiogenesis and vessel maturation. *Nat. Commun.* **2017**, *8*, 16106. [CrossRef] [PubMed]
12. Eilken, H.M.; Diéguez-Hurtado, R.; Schmidt, I.; Nakayama, M.; Jeong, H.W.; Arf, H.; Adams, S.; Ferrara, N.; Adams, R.H. Pericytes regulate VEGF-induced endothelial sprouting through VEGFR1. *Nat. Commun.* **2017**, *8*, 1574. [CrossRef] [PubMed]
13. Barlow, K.D.; Sanders, A.M.; Soker, S.; Ergun, S.; Metheny-Barlow, L.J. Pericytes on the tumor vasculature: Jekyll or Hyde? *Cancer Microenviron.* **2013**, *6*, 1–17. [CrossRef] [PubMed]
14. Chang, W.G.; Andrejecsk, J.W.; Kluger, M.S.; Saltzman, W.M.; Pober, J.S. Pericytes modulate endothelial sprouting. *Cardiovasc. Res.* **2013**, *100*, 492–500. [CrossRef]
15. Morikawa, S.; Baluk, P.; Kaidoh, T.; Haskell, A.; Jain, R.K.; McDonald, D.M. Abnormalities in pericytes on blood vessels and endothelial sprouts in tumors. *Am. J. Pathol.* **2002**, *10*, 885–1000. [CrossRef]
16. Sweeney, M.D.; Ayyadurai, S.; Zlokovic, B.V. Pericytes of the neurovascular unit: Key functions and signaling pathways. *Nat. Neurosci.* **2016**, *19*, 771–783. [CrossRef]
17. Wu, C.C.; Liu, F.L.; Sytwu, H.K.; Tsai, C.Y.; Chang, D.M. CD146+ mesenchymal stem cells display greater therapeutic potential than CD146- cells for treating collagen-induced arthritis in mice. *Stem Cell Res. Ther.* **2016**, *7*, 23. [CrossRef]

18. Espagnolle, N.; Guilloton, F.; Deschaseaux, F.; Gadelorge, M.; Sensébé, L.; Bourin, P. CD146 expression on mesenchymal stem cells is associated with their vascular smooth muscle commitment. *J. Cell Mol. Med.* **2014**, *18*, 104–114. [CrossRef]
19. Nava, S.; Sordi, V.; Pascucci, L.; Tremolada, C.; Ciusani, E.; Zeira, O.; Cadei, M.; Soldati, G.; Pessina, A.; Parati, E.; et al. Long-Lasting Anti-Inflammatory Activity of Human Microfragmented Adipose Tissue. *Stem Cells Int.* **2019**, *2019*, 5901479. [CrossRef]
20. Ceserani, V.; Ferri, A.; Berenzi, A.; Benetti, A.; Ciusani, E.; Pascucci, L.; Bazzucchi, C.; Coccè, V.; Bonomi, A.; Pessina, A.; et al. Angiogenic and anti-inflammatory properties of micro-fragmented fat tissue and its derived mesenchymal stromal cells. *Vasc. Cell* **2016**, *8*, 3. [CrossRef]
21. Leroyer, A.S.; Blin, M.G.; Bachelier, R.; Bardin, N.; Blot-Chabaud, M.; Dignat-George, F. CD146 (Cluster of Differentiation 146). *Arter. Thromb Vasc. Biol.* **2019**, *39*, 1026–1033. [CrossRef] [PubMed]
22. Hirschi, K.K.; Rohovsky, S.A.; D'Amore, P.A. PDGF, TGF-beta, and heterotypic cell-cell interactions mediate endothelial cell-induced recruitment of 10T1/2 cells and their differentiation to a smooth muscle fate. *J. Cell Biol.* **1998**, *141*, 805–814, Erratum in *J. Cell Biol.* **1998**, *141*, 1287. [CrossRef] [PubMed]
23. Benedito, R.; Rocha, S.F.; Woeste, M.; Zamykal, M.; Radtke, F.; Casanovas, O.; Duarte, A.; Pytowski, B.; Adams, R.H. Notch-dependent VEGFR3 upregulation allows angiogenesis without VEGF-VEGFR2 signalling. *Nature* **2012**, *484*, 110–114. [CrossRef] [PubMed]
24. Hosaka, K.; Yang, Y.; Nakamura, M.; Andersson, P.; Yang, X.; Zhang, Y.; Seki, T.; Scherzer, M.; Dubey, O.; Wang, X.; et al. Dual roles of endothelial FGF-2-FGFR1-PDGF-BB and perivascular FGF-2-FGFR2-PDGFRβ signaling pathways in tumor vascular remodeling. *Cell Discov.* **2018**, *4*, 3. [CrossRef] [PubMed]
25. Balzarini, P.; Benetti, A.; Invernici, G.; Cristini, S.; Zicari, S.; Caruso, A.; Gatta, L.B.; Berenzi, A.; Imberti, L.; Zanotti, C.; et al. Transforming growth factor-beta1 induces microvascular abnormalities through a down-modulation of neural cell adhesion molecule in human hepatocellular carcinoma. *Lab. Investig.* **2012**, *92*, 1297–1309. [CrossRef] [PubMed]
26. Raza, A.; Franklin, M.J.; Dudek, A.Z. Pericytes and vessel maturation during tumor angiogenesis and metastasis. *Am. J. Hematol.* **2010**, *85*, 593–598. [CrossRef] [PubMed]
27. Carmeliet, P.; Jain, R.K. Molecular mechanisms and clinical applications of angiogenesis. *Nature* **2011**, *473*, 298–307. [CrossRef]
28. Tremolada, C. Mesenchymal Stromal Cells and Micro Fragmented Adipose Tissue: New Horizons of Effectiveness of Lipogems. *J. Stem Cells Res. Dev. Ther.* **2019**, *5*, 017. [CrossRef]
29. Zimmerlin, L.; Donnenberg, V.S.; Rubin, J.P.; Donnenberg, A.D. Mesenchymal markers on human adipose stem/progenitor cells. *Cytom. A.* **2013**, *83*, 134–140. [CrossRef]
30. Lindblom, P.; Gerhardt, H.; Liebner, S.; Abramsson, A.; Enge, M.; Hellström, M.; Bäckström, G.; Fredriksson, S.; Landegren, U.; Nyström, H.C.; et al. Endothelial PDGF-B retention is required for proper investment of pericytes in the microvessel wall. *Genes Dev.* **2003**, *17*, 1835–1840. [CrossRef]
31. Bussolino, F.; Di Renzo, M.F.; Ziche, M.; Bocchietto, E.; Olivero, M.; Naldini, L.; Gaudino, G.; Tamagnone, L.; Coffer, A.; Comoglio, P.M. Hepatocyte growth factor is a potent angiogenic factor which stimulates endothelial cell motility and growth. *J. Cell Biol.* **1992**, *119*, 629–641. [CrossRef] [PubMed]
32. Stratman, A.N.; Schwindt, A.E.; Malotte, K.M.; Davis, G.E. Endothelial-derived PDGF-BB and HB-EGF coordinately regulate pericyte recruitment during vasculogenic tube assembly and stabilization. *Blood* **2010**, *116*, 4720–4730. [CrossRef] [PubMed]
33. Kang, T.Y.; Bocci, F.; Jolly, M.K.; Levine, H.; Onuchic, J.N.; Levchenko, A. Pericytes enable effective angiogenesis in the presence of proinflammatory signals. *Proc. Natl. Acad. Sci. USA* **2019**, *116*, 23551–23561. [CrossRef] [PubMed]
34. Esteves, C.L.; Sheldrake, T.A.; Mesquita, S.P.; Pesántez, J.J.; Menghini, T.; Dawson, L.; Péault, B.; Donadeu, F.X. Isolation and characterization of equine native MSC populations. *Stem Cell Res. Ther.* **2017**, *8*, 80. [CrossRef] [PubMed]
35. Hansen-Smith, F.M.; Hudlicka, O.; Egginton, S. In vivo angiogenesis in adult rat skeletal muscle: Early changes in capillary network architecture and ultrastructure. *Cell Tissue Res.* **1996**, *286*, 123–136. [CrossRef] [PubMed]
36. Xian, X.; Håkansson, J.; Ståhlberg, A.; Lindblom, P.; Betsholtz, C.; Gerhardt, H.; Semb, H. Pericytes limit tumor cell metastasis. *J. Clin. Investig.* **2006**, *116*, 642–651. [CrossRef]
37. Chen, J.; Luo, Y.; Huang, H.; Wu, S.; Feng, J.; Zhang, J.; Yan, X. CD146 is essential for PDGFRβ-induced pericyte recruitment. *Protein Cell* **2018**, *9*, 743–747. [CrossRef]
38. Hosaka, K.; Yang, Y.; Seki, T.; Fischer, C.; Dubey, O.; Fredlund, E.; Hartman, J.; Religa, P.; Morikawa, H.; Ishii, Y.; et al. Pericyte-fibroblast transition promotes tumor growth and metastasis. *Proc. Natl. Acad. Sci. USA* **2016**, *13*, E5618–E5627. [CrossRef]
39. Alessandri, G.; Coccè, V.; Pastorino, F.; Paroni, R.; Dei Cas, M.; Restelli, F.; Pollo, B.; Gatti, L.; Tremolada, C.; Berenzi, A.; et al. Microfragmented human fat tissue is a natural scaffold for drug delivery: Potential application in cancer chemotherapy. *J. Control. Release* **2019**, *302*, 2–18. [CrossRef]
40. Tremolada, C.; Colombo, V.; Ventura, C. Adipose Tissue and Mesenchymal Stem Cells: State of the Art and Lipogems®Technology Development. *Curr. Stem Cell Rep.* **2016**, *2*, 304–312. [CrossRef]
41. Alessandri, G.; Raju, K.S.; Gullino, P.M. Interaction of gangliosides with fibronectin in mobilization of capillary endothelium. *Invasion Metastasis* **1986**, *6*, 145–165. [PubMed]

42. Schindelin, J.; Arganda-Carreras, I.; Frise, E.; Kaynig, V.; Longair, M.; Pietzsch, T.; Preibisch, S.; Rueden, C.; Saalfeld, S.; Schmid, B.; et al. Fiji: An open-source platform for biological-image analysis. *Nat. Methods* **2012**, *9*, 676–682. [CrossRef] [PubMed]
43. Meirelles Lda, S.; Fontes, A.M.; Covas, D.T.; Caplan, A.I. Mechanisms involved in the therapeutic properties of mesenchymal stem cells. *Cytokine Growth Factor Rev.* **2009**, *20*, 5–6. [CrossRef] [PubMed]

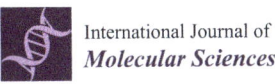

Article

Exosomal Carboxypeptidase E (CPE) and CPE-shRNA-Loaded Exosomes Regulate Metastatic Phenotype of Tumor Cells

Sangeetha Hareendran [1], Bassam Albraidy [1], Xuyu Yang [1], Aiyi Liu [2], Anne Breggia [3], Clark C. Chen [4] and Y. Peng Loh [1,*]

1. Section on Cellular Neurobiology, *Eunice Kennedy Shriver* National Institute of Child Health and Human Development, National Institutes of Health, Bethesda, MD 20892, USA; sangeetha.hareendran@nih.gov (S.H.); balbr025@uottawa.ca (B.A.); xuyu.yang@nih.gov (X.Y.)
2. Biostatistics & Bioinformatics Branch, *Eunice Kennedy Shriver National* Institute of Child Health and Human Development, National Institutes of Health, Bethesda, MD 20892, USA; liua@mail.nih.gov
3. Maine Medical Center BioBank, Portland, ME 04074, USA; bregga@mmc.org
4. Department of Neurosurgery, University of Minnesota Medical School, Minneapolis, MN 55455, USA; ccchen@umn.edu
* Correspondence: author: lohp@mail.nih.gov

Abstract: Background: Exosomes promote tumor growth and metastasis through intercellular communication, although the mechanism remains elusive. Carboxypeptidase E (CPE) supports the progression of different cancers, including hepatocellular carcinoma (HCC). Here, we investigated whether CPE is the bioactive cargo within exosomes, and whether it contributes to tumorigenesis, using HCC cell lines as a cancer model. Methods: Exosomes were isolated from supernatant media of cancer cells, or human sera. mRNA and protein expression were analyzed using PCR and Western blot. Low-metastatic HCC97L cells were incubated with exosomes derived from high-metastatic HCC97H cells. In other experiments, HCC97H cells were incubated with CPE-shRNA-loaded exosomes. Cell proliferation and invasion were assessed using MTT, colony formation, and matrigel invasion assays. Results: Exosomes released from cancer cells contain *CPE* mRNA and protein. *CPE* mRNA levels are enriched in exosomes secreted from high- versus low-metastatic cells, across various cancer types. In a pilot study, significantly higher *CPE* copy numbers were found in serum exosomes from cancer patients compared to healthy subjects. HCC97L cells, treated with exosomes derived from HCC97H cells, displayed enhanced proliferation and invasion; however, exosomes from HCC97H cells pre-treated with CPE-shRNA failed to promote proliferation. When HEK293T exosomes loaded with CPE-shRNA were incubated with HCC97H cells, the expression of CPE, Cyclin D1, a cell-cycle regulatory protein and *c-myc*, a proto-oncogene, were suppressed, resulting in the diminished proliferation of HCC97H cells. Conclusions: We identified CPE as an exosomal bioactive molecule driving the growth and invasion of low-metastatic HCC cells. CPE-shRNA loaded exosomes can inhibit malignant tumor cell proliferation via Cyclin D1 and c-MYC suppression. Thus, CPE is a key player in the exosome transmission of tumorigenesis, and the exosome-based delivery of CPE-shRNA offers a potential treatment for tumor progression. Notably, measuring CPE transcript levels in serum exosomes from cancer patients could have potential liquid biopsy applications.

Keywords: cancer proliferation; hepatocellular carcinoma; metastasis; engineered exosomes; diagnostic biomarker; cancer therapy

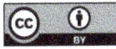

1. Introduction

Exosomes are nano-sized extracellular vesicles (30–140 nm in diameter), which facilitate critical intercellular communication by way of transferring bioactive molecules. While exosomes are secreted by most cells, it is important to note that exosomes derived from tumor cells have a distinctly different composition to those released from healthy cells [1]. Tumor-derived exosomes are known to promote the tumorigenesis, metastasis, and modulation of the tumor microenvironment [2–4]. Recent reports have shown that exosomes released from malignant hepatocellular carcinoma (HCC) cells can increase the tumorigenic and migratory functions of low-metastatic HCC cells by inducing EMT (epithelial- mesenchymal transition), via the MAPK/ERK pathway [5], or by transferring miR-92a-3p to target PTEN and activating downstream Akt/Snail pathway [6]. Primary HCC-derived exosomes support metastases by enhancing SMAD3 signaling in circulating tumor cells to promote their adhesion [7]. Circular RNAs transferred through exosomes have also been shown to influence HCC metastasis by downregulating the miR-449a–MET pathway [8]. Similar exosome-mediated transfers of invasive and metastatic properties between cancer cells have been documented in breast cancer and ovarian cancer [9,10]. Additionally, exosomes can serve as a safe delivery system for siRNA-/shRNA-related interventions [11]. The intravenous administration of targeted exosomes can successfully deliver siRNA to the mouse brain [12]. Using orthotopic pancreatic cancer mouse models, it was demonstrated that exosomes carrying *KRAS* specific siRNA can suppress tumor growth, inhibit metastasis, and improve overall survival [13]. It remains to be determined what exosomal factors induce tumor growth and metastasis in HCC and other cancers, and whether exosomes can be exploited for targeted cancer therapy.

Recently, serum-derived and urinary exosomes have attracted much attention as an analyte in liquid biopsy for diagnosis and monitoring treatment response in cancer. Various exosomal cargoes have now been identified as candidate biomarkers for cancer diagnosis [1,14]. For example, Glypican-1 is enriched in circulating exosomes in pancreatic cancer patients and correlates with tumor burden [15]; LRG1 in urinary exosomes is a potential biomarker for detecting NSCLC [16]. Besides proteins, certain exosomal miRNAs have been correlated with poor prognosis [17]. Urinary exosomal miR-2909 was associated with prostate cancer severity [18], while exosomal miR-141 was found to be up-regulated in patients with prostate cancer [19]. However, despite having many candidate biomarkers, few exosome-based diagnostic assays have been developed for clinical use. Ideally, finding a common exosomal biomarker for diagnosis across many cancer types would be very useful, but remains challenging. Thus far, studies have suggested that serum/plasma exosomal Glypican-1 could be a potential multi-cancer diagnostic biomarker for pancreatic, colorectal, and breast cancer [14].

Carboxypeptidase E (CPE) is an exopeptidase, initially discovered as a prohormone processing enzyme [20,21]. Subsequently, non-enzymatic functions of CPE as a sorting receptor for prohormones and a trophic factor in mediating cell survival have been reported [22–24]. In cancer, the aberrant upregulation of CPE is found in endocrine tumors (pituitary adenomas) [25], as well as non-endocrine tumors (cervical, colorectal, ovarian and pancreatic cancer, HCC, and glioblastoma) [26–30]. CPE promotes cell proliferation and migration in osteosarcoma, colorectal, and pancreatic cancer cell lines [28,31,32]. Besides the full length wild-type CPE (WT-CPE), a 40 kDa splice variant of CPE (CPE-ΔN) has been cloned and shown to promote tumor cell proliferation and invasion, by a distinct mechanism [33,34]. This 40 kDa CPE-ΔN variant is an N-terminal truncated form of the CPE protein, and is translocated into the nucleus to induce the expression of metastasis-associated genes [34]. Given the multi-faceted role of CPE in tumorigenesis, we investigated whether CPE could play a critical role in the exosomal transmission of tumorigenesis.

In this study, we investigated (1) if *CPE* mRNA and protein are present within exosomes secreted from cancer cells, and if exosomal CPE can confer the growth and metastasis of cancer cells; and (2) whether CPE-shRNA-loaded exosomes could be taken up by malignant cancer cells to inhibit tumor growth as a potential therapeutic strategy. We found that *CPE* mRNA is enriched in exosomes released from highly malignant cells of different cancer origins. Moreover, we carried out a pilot study using patient-derived sera exosomes and showed that *CPE* mRNA in circulating exosomes could be developed as a diagnostic cancer biomarker. We characterized the *CPE* mRNA and protein within exosomes from HCC cells, and showed that the down-regulation of CPE in the parental HCC97H (high-metastatic) cells prior to exosome isolation prevented the exosomal transfer of malignant properties from HCC97H to HCC97L (low-metastatic) cells. We also tested whether the exosomal route could be used to deliver CPE-shRNA to target HCC cells to inhibit proliferation, and determined the possible mechanism involved. Notably, the exosomes loaded with CPE-shRNA inhibited the growth of recipient HCC cells by suppressing Cyclin-D1 and c-MYC expression. These findings indicate that exosomal CPE and modified exosomes enclosing CPE-specific shRNA can modulate the malignant properties of cancer cells.

2. Results
2.1. Presence of CPE in Exosomes Derived from Cancer Cells

Particle analyses revealed that exosomes derived from HCC cells exhibiting high metastasis, were approximately 100 nm in diameter, as depicted in the representative graphs in Figure 1A. These vesicles were characterized by the presence of exosome-specific markers CD63 and TSG101, along with the presence of CPE (Figure 1B). The Western blot band of ~50 kDa corresponded to the size of WT-CPE (~50–53 kDa). To determine if CPE mRNA and its splice variant, CPE-ΔN (which encodes a 40 kDa protein), are present within exosomes derived from three different cancer cell lines, we used a specific primer set ΔF/ΔR which flanks the region of deletion in exon1 to differentiate CPE-ΔN mRNA sequence, in addition to primers flanking the rest of the CPE mRNA. The primer sequences used are given in Supplementary Table S1. The position of the deletion in CPE-ΔN and the primer sets used for PCR are shown in Figure 1C. As shown in Figure 1D, the amplified PCR region in exosomes derived from CAOV3 (ovarian cancer), HCC97H (liver cancer), and MDA-MB-231 (breast cancer) cell lines corresponds to WT-CPE gene segments, and not CPE-ΔN. Using overlapping primer sets, we could amplify close to 1 kb from the 5′ end to the middle portion of CPE mRNA, while parts of 3′ region were missing, as shown in Supplementary Figure S1. Although we were unable to amplify the full-length mRNA of CPE, the contiguous portion of the mRNA that we amplified, in fact, encodes the entire coding sequence of CPE mRNA. Our results indicate that exosomes derived from HCC, breast, and ovarian cancer cell lines contain CPE mRNA. An analysis of HCC exosomes showed the presence of WT-CPE protein.

2.2. Exosomes Isolated from Highly Malignant Cancer Cells Show Elevated CPE mRNA Levels

Elevated expression levels of CPE have been associated with malignancy in various types of cancer cell lines in in vitro and patient tumors [26–29,31,32]. We have previously shown, using Northern blot and RT-PCR, that high-metastatic HCC97H cells have more abundant CPE mRNA levels compared to low-metastatic HCC97L cells [34]. Similarly, we also found that aggressive glioblastoma cells LN-18 express higher CPE mRNA levels than less aggressive U-118 cells. Previous reports further provide evidence that high-metastatic colon, prostate and pancreatic cells are associated with increased levels of CPE mRNA compared to the corresponding low-metastatic cell [32,33]. Based on these observations and our finding that cancer cell exosomes contain CPE, we then determined if the levels of CPE mRNA within exosomes released from these parental cancer cells (Supplementary Table S2) correlate with their malignancy. CPE mRNA copy numbers in the exosomes were measured using the standard curve method. Figure 2A–E shows that significantly higher CPE mRNA copy numbers are present in exosomes released from malignant cancer cells compared to those released from cancer cell lines with low malignancy, across various types of cancer, such as HCC, glioblastoma, prostate cancer, colon cancer, and pancreatic cancer. These data indicate that exosomes secreted by malignant cancer cells have elevated levels of CPE mRNA copy numbers compared to their low-malignant counterpart.

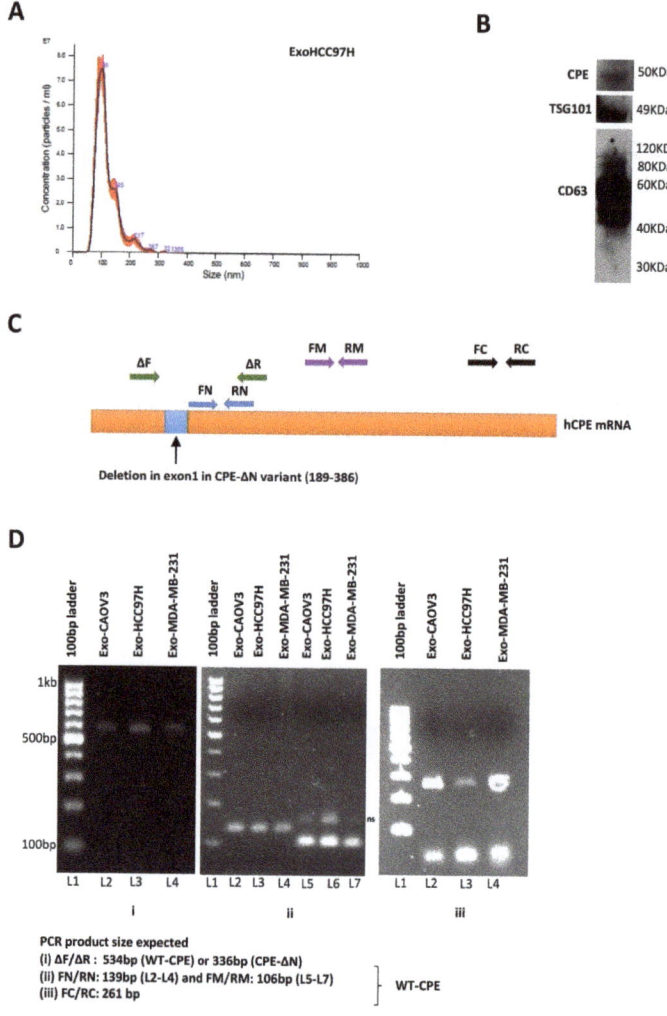

Figure 1. Detection of CPE in cancer cell exosomes. (**A**) Characterization of metastatic liver cancer cell derived exosomes: Representative graph (left panel) showing the concentration plotted against particle size of exosomes released from HCC97H cells, determined using NanoSight analysis. (**B**) Western blot showing WT-CPE and exosomal markers TSG101 and CD63 in exosomes released from HCC97H cells. (**C**) Schematic showing human *CPE* mRNA with the position of RT-PCR primers used to detect *CPE* gene fragments. The region of deletion seen in exon 1 of *CPE-ΔN* variant, another isoform of CPE detected in cancer cells is marked as a blue box and the ΔF/ΔR primer set used to distinguish *WT-CPE* and *CPE-ΔN* sequences are denoted by green arrows. (**D**) Exosomes isolated from CAOV3, HCC97H and MDA-MB-231 cells were analyzed using RT-PCR to determine the presence of *CPE* transcripts. Images of agarose gels showing the amplicons generated using the primers specific for 5′-end (**Di**), middle (**Dii**) or 3′-end parts of *CPE* mRNA (**Diii**), besides the region flanking the exon 1 deletion in *CPE-ΔN* sequence (**Di**). The expected PCR product sizes are given below the gel images. Major band sizes represented by the 100 bp DNA ladder are shown in (**Di**). 'ns' refers to non-specific band in (**Dii**).

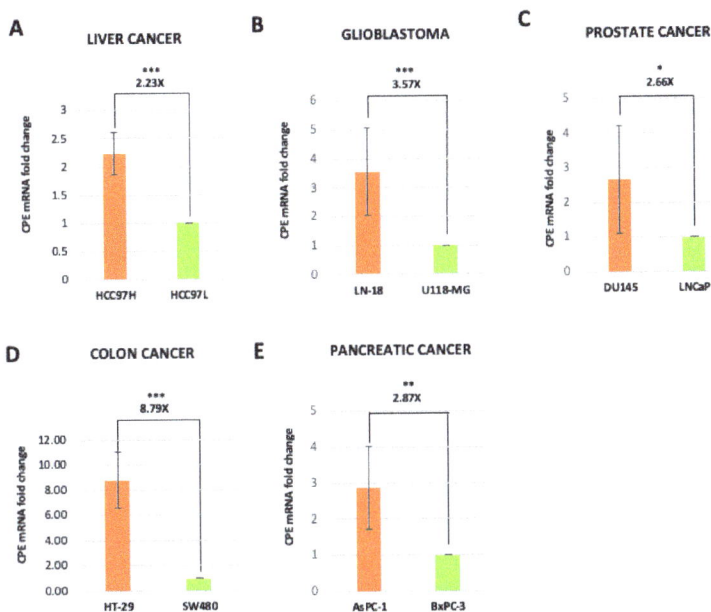

Figure 2. Malignant cancer cells release exosomes with elevated *CPE* copy numbers. (**A–E**) Bar graph showing the fold change of *CPE* mRNA copy numbers measured in exosomes derived from malignant/aggressive cells (orange bars) versus low-malignant cells (green bars) from different types of cancer as denoted in the figure (N = 3 for (**B,C,E**) and N = 2 for (**A,D**)). Standard curve method using CPE 5′-DNA fragment of known concentration was used to perform quantitation of *CPE* mRNA copy numbers. Data represents mean ± SD of 2 or 3 independent experiments. Error bars denote SD. Statistical analysis for all panels was performed by Student's *t*-test: *, $p < 0.05$; **, $p < 0.01$; ***, $p < 0.001$.

2.3. Serum Exosomes from Cancer Patients Have Higher CPE Transcript Copy Numbers than Healthy Controls

Given that elevated *CPE* mRNA level is correlated with malignancy in cancer cell lines, we then examined the *CPE* mRNA copy number in human sera exosomes derived from patients with different types of cancer and healthy controls (see Supplementary Table S3 for subject details) in a pilot study. *CPE* mRNA copy numbers in the sera exosomes were determined using the standard curve method. The *CPE* copy numbers in serum-derived exosomes are summarized using mean (standard deviation, SD) and median (interquartile range, IQR). For the cancer cases, the mean is 670.08 (SD = 1176.98) and the median is 365.30 (IQR = 490.97−241.02 = 249.95); for the normal cases, the mean is 132.91 (SD = 72.75) and the median is 115.20 (IQR = 178.06−88.76 = 89.30). The Shapiro–Wilk normality test on the *CPE* copy number data in cancer cases showed a significant departure from normality ($p < 0.001$). Therefore, the log10 transformed data, presented in Figure 3A using box plots, are used for analysis. Logistic regression performed on the log10-transformed data showed that *CPE* copy number in sera exosomes is significantly associated with cancer (beta = 5.924, $p = 0.0007$). The empirical receiver operating characteristics (ROC) curve (Figure 3B) and its relatively large area under the curve (AUC = 0.872) corroborates the logistic regression analysis.

Box plots showing the log-transformed data of CPE copy numbers in sera exosomes from 3 major cancer types (breast cancer, ovarian cancer and glioblastoma) with $n \geq 5$, compared to controls, are shown in the Supplementary Figure S2. The results from this pilot study indicate that higher *CPE* copy numbers are found in sera exosomes from cancer patients versus healthy subjects. Due to limited availability of samples, a more detailed analysis of correlation with stage/disease type has not been performed. Our current data suggest that high CPE mRNA levels in serum exosomes is indicative of cancer. This will be the basis of future research, where one can measure and compare exosomal CPE mRNA in stage-stratified patients to further explore the clinical value of its application as a biomarker.

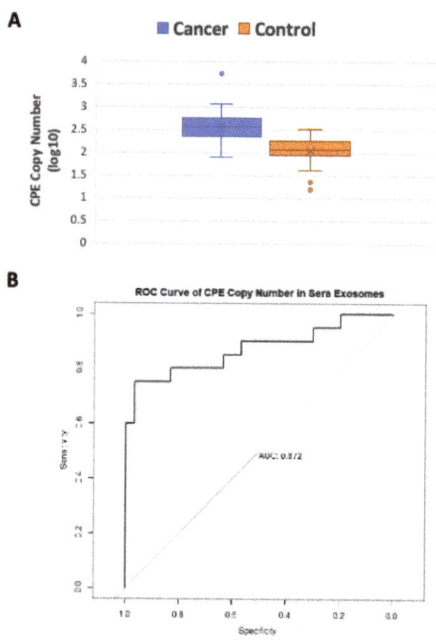

Figure 3. Serum exosomes from cancer patients are enriched in *CPE* mRNA. (**A**) Box plot showing the log-transformed data of CPE copy numbers in sera exosomes derived from 20 cancer patients versus 30 healthy subjects ($p = 0.0007$). (**B**) ROC curve of *CPE* copy numbers in exosomes from cancer patients' sera compared to control sera, showing the AUC. Types of cancer included (in cases): Breast cancer (n = 5), Ovarian cancer (n = 5), Glioblastoma (n = 5), Colon cancer (n = 1), Cervical cancer (n = 1), Kidney cancer (n = 1), Pancreatic cancer (n = 1) and Prostate cancer (n = 1). Quantitation of *CPE* mRNA copy numbers was perfomed by standard curve method using CPE 5'-DNA fragment of known concentration. Logistic regression and receiver operating characteristics (ROC) curve analysis was used to determine the association of cancers with *CPE* copy number in sera exosomes.

2.4. HCC97H Exosomes Enhance Proliferation and Invasion of HCC97L Cells in a CPE-Dependent Manner

As exosomes mediate cell–cell communication by the transfer of cargo, we investigated whether exosomal CPE taken up by recipient cells can modulate their proliferation and invasion. HCC97H and HCC97L cell lines were used as a model system to test exosomal CPE function because they exhibit high- versus low-metastatic potential respectively, and are derived from the same parental cell line [35]. We found that the incubation of HCC97L cells with HCC97H-derived exosomes increased their proliferation by ~36% ($p = 0.03$) in the MTT assay (Figure 4A) and invasion through matrigel ~2-fold ($p < 0.0001$) (Figure 4D). However, the downregulation of CPE by specific shRNA in HCC97H cells prior to exosome isolation abolished the effect of these exosomes on growth (Figure 4B, decreased by 32.64%; $p = 0.015$) and the invasion of HCC97L cells by 1.9-fold (Figure 4E). Moreover, treatment with exosomes isolated from HCC97H after the silencing of CPE expression resulted in downregulation of *CPE* mRNA levels in the recipient HCC97L cells. The gene expression was quantified using the 2−ΔΔCt method (Figure 4C). Although we used the MTT assay as a measure of cell viability, it basically indicates the metabolic activity of the cells, which could be affected by the culture conditions (e.g., media pH) and the physiological state of the cells. Nevertheless, these results indicate that exosomes isolated from HCC cells with high metastasis, when incubated with low-metastatic HCC cells, can enhance their growth and metastatic properties, and that CPE plays an important role in this process.

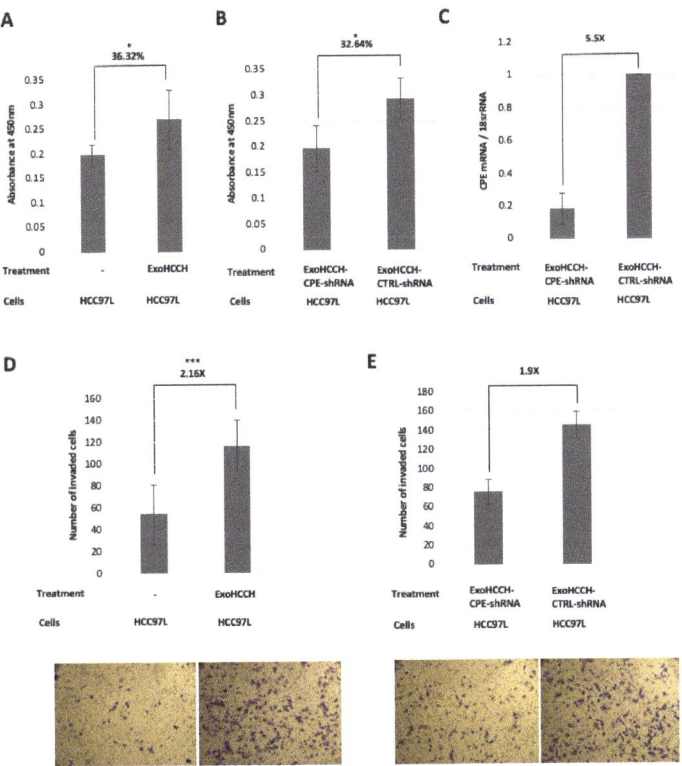

Figure 4. Exosomes from HCC97H cells enhance proliferation and invasion of recipient HCC97L cells in a CPE-dependent manner. (**A,B**) Bar graph showing the absorbance values obtained in the MTT cell proliferation assay on day 5 of HCC97L cells treated with exosomes (corresponding to 75 µg of exosomal protein) from HCC97H cells (ExoHCCH, **A**) or with exosomes isolated 48 h after lipofectamine- mediated transfection of HCC97H cells with either 25 nM of CPE targeting shRNA or control shRNA, (ExoHCCH-CPE-shRNA/ExoHCCH-CTRL-shRNA, **B**) (N = 2, n = 3). ExoHCCH increase the proliferation of HCC97L cells, however downregulation of CPE expression in HCC97H cells before exosome isolation abolishes this effect. Data represents mean ± SD of 2 independent experiments. (**C**) Bar graph showing the fold change in knockdown of *CPE* mRNA levels in HCC97L cells treated with ExoHCCH-CPE-shRNA relative to cells treated with ExoHCCH-CTRL-shRNA (N = 2). Data represents mean ± SD of 2 independent experiments. The 2−ΔΔCt method was used for gene expression analysis and 18s rRNA was the internal control. (**D,E**) Bar graph and representative images of wells showing the number of HCC97L cells that invaded through matrigel after treatment with ExoHCCH (**D**) (N = 2, n = 2), or with either ExoHCCH-CPE-shRNA or ExoHCCH-CTRL-shRNA (**E**) (N = 1, n = 2). Data represents mean ± SD of 2 independent experiments (**D**) and mean ± SD of technical replicates (**E**). HCCH97L cells treated with ExoHCCH exhibit enhanced invasion through matrigel, and this effect is abolished if HCC97H cells are transfected with CPE-shRNA before exosome isolation. Scale bar = 100µm. Statistical analysis for all panels was performed by Student's *t*-test: *, $p < 0.05$; ***, $p < 0.001$.

2.5. Exosomes Loaded with CPE-shRNA Inhibit Proliferation of Malignant HCC Cells

Previous reports have shown that the injection of exosomes carrying *KRAS* siRNA could impede tumor growth and metastasis in pancreatic cancer mouse models [13]. Here, we tested if we could load HEK293T cell-derived exosomes with CPE-shRNA using adenovirus infection and then transfer the shRNA via the exosomes to target the proliferation of recipient HCC97H cells. Indeed, we detected a fluorescence signal of the GFP protein fused to the CPE-shRNA in the recipient HCC97H cells, after incubation with the exosomes isolated from HEK293T cells (ExoHEK) infected with adenovirus encoding CPE-shRNA-GFP (schematic of exosome loading and transfer is shown in Figure 5A, and the adenovirus vector map and CPE-shRNA sequence are depicted in Figure S3). These shRNA-loaded ExoHEK were characterized by NanoSight analysis and visualized using TEM, as shown in Figures 5B and S4, and Table S4. No viral particles were observed in the exosome preparation, when visualized using TEM. Following treatment with ExoHEK-CPE-shRNA, a 4.74-fold reduction in *CPE* mRNA levels (Figure 6A) and a 70% reduction of secreted CPE protein (Figure 6B) were observed in the HCC97H cells, concomitant with a 3-fold decrease in cell proliferation at D7/8 ($p < 0.0001$) (Figure 6C, MTT assay) and a 5.3-fold reduction in the number of colonies formed ($p = 0.0001$) (Figure 6D,E). By co-treating HCC97H cells with AdCPE-shRNA and unloaded ExoHEK, we were able to ascertain that the growth inhibition effect seen on HCC97H cells was mediated by the transfer of CPE-shRNA by the HEK293 exosomes, and not due to any modification of exosomal content of CPE-suppressed HEK293 cells (data not shown). Furthermore, there was a 3-fold downregulation of expression of the cell cycle regulator, Cyclin D1, at the mRNA level ($p = 0.0089$) (Figure 6F), and a 23% reduction in Cyclin D1 protein (Figure 6G) in HCC97H cells treated with CPE-shRNA-loaded exosomes, consistent with the decrease in proliferation. Importantly, the expression of c-MYC, a transcription factor and proto-oncogene, was found to be significantly reduced by 2-fold ($p = 0.0003$) in the ExoHEK-CPE-shRNA-treated HCC97H cells (Figure 6H). The $2-\Delta\Delta Ct$ method was used for qRT-PCR-based expression analyses of CPE, Cyclin D1 and c-MYC transcripts in the HCC97H cells, with 18s rRNA as the internal control. These results show that the downregulation of CPE through exosome-mediated shRNA delivery can inhibit the proliferation of malignant liver cancer cells.

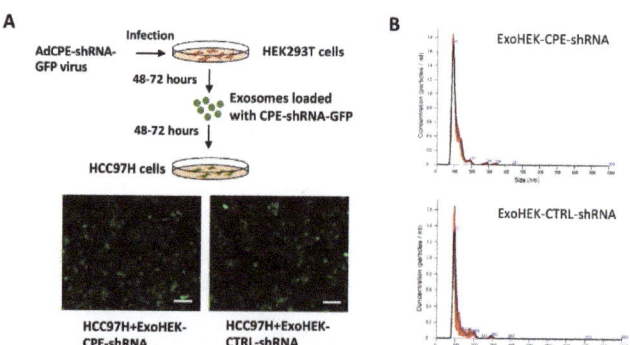

Figure 5. Characterization of exosomes loaded with CPE-shRNA. (**A**) Schematic showing the strategy of loading and transfer of CPE-shRNA via exosomes. Exosomes were isolated from supernatant media of HEK293T cells (ExoHEK) infected with adenovirus encoding either CPE-shRNA or CTRL-shRNA, fused to GFP. HCC97H cells treated with these modified exosomes exhibited green fluorescence, validating the transfer of CPE-shRNA through the exosomes. Representative images showing GFP fluorescence in target HCC97H cells, treated with either ExoHEK-CPE-shRNA or ExoHEK-CTRL-shRNA are included. Scale bar = 100 μm. (**B**) Graph showing the concentration and size distribution of ExoHEK-CPE-shRNA and ExoHEK-CTRL-shRNA, as determined by NanoSight analysis.

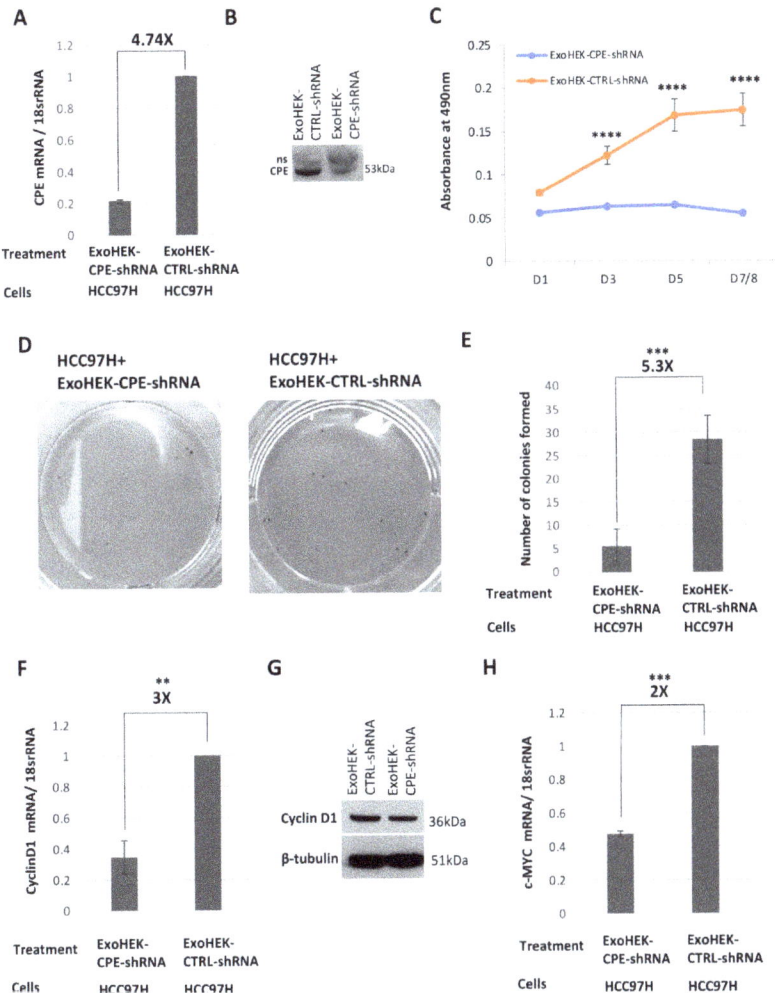

Figure 6. CPE-shRNA-loaded exosomes inhibit proliferation of malignant HCC cells. (**A**) Bar graph showing the fold change in downregulation of *CPE* mRNA levels in HCC97H cells treated for 48h with ExoHEK-CPE-shRNA in comparison to cells treated with ExoHEK-CTRL-shRNA (N = 2). The 2−ΔΔCt method was used for *CPE* mRNA expression analysis and 18s rRNA was used as the reference. Data represents mean ± SD of 2 independent experiments. (**B**) Western blot showing suppressed secreted CPE levels (70.91% ± 0.003 [SD] decrease) in the media of HCC97H cells treated with ExoHEK-CPE-shRNA relative to the media of cells treated with ExoHEK-CTRL-shRNA (N = 2). ns: non-specific. (**C**) Representative line graph showing the absorbance values obtained in the MTT cell proliferation assay from D1- D7/8 of HCC97H cells treated with HEK293T exosomes loaded with either CPE-shRNA or Control shRNA. CPE-shRNA loaded exosomes inhibit the proliferation of HCC97H cells (N = 3, n = 3). Data represents mean ± SD of the triplicate wells of the representative experiment. Statistical analysis was performed by Two-way ANOVA with Sidak's multiple comparisons test. ****, $p < 0.0001$. (**D,E**) Representative images and bar graph showing the number of colonies formed by HCC97H cells treated with ExoHEK-CPE-shRNA or ExoHEK-CTRL shRNA. Exosomes loaded with CPE-shRNA significantly decreased the colony formation ability of HCC97H cells (N = 2, n = 3). Data represents mean ± SD of 2 independent experiments. Error bars denote SD

(**F**) Bar graph showing the downregulation of *Cyclin D1* mRNA expression in HCC97H cells incubated with ExoHEK-CPE-shRNA compared to the control (N = 3). Relative qRT-PCR was performed for *Cyclin D1* mRNA quantification by 2−ΔΔCt method, and 18s rRNA was used as the reference. Data represents mean ± SD of 3 independent experiments. (**G**) Representative western blot showing reduced levels of Cyclin D1 (23.17% ± 0.022 [SD] decrease) in HCC97H cells treated with ExoHEK-CPE-shRNA compared to cells treated with ExoHEK-CTRL-shRNA (N = 2). (**H**) Bar graph showing the suppression of *c-MYC* mRNA levels in HCC97H cells after treating with ExoHEK-CPE-shRNA relative to cells treated with ExoHEK-CTRL-shRNA (N = 3). Relative qRT-PCR was performed for *c-MYC* mRNA quantification by 2−ΔΔCt method, and 18s rRNA was used as the reference. Data represents mean ± SD of 3 independent experiments. Statistical analysis for E, F and G panels was performed by Student's *t*-test: **, $p < 0.01$, ***, $p < 0.001$.

3. Discussion

Exosomes or extracellular vesicles are known to promote the growth and metastasis of liver and other cancers, through intercellular communication, but their internal cargo driving these effects remain unclear. Liquid biopsy assays utilizing tumor exosomes, present in many biological fluids, are being developed to diagnose and predict the prognosis of cancers such as melanoma, prostate cancer, glioblastoma and pancreatic cancer [19,36–38]. Serum levels of exosomal miRNAs such as miR-21, miR-141, and miR-718 have been correlated with advanced stages of squamous cell carcinoma, prostate cancer and HCC recurrence after liver transplant, respectively [19,39]. The elevated expression of CPE in tumors has been correlated with poor outcomes in patients with lung, cervical, and pancreatic cancer, and hepatocellular carcinoma [27–29,40]. Furthermore, CPE has been shown to promote the survival, growth, and invasion of tumor cells [26,28,32,41,42]. We therefore investigated whether CPE is present within cancer cell exosomes, and if so, if it plays a pivotal role in promoting tumor cell proliferation and invasion in recipient cells. Indeed, we found *CPE-WT* mRNA, but not the *CPE-ΔN* variant within the exosomes derived from liver, breast and ovarian cancer cells. Interestingly, the contiguous portion of the mRNA (~1.2 kb) that we detected encodes the entire coding region of *CPE*, with some of the noncoding 3′ end missing. Full-length *CPE* in HCC and other cancer cells is ~2.4 kb [34], but whether this 1.2 kb transcript of *CPE* mRNA could be successfully translated to yield a functional protein awaits future studies. Within the exosomes derived from HCC97H cells, we found a ~50 kDa CPE protein approximating the size reported for WT-CPE. These data reveal that both *CPE* mRNA and protein are packaged inside cancer cell exosomes.

Consistent with reports that elevated CPE expression levels in tumors correlate with the progression of the disease [26–29,31,32], we demonstrated that *CPE* mRNA copy numbers are significantly higher in exosomes isolated from malignant cancer cells compared to low-malignant cancer cell exosomes, across different cancer types. The finding of a positive correlation of *CPE* mRNA copy numbers with malignancy suggests that circulating exosomal CPE could potentially serve as a useful biomarker to detect cancer in patients. To this end, as a proof of concept, we showed that significantly high *CPE* mRNA copy numbers are present in serum-derived exosomes from patients with various types of cancer versus normal healthy controls. However, while the results are promising, this remains a pilot clinical study, as the sample size is small, and extensive studies with more patients with different cancer types are necessary to develop the use of exosomal CPE as a cancer biomarker.

Accumulating evidence suggest that transfer of exosomal cargo is linked to cellular communication within the tumor microenvironment and metastatic disease development. Exosomes from highly metastatic melanoma 'educate' bone marrow progenitors by elevating their MET receptor (hepatocyte growth factor receptor) expression, thereby facilitating primary tumor growth and metastasis [4]. Previous studies have shown that it is possible to transfer the metastatic behavior of highly malignant cancer cells to those with low malignancy through exosomes [43]. We have previously shown, by Northern blot analysis, that CPE mRNA levels in HCC97L cells are extremely low, when compared to HCC97H cells [34], and hence, we used HCC97L cells to examine if CPE could be potentially involved in the phenotypic transformation of these cells on treatment with exosomes secreted by HCC97H cells. Our study demonstrated that both the proliferation and invasion of HCC97L cells were significantly increased by incubation with HCC97H exosomes. Most importantly, we showed that this phenocopying of malignant behavior in HCC cells via exosomes was dependent on CPE. Thus, our data indicate that the exosomal cargo, CPE, plays a key role in exosome-mediated cell–cell communication to promote liver cancer proliferation and invasion. Future research will determine the mechanism of how exosomal CPE mRNA/protein derived from HCC97H cells mediates the tumor enhancing effect in HCC97L cells. As we stated in our previous publication [34], CPE is primarily secreted in HCC and other cancer cell lines. It is therefore difficult to detect and quantify CPE protein in cancer cell extract, as it is rapidly secreted after biosynthesis. This poses a challenge for quantifying any increase in CPE protein levels, in the ExoHCCH-treated HCC97L cells. In addition, we do not yet understand how the CPE mRNA/protein in exosomes is taken up by the recipient cells or the CPE protein's intracellular route and fate after uptake. Similarly, the exact mechanism of how the silencing of CPE expression in the HCC97H cells, prior to exosome isolation, blocks the pro-tumorigenic effect on the HCC97L cells is also not clear. It could be through the modulation of intrinsic cell properties of HCC97H cells, which later impact the exosomal content, and not necessarily a direct effect of CPE content in the exosomes. This speculation can also be extended to the observation that the treatment of HCC97L cells with ExoHCCH induces tumor enhancing effects by way of either the transfer of CPE mRNA/protein to the recipient HCC97L cells or by other CPE-regulated target genes/proteins present within the milieu of the HCC97H derived exosomes. The suppression of CPE in the exosome producer HCC97H cells clearly abolishes the tumor enhancing effects on low-metastatic HCC cells, strongly supporting that CPE is important for exosome-mediated malignant transformation. Interestingly, we observed that CPE mRNA levels are downregulated in the HCC97L cells when incubated with exosomes derived from CPE-shRNA treated HCC97H cells, but not when treated with control-shRNA. This result suggests that the suppression of CPE mRNA expression in the recipient cells after exosome treatment could have caused the repressive effects on proliferation and invasion.

As we found correlation of elevated *CPE* mRNA levels with high malignancy in many other cancer cells, including breast cancer, prostate cancer, pancreatic cancer, and glioblastoma, we speculate that exosomal CPE could also likely promote the proliferation and invasion of these cancer types. The mechanism by which exosome associated CPE transfers the malignant phenotype to recipient cells requires more investigation.

Exosomes have been shown to act as vehicles to safely deliver cargo such as siRNA to the brain and pancreas [12,13]. We showed that CPE-shRNA transferred via exosomes to HCC97H cells can downregulate their tumorigenic propensity, through the suppression of Cyclin-D1 and c-MYC levels. In general, the over-expression of Cyclin D1 is associated with tumor progression, chemotherapeutic resistance, and metastasis [44,45], while the upregulation of c-MYC, a transcription factor that regulates proliferation and cell-cycle progression, is strongly correlated with poor prognosis in liver cancer patients, including metastasis [46]. p53 mutations, when combined with the constitutive activation of c-MYC, can lead to DNA damage and induce liver tumorigenesis [47]. Indeed, earlier reports have suggested that Cyclin D1 acts downstream of CPE in colorectal cancer and osteosarcoma cells, to promote the proliferation of these cells [7,31,32]. c-MYC was identified as one of the genes that showed 2-fold downregulation in HCC97H cells treated with ExoHEK-CPE-shRNA versus ExoHEK-CTRL-shRNA, using a Human Tumor Metastasis $-RT^2$ Profiler PCR Array (QIAGEN, Cat# 330231 PAHS-028ZA; data not shown), and hence, was chosen for further validation in this study. We propose that CPE controls its targets, such as c-MYC and Cyclin D1, through binding a receptor to activate downstream signaling. We have recently found that CPE activates a receptor HTR1E to activate the ERK pathway [48]. ERK/c-MYC and ERK/Cyclin D1 signaling are well known in promoting proliferation and migration in cancer cells, and HTR1E has been found in human cancer cells. This is one possible way for secreted soluble CPE to promote tumor cell growth, although CPE may activate other signaling pathways to regulate cancer growth and metastasis [49]. At the present time, we do not know how exosomes which release their cargo, including CPE into the cytoplasm of the cell, activate their downstream targets. However, extrapolating from our studies of 40kD CPE-ΔN, the splice variant lacking the N-terminus signal peptide, which does not go into the RER/Golgi secretory pathway, but is translocated from the cytoplasm into the nucleus where it acts as a transcription factor to activate many genes including β-catenin, c-MYC and Cyclin D1 [50], we speculate that exosomal WT-CPE released into the cytoplasm could up-regulate c-Myc and Cyclin D1 expression in a similar manner. Our results highlight the potential of exosomes harboring CPE-shRNA to be developed as a therapeutic agent for treating HCC. Interestingly, treatment with exosomes carrying shRNA to target *KRAS* has suppressed tumor progression and enhanced survival in pancreatic cancer mouse models [13]. A similar strategy using CPE-shRNA loaded exosomes could also be applied to other tumors such as glioblastoma, osteosarcoma, colorectal cancer, and pancreatic cancer, where CPE plays a pro-tumorigenic role.

4. Materials and Methods

4.1. Cell Culture

Human cancer cell lines HCC97H, HCC97L (liver cancer); MDA-MD-231, MCF-7 (breast cancer); AsPC-1, BxPC-3 (pancreatic cancer), HT-29, SW480 (colorectal cancer), DU145, LNCaP (prostate cancer) and LN-18, U118-MG (glioblastoma), exhibiting either malignant or low-malignant potential, respectively, and malignant CAOV3 cells (ovarian cancer), were cultured in DMEM medium supplemented with 10% fetal bovine serum at 37 °C in a humidified 5% CO_2 incubator. The various cancer cell lines were seeded at approximately equal numbers in the culture dish and maintained at similar conditions, such as volume of growth media and incubation time. All cell lines, except HCC cells, were obtained from ATCC (Manassas, VA, USA). Human HCC cell lines with low- and high-metastatic potential, MHCC97L and MHCC97H (referred to in this study as HCC97L or low-metastatic HCC and HCC97H or high-metastatic HCC), respectively, derived from the same parental cell line, were obtained from Liver Cancer Institute, Fudan University (Shanghai, China).

4.2. Patient Serum Samples

Blood samples were collected from 22 patients diagnosed with different types of cancers prior to surgery, and the serum was prepared and stored at −80 °C till exosome isolation. Sera were obtained from glioblastoma patients diagnosed with WHO Grade IV Glioblastomas (IDH wild type) prior to surgery, from UCSD Medical Center, San Diego, CA (IRB 120345). All other cancer serum samples were from patients with Stage I and II tumors, except 2 stage III (colon and ovarian), 2 benign (breast and colon), 1 unknown (ovarian) and 2 invasive but stage not known (breast), and were obtained from Maine Medical Center BioBank (Portland, ME, USA), which operates under an Institutional Review Board (IRB) approved protocol, and is overseen by the MMCRI Office of Research Compliance (FWA00003993). Sera from 30 healthy donors were obtained at the National Institutes of Health from The Blood Bank and under protocol 00-CH-0093, approved by IRB of the Eunice Kennedy Shriver National Institute of Child Health and Human Development, Bethesda, MD, USA. All serum samples were coded and unidentified.

4.3. Isolation of Exosomes

When cells seeded in a 60 mm dish reached 75% confluency (~2.5 × 10^6 cells), the supernatant media were collected and pre-cleared of cell debris by centrifugation at 2500 rpm for 10 min at 4 °C. Exosomes were isolated from the pre-cleared supernatant culture media of cells using ExoQuick TC reagent (System Biosciences, EXOTC50A-1, Palo Alto, CA, USA), according to manufacturer's instructions. Briefly, 1 mL of reagent was added per 5 mL of culture media, and incubated at 4 °C for at least 12 h. Exosomes present in the incubated media were then pelleted down by centrifugation at 1500× g for 30 min and resuspended in either 50 µL of PBS or TRIzol reagent (Sigma, St. Louis, MO, USA) for RNA isolation or in RIPA protein lysis buffer for Western blot, and stored in −80 °C until further use. Serum exosomes were isolated from 250 µL serum using ExoCap composite kit (MBL International, Woburn, MA, USA) per instruction manual, which is based on an antibody coupled magnetic capture bead-based procedure. The kit contains a mixture of CD9, CD63, CD81 and EpCAM capture beads. This step was followed by the purification of exosomal RNA using ExoCap Nucleic acid elution buffer (MBL International, MEX-E kit, Woburn, MA, USA), according to the kit protocol.

4.4. NanoSight Analysis

A nanoparticle tracking analysis (NTA) was performed to determine size distribution and concentration of exosomes using NanoSight LM10 instrument (Malvern Panalytical, Malvern, UK), equipped with a 405 nm LM12 module and EM-CCD camera (DL-658-OEM-630, Andor Technology, Belfast, UK) and NTAv3.1 software (Malvern Panalytical, Malvern, UK). Two microlitres of exosomes were diluted with 500 µL of PBS before analysis. The dilution factor was accounted to obtain the final exosome concentrations. Results are displayed as a graph with size (nm) vs. concentration (particles/mL) measurements, and a scatter plot with size (nm) vs. intensity (a.u).

4.5. RT-PCR

cDNA was synthesized from 3–6 µg of RNA from exosomes using sensiFAST cDNA synthesis kit (BIOLINE Meridian Bioscience, BIO-65053, Memphis, TN, USA) based on manufacturer's instructions. CPE transcript was amplified using SeqAMP DNA polymerase (Clonetech, catalog no: 638509, Mountain View, CA, USA) and different primer sets, as indicated in the corresponding figure. Primer sequences are given in Supplementary Table S1. The PCR cycle consisted of an initial 'hot start' at 94 °C for 3 min, followed by 35 cycles of amplification (94 °C 30 s, 60 °C 30 s, 72 °C 30 s), with a final extension step of 72 °C for 5 min. PCR products were analyzed on 1.8% agarose gels.

4.6. Quantitative Real-Time PCR

Exosomal RNA was purified from supernatant media of cells using SeraMir kits (System Biosciences, RA800A, Palo Alto, CA, USA) or TRIzol reagent (Sigma-Aldrich, St. Louis, MO, USA), and from serum using ExoCap composite kits. TRIzol isolated RNA from exosomes was used only for RT-PCR experiments shown in Figure 1C,D and Supplementary Figure S1. The first-strand cDNA was synthesized with 0.1 µg of total RNA using SensiFast cDNA Synthesis kit (BIOLINE Meridian Bioscience, Memphis, TN, USA). qRT-PCR was performed using SYBR Green PCR Matrix Mix (Applied BioSystem, #4367659, Waltham, MA, USA) in an ABI PRISM 7900 Sequence Detector (Applied Biosystems, Waltham, MA, USA), with cycling conditions as: 95 °C for 5 min, followed by 40 amplification cycles of denaturation 95 °C for 15 s, annealing 60 °C for 60 s, and extension 72 °C for 30 s, and final extension at 72 °C for 10 min. In the absence of a good internal control for exosomal mRNA normalization, the standard curve method using a CPE 5′-DNA fragment of known concentration was used to perform quantitation of *CPE* mRNA copy numbers in exosomes using FN/RN primer set. All samples for sera copy number determination including the standard curve were run together in a 384-well PCR plate. For cancer cell exosomes, the fold change in exosomal CPE mRNA copy number of high-metastatic cells with respect to the exosomal CPE mRNA copy number of low-metastatic cells was determined by dividing the first number with the latter. The mean fold change ± SD of the independent experiments is shown in the bar graph. This was done across the different cancer types. TRIzol was used to isolate RNA from HCC cells. The $2-\Delta\Delta Ct$ method was used to calculate the relative fold difference of mRNA expression of *CPE*, *Cyclin D1*, and *c-MYC* in HCC97L and HCC97H cells. 18s rRNA was used for data normalization. Primer sequences used are listed in Supplementary Table S1. All qRT-PCR assays were run in triplicate.

4.7. Western Blot

Exosome/cellular protein lysates were prepared using RIPA lysis and extraction buffer (Thermo Fisher Scientific, #89901, Waltham, MA, USA) supplemented with Halt Protease inhibitor cocktail (Thermo Scientific, #87786, Waltham, MA, USA). Forty-five µg of exosomal protein or 25 µg of cellular protein was loaded per lane of the SDS-PAGE gel, and Western blot was performed, as described previously [42]. For the analysis of secreted WT-CPE, the supernatant media of cells were concentrated using Amicon Ultra 10k MWCO centrifugal filter (Millipore Sigma, St. Louis, MO, USA). Monoclonal antibody against CPE (#610758, 1:2000 dilution) was purchased from BD Biosciences (Franklin Lakes, NJ, USA), and primary antibodies to TSG101 (ab612696, 1:500 dilution) and CD63 (ab68418, 1:1000 dilution) were from Abcam (Cambridge, MA, USA). Cyclin D1 (#92G2, 1:500) antibody was from Cell Signaling Technology (Danvers, MA, USA) and β-tubulin (#T5168, 1:2000) was procured from Sigma-Aldrich (St. Louis, MO, USA).

4.8. In Vitro Exosome Transfer Experiments

To perform exosome transfer experiments using HCC97H-derived exosomes, HCC97H cells were seeded in a 60 mm dish and transfected with either 25 nM CPE-shRNA, which is a pool of three target-specific lentiviral vector constructs (each encoding 19–25 nt shRNAs) or control shRNA plasmids (Santa Cruz Biotechnology Inc, Cat#sc-45378-SH, sc-108060, Dallas, TX, USA) using Lipofectamine 2000 reagent (Thermo Fisher Scientific, Waltham, MA, USA). Forty-eight hours later, the supernatant media of the transfected cells were collected, and exosomes were isolated. Exosomes were also isolated from the culture media of untransfected HCC97H cells (ExoHCCH) for some experiments. After dissolving the exosome pellet in 50 µL of PBS, the exosomal protein was estimated using protein assay (Bio-Rad Laboratories, Cat#500-0006, Hercules, CA, USA). HCC97L cells seeded in a 6-well plate were treated with 75 µg of exosomal protein/well for 48 h, after which the cells were harvested, and seeded for MTT and cell invasion assays. Based on the NanoSight analyses of ExoHCCH, ExoHCCH-CPE-shRNA and ExoHCCH-CTRL-shRNA, the number of particles added was quantitated to be approximately equal to $55–70 \times 10^{10}$ particles/well.

For experiments targeting HCC97H with CPE-shRNA-loaded exosomes, HEK293T cells were infected with adenovirus carrying either CPE-shRNA-GFP or control-shRNA-GFP (Vector Biolabs, Cat# shADV-229236, Malvern, PA, USA) at MOI 25 for 48–72 h. After 5–6 h of infection, the culture media were replaced to remove viral particles present in the infection media. Exosomes were isolated from the supernatant media of the infected cells, and the exosomal protein was estimated. To compare and standardize exosome loading, 25 µg of the exosomal protein (exoHEK), either exoHEK-CPE-shRNA or exoHEK-CTRL-shRNA, were used to treat HCC97H cells, seeded in 4-well chamber slides. Moreover, 48 h later, the GFP (green fluorescent protein) fluorescence of the cells, which is an indirect measurement of shRNA loading and transfer via exosomes, was documented using a fluorescent microscope (Eclipse 80i, Nikon or Zeiss Wide-Field), and the GFP levels were quantitated using Image J software using the following formula:

$$\text{CTCF (corrected total cell fluorescence)} = \text{Integrated Density} - (\text{Area of selected cell} \times \text{Mean fluorescence of background readings})$$

Area, mean fluorescence, and integrated density values are obtained from the Image J software (http://imagej.nih.gov/ij/, accessed on 15 March 2019). The fold change difference in the GFP levels between ExoHEK-CPE-shRNA and ExoHEK-CTRL-shRNA treated HCC97H cells, if any, is determined. Subsequently, HCC97H cells seeded in a 30 mm dish were treated with 100 µg of ExoHEK-CPEshRNA. The amount of ExoHEK-CTRL-shRNA to be added was calculated based on the fold change difference in the GFP levels, determined by Image J software analysis of fluorescent images, performed in the prior standardization step, such that the GFP levels between the ExoHEK-CPE-shRNA and

ExoHEK-CTRL-shRNA treatment groups are comparable. After 48 h, the cells were seeded for MTT and colony formation assays.

4.9. Cell Proliferation Assay

To assess the proliferation of cells, 2000 cells/well were seeded in a 96-well plate and the MTT (3-(4,5-dimethylthiazol-2-yl)-2,5-diphenyltetrazolium bromide) assay was performed on days 1, 3, 5 and 7/8, as reported previously [51]. Absorbance reading was taken at 490 nm or 450 nm in a microplate reader (BioTek, Winooski, VT, USA).

4.10. Matrigel Invasion Assay

Furthermore, a 24-well Corning Matrigel invasion chamber (Corning, NY, USA) with 8-μm pores was used to perform the cell invasion assay. Briefly, 500 μL of cell suspension (1×10^5 cells/mL) in serum-free media was added to the top chamber, while serum supplemented media were added to the lower chamber. After 24 h, invaded cells were fixed with 100% methanol and stained with 1% crystal violet solution. Images from five different fields/well were captured, and cells were counted.

4.11. Colony Formation Assay

Cells were seeded in a 6-well plate at a density of 2000 cells/well and cultured for 11–15 days to allow colonies to form, following which, they were fixed using 100% methanol and stained with 1% crystal violet solution. Representative images of wells were taken, and a number of colonies containing at least 50 cells were counted using Image J software (http://imagej.nih.gov/ij/, accessed on 15 March 2019).

4.12. Statistical Analysis

The data represent mean ± SD (standard deviation) of independent experiments (N), performed in triplicate (n = 3), or as stated in the figure legend. Statistical significance was determined using Student's *t*-test or two-way ANOVA, and p values are denoted as * $p < 0.05$, ** $p < 0.01$, *** $p < 0.001$ and **** $p < 0.0001$, and are specified in the figure legend. A two-way ANOVA with Sidak's multiple comparisons test was performed using GraphPAD PRISM. Box plot and Shapiro-Wilk normality test were used to examine the distribution of *CPE* copy numbers in human sera exosomes. A logistic regression and a receiver operating characteristics (ROC) curve analysis were performed to investigate the association of cancers with *CPE* copy number in sera-derived exosomes.

5. Conclusions

We have identified a new bioactive molecule, CPE, in exosomes, that has the ability to transfer the malignant phenotype from low- to high-metastatic HCC cells, suggesting that circulating exosomes carrying CPE may represent a novel mechanism for promoting tumor metastasis in the body. Our data show that exosomes modified to carry CPE-shRNA could suppress tumor growth and be a potentially exciting new therapy for treating liver and other cancers, since CPE expression is upregulated in many cancer types. Our pilot clinical study suggests that *CPE* mRNA in circulating exosomes could be developed as a biomarker for diagnosing cancer. Future investigations will focus on translating our findings to preclinical models and advancing the potential clinical use of the exosome-based delivery of CPE-shRNA in the treatment of different types of cancer.

Supplementary Materials: The following supporting information can be downloaded at: https://www.mdpi.com/article/10.3390/ijms23063113/s1.

Author Contributions: Conceptualization, Y.P.L. and X.Y.; methodology, S.H., B.A. and A.L.; software, S.H.; validation, S.H., X.Y., A.L., A.B., C.C.C. and Y.P.L.; formal analysis, S.H., B.A., X.Y. and A.L.; investigation, S.H., B.A., X.Y., A.B. and C.C.C.; resources, Y.P.L., A.B. and C.C.C.; data curation, S.H. and Y.P.L.; writing—original draft preparation, S.H.; writing—review and editing, X.Y., B.A., A.L.,

A.B., C.C.C. and Y.P.L.; supervision, Y.P.L. and X.Y.; project administration, Y.P.L.; funding acquisition, Y.P.L. All authors have read and agreed to the published version of the manuscript.

Funding: This research was supported by the Intramural Research Program of the Eunice Kennedy Shriver National Institute of Child Health and Human Development (NICHD) (grant number: ZIA HD000056), National Institutes of Health and the National Cancer Institute, USA.

Institutional Review Board Statement: Serum samples from patients diagnosed with different types of cancers were obtained from Maine Medical Center BioBank, Portland, ME, which operates under an Institutional Review Board (IRB)-approved protocol #2526 on 31 May 2016, and is overseen by the MMCRI Office of Research Compliance (FWA00003993 approved on 23 April 2019) and UCSD Medical Center, San Diego, CA, USA (IRB 120345 approved 5 February 2015 and renewed annually). Sera from healthy donors were obtained at the National Institutes of Health Blood Bank under protocol 00-CH-0093, approved on 27 March 2013 and renewed annually by IRB of the *Eunice Kennedy Shriver* National Institute of Child Health and Human Development, Bethesda, MD, USA. All serum samples were coded and unidentified. Consent to participate—not applicable.

Informed Consent Statement: Informed consent was obtained from all subjects involved in the study.

Data Availability Statement: Data supporting the findings of this study are contained within the article and the additional supplemental files. All data discussed in the paper and all materials will be made available to readers upon request from the corresponding author.

Acknowledgments: We thank Jennifer Clare Jones and Bryce Killingsworth (Center for Cancer Research, NCI) for their contributions towards NanoSight and NanoFACS analyses; Louis Dye, Lynne Holtzclaw and Vincent Schram (NICHD Microscopy Core Facility) for their assistance in electron microscopy and Wei Zhang, Biostatistics & Bioinformatics Branch (NICHD) for help with statistical analysis. We thank Karel Pacak (NICHD) and the NIH blood bank for providing sera from healthy volunteers.

Conflicts of Interest: The authors declare no conflict of interest.

Abbreviations

CPE	Carboxypeptidase E
HCC	Hepatocellular carcinoma
HEK	Human embryonic kidney
TSG101	Tumor susceptibility gene 101
AUC	Area under the curve
ROC	Receiver operating characteristics
GFP	Green fluorescent protein
NTA	Nanoparticle tracking analysis
EMT	Epithelial-Mesenchymal Transition

References

1. Tamura, T.; Yoshioka, Y.; Sakamoto, S.; Ichikawa, T.; Ochiya, T. Extracellular vesicles as a promising biomarker resource in liquid biopsy for cancer. *Extracell. Vesicles Circ. Nucleic Acids* **2021**, *2*, 148–174. [CrossRef]
2. Hoshino, A.; Costa-Silva, B.; Shen, T.L.; Rodrigues, G.; Hashimoto, A.; Tesic Mark, M.; Molina, H.; Kohsaka, S.; Di Giannatale, A.; Ceder, S.; et al. Tumour exosome integrins determine organotropic metastasis. *Nature* **2015**, *527*, 329–335. [CrossRef] [PubMed]
3. Luga, V.; Wrana, J.L. Tumor-stroma interaction: Revealing fibroblast-secreted exosomes as potent regulators of Wnt-planar cell polarity signaling in cancer metastasis. *Cancer Res.* **2013**, *73*, 6843–6847. [CrossRef] [PubMed]
4. Peinado, H.; Aleckovic, M.; Lavotshkin, S.; Matei, I.; Costa-Silva, B.; Moreno-Bueno, G.; Hergueta-Redondo, M.; Williams, C.; Garcia-Santos, G.; Ghajar, C.; et al. Melanoma exosomes educate bone marrow progenitor cells toward a pro-metastatic phenotype through MET. *Nat. Med.* **2012**, *18*, 883–891. [CrossRef] [PubMed]
5. Chen, L.; Guo, P.; He, Y.; Chen, Z.; Chen, L.; Luo, Y.; Qi, L.; Liu, Y.; Wu, Q.; Cui, Y.; et al. HCC-derived exosomes elicit HCC progression and recurrence by epithelial-mesenchymal transition through MAPK/ERK signalling pathway. *Cell Death Dis.* **2018**, *9*, 513. [CrossRef]
6. Yang, B.; Feng, X.; Liu, H.; Tong, R.; Wu, J.; Li, C.; Yu, H.; Chen, Y.; Cheng, Q.; Chen, J.; et al. High-metastatic cancer cells derived exosomal miR92a-3p promotes epithelial-mesenchymal transition and metastasis of low-metastatic cancer cells by regulating PTEN/Akt pathway in hepatocellular carcinoma. *Oncogene* **2020**, *39*, 6529–6543. [CrossRef]

7. Fu, Q.; Zhang, Q.; Lou, Y.; Yang, J.; Nie, G.; Chen, Q.; Chen, Y.; Zhang, J.; Wang, J.; Wei, T.; et al. Primary tumor-derived exosomes facilitate metastasis by regulating adhesion of circulating tumor cells via SMAD3 in liver cancer. *Oncogene* **2018**, *37*, 6105–6118. [CrossRef]
8. Wang, G.; Liu, W.; Zou, Y.; Wang, G.; Deng, Y.; Luo, J.; Zhang, Y.; Li, H.; Zhang, Q.; Yang, Y.; et al. Three isoforms of exosomal circPTGR1 promote hepatocellular carcinoma metastasis via the miR449a-MET pathway. *EBioMedicine* **2019**, *40*, 432–445. [CrossRef]
9. Kia, V.; Paryan, M.; Mortazavi, Y.; Biglari, A.; Mohammadi-Yeganeh, S. Evaluation of exosomal miR-9 and miR-155 targeting PTEN and DUSP14 in highly metastatic breast cancer and their effect on low metastatic cells. *J. Cell. Biochem.* **2019**, *120*, 5666–5676. [CrossRef]
10. Shen, X.; Wang, C.; Zhu, H.; Wang, Y.; Wang, X.; Cheng, X.; Ge, W.; Lu, W. Exosome-mediated transfer of CD44 from high-metastatic ovarian cancer cells promotes migration and invasion of low-metastatic ovarian cancer cells. *J. Ovarian Res.* **2021**, *14*, 38. [CrossRef]
11. El-Andaloussi, S.; Lee, Y.; Lakhal-Littleton, S.; Li, J.; Seow, Y.; Gardiner, C.; Alvarez-Erviti, L.; Sargent, I.L.; Wood, M.J. Exosome-mediated delivery of siRNA in vitro and in vivo. *Nat. Protoc.* **2012**, *7*, 2112–2126. [CrossRef] [PubMed]
12. Alvarez-Erviti, L.; Seow, Y.; Yin, H.; Betts, C.; Lakhal, S.; Wood, M.J. Delivery of siRNA to the mouse brain by systemic injection of targeted exosomes. *Nat. Biotechnol.* **2011**, *29*, 341–345. [CrossRef] [PubMed]
13. Kamerkar, S.; LeBleu, V.S.; Sugimoto, H.; Yang, S.; Ruivo, C.F.; Melo, S.A.; Lee, J.J.; Kalluri, R. Exosomes facilitate therapeutic targeting of oncogenic KRAS in pancreatic cancer. *Nature* **2017**, *546*, 498–503. [CrossRef] [PubMed]
14. Logozzi, M.; Mizzoni, D.; Di Raimo, R.; Fais, S. Exosomes: A Source for New and Old Biomarkers in Cancer. *Cancers* **2020**, *12*, 2566. [CrossRef] [PubMed]
15. Frampton, A.E.; Prado, M.M.; Lopez-Jimenez, E.; Fajardo-Puerta, A.B.; Jawad, Z.A.R.; Lawton, P.; Giovannetti, E.; Habib, N.A.; Castellano, L.; Stebbing, J.; et al. Glypican-1 is enriched in circulating-exosomes in pancreatic cancer and correlates with tumor burden. *Oncotarget* **2018**, *9*, 19006–19013. [CrossRef]
16. Li, Y.; Zhang, Y.; Qiu, F.; Qiu, Z. Proteomic identification of exosomal LRG1: A potential urinary biomarker for detecting NSCLC. *Electrophoresis* **2011**, *32*, 1976–1983. [CrossRef]
17. Hessvik, N.P.; Sandvig, K.; Llorente, A. Exosomal miRNAs as Biomarkers for Prostate Cancer. *Front. Genet.* **2013**, *4*, 36. [CrossRef]
18. Wani, S.; Kaul, D.; Mavuduru, R.S.; Kakkar, N.; Bhatia, A. Urinary-exosomal miR-2909: A novel pathognomonic trait of prostate cancer severity. *J. Biotechnol.* **2017**, *259*, 135–139. [CrossRef]
19. Li, Z.; Ma, Y.Y.; Wang, J.; Zeng, X.F.; Li, R.; Kang, W.; Hao, X.K. Exosomal microRNA-141 is upregulated in the serum of prostate cancer patients. *OncoTargets Ther.* **2016**, *9*, 139–148. [CrossRef]
20. Fricker, L.D.; Snyder, S.H. Purification and characterization of enkephalin convertase, an enkephalin-synthesizing carboxypeptidase. *J. Biol. Chem.* **1983**, *258*, 10950–10955. [CrossRef]
21. Hook, V.Y.; Loh, Y.P. Carboxypeptidase B-like converting enzyme activity in secretory granules of rat pituitary. *Proc. Natl. Acad. Sci. USA* **1984**, *81*, 2776–2780. [CrossRef] [PubMed]
22. Cheng, Y.; Cawley, N.X.; Loh, Y.P. Carboxypeptidase E/NFalpha1: A new neurotrophic factor against oxidative stress-induced apoptotic cell death mediated by ERK and PI3-K/AKT pathways. *PLoS ONE* **2013**, *8*, e71578. [CrossRef]
23. Cool, D.R.; Normant, E.; Shen, F.; Chen, H.C.; Pannell, L.; Zhang, Y.; Loh, Y.P. Carboxypeptidase E is a regulated secretory pathway sorting receptor: Genetic obliteration leads to endocrine disorders in Cpe(fat) mice. *Cell* **1997**, *88*, 73–83. [CrossRef]
24. Dhanvantari, S.; Loh, Y.P. Lipid raft association of carboxypeptidase E is necessary for its function as a regulated secretory pathway sorting receptor. *J. Biol. Chem.* **2000**, *275*, 29887–29893. [CrossRef]
25. Morris, D.G.; Musat, M.; Czirjak, S.; Hanzely, Z.; Lillington, D.M.; Korbonits, M.; Grossman, A.B. Differential gene expression in pituitary adenomas by oligonucleotide array analysis. *Eur. J. Endocrinol.* **2005**, *153*, 143–151. [CrossRef]
26. Armento, A.; Ilina, E.I.; Kaoma, T.; Muller, A.; Vallar, L.; Niclou, S.P.; Kruger, M.A.; Mittelbronn, M.; Naumann, U. Carboxypeptidase E transmits its anti-migratory function in glioma cells via transcriptional regulation of cell architecture and motility regulating factors. *Int. J. Oncol.* **2017**, *51*, 702–714. [CrossRef]
27. Huang, S.F.; Wu, H.D.; Chen, Y.T.; Murthy, S.R.; Chiu, Y.T.; Chang, Y.; Chang, I.C.; Yang, X.; Loh, Y.P. Carboxypeptidase E is a prediction marker for tumor recurrence in early-stage hepatocellular carcinoma. *Tumour Biol.* **2016**, *37*, 9745–9753. [CrossRef]
28. Liu, A.; Shao, C.; Jin, G.; Liu, R.; Hao, J.; Shao, Z.; Liu, Q.; Hu, X. Downregulation of CPE regulates cell proliferation and chemosensitivity in pancreatic cancer. *Tumour Biol.* **2014**, *35*, 12459–12465. [CrossRef]
29. Shen, H.W.; Tan, J.F.; Shang, J.H.; Hou, M.Z.; Liu, J.; He, L.; Yao, S.Z.; He, S.Y. CPE overexpression is correlated with pelvic lymph node metastasis and poor prognosis in patients with early-stage cervical cancer. *Arch. Gynecol. Obstet.* **2016**, *294*, 333–342. [CrossRef]
30. Wang, Z.Q.; Faddaoui, A.; Bachvarova, M.; Plante, M.; Gregoire, J.; Renaud, M.C.; Sebastianelli, A.; Guillemette, C.; Gobeil, S.; Macdonald, E.; et al. BCAT1 expression associates with ovarian cancer progression: Possible implications in altered disease metabolism. *Oncotarget* **2015**, *6*, 31522–31543. [CrossRef]
31. Fan, S.; Li, X.; Li, L.; Wang, L.; Du, Z.; Yang, Y.; Zhao, J.; Li, Y. Silencing of carboxypeptidase E inhibits cell proliferation, tumorigenicity, and metastasis of osteosarcoma cells. *OncoTargets Ther.* **2016**, *9*, 2795–2803. [CrossRef]
32. Liang, X.H.; Li, L.L.; Wu, G.G.; Xie, Y.C.; Zhang, G.X.; Chen, W.; Yang, H.F.; Liu, Q.L.; Li, W.H.; He, W.G.; et al. Upregulation of CPE promotes cell proliferation and tumorigenicity in colorectal cancer. *BMC Cancer* **2013**, *13*, 412. [CrossRef] [PubMed]

33. Hareendran, S.; Yang, X.; Lou, H.; Xiao, L.; Loh, Y.P. Carboxypeptidase E-N Promotes Proliferation and Invasion of Pancreatic Cancer Cells via Upregulation of CXCR2 Gene Expression. *Int. J. Mol. Sci.* **2019**, *20*, 5725. [CrossRef] [PubMed]
34. Yang, X.; Lou, H.; Chen, Y.T.; Huang, S.F.; Loh, Y.P. A novel 40kDa N-terminal truncated carboxypeptidase E splice variant: Cloning, cDNA sequence analysis and role in regulation of metastatic genes in human cancers. *Genes Cancer* **2019**, *10*, 160–170. [CrossRef]
35. Li, Y.; Tang, Z.Y.; Ye, S.L.; Liu, Y.K.; Chen, J.; Xue, Q.; Chen, J.; Gao, D.M.; Bao, W.H. Establishment of cell clones with different metastatic potential from the metastatic hepatocellular carcinoma cell line MHCC97. *World J. Gastroenterol.* **2001**, *7*, 630–636. [CrossRef]
36. Logozzi, M.; De Milito, A.; Lugini, L.; Borghi, M.; Calabro, L.; Spada, M.; Perdicchio, M.; Marino, M.L.; Federici, C.; Iessi, E.; et al. High levels of exosomes expressing CD63 and caveolin-1 in plasma of melanoma patients. *PLoS ONE* **2009**, *4*, e5219. [CrossRef]
37. Nilsson, J.; Skog, J.; Nordstrand, A.; Baranov, V.; Mincheva-Nilsson, L.; Breakefield, X.O.; Widmark, A. Prostate cancer-derived urine exosomes: A novel approach to biomarkers for prostate cancer. *Br. J. Cancer* **2009**, *100*, 1603–1607. [CrossRef]
38. Skog, J.; Wurdinger, T.; van Rijn, S.; Meijer, D.H.; Gainche, L.; Sena-Esteves, M.; Curry, W.T., Jr.; Carter, B.S.; Krichevsky, A.M.; Breakefield, X.O. Glioblastoma microvesicles transport RNA and proteins that promote tumour growth and provide diagnostic biomarkers. *Nat. Cell Biol.* **2008**, *10*, 1470–1476. [CrossRef]
39. Tanaka, Y.; Kamohara, H.; Kinoshita, K.; Kurashige, J.; Ishimoto, T.; Iwatsuki, M.; Watanabe, M.; Baba, H. Clinical impact of serum exosomal microRNA-21 as a clinical biomarker in human esophageal squamous cell carcinoma. *Cancer* **2013**, *119*, 1159–1167. [CrossRef]
40. Kuo, I.Y.; Liu, D.; Lai, W.W.; Wang, Y.C.; Loh, Y.P. Carboxypeptidase E mRNA: Overexpression predicts recurrence and death in lung adenocarcinoma cancer patients. *Cancer Biomark.* **2021**, 1–9. [CrossRef]
41. Fan, S.; Gao, X.; Chen, P.; Li, X. Carboxypeptidase E-DeltaN promotes migration, invasiveness, and epithelial-mesenchymal transition of human osteosarcoma cells via the Wnt-beta-catenin pathway. *Biochem. Cell Biol.* **2019**, *97*, 446–453. [CrossRef] [PubMed]
42. Murthy, S.R.K.; Dupart, E.; Al-Sweel, N.; Chen, A.; Cawley, N.X.; Loh, Y.P. Carboxypeptidase E promotes cancer cell survival, but inhibits migration and invasion. *Cancer Lett.* **2013**, *341*, 204–213. [CrossRef] [PubMed]
43. Zomer, A.; Maynard, C.; Verweij, F.J.; Kamermans, A.; Schafer, R.; Beerling, E.; Schiffelers, R.M.; de Wit, E.; Berenguer, J.; Ellenbroek, S.I.J.; et al. In vivo imaging reveals extracellular vesicle-mediated phenocopying of metastatic behavior. *Cell* **2015**, *161*, 1046–1057. [CrossRef] [PubMed]
44. Diehl, J.A. Cycling to cancer with cyclin D1. *Cancer Biol. Ther.* **2002**, *1*, 226–231. [CrossRef]
45. Shintani, M.; Okazaki, A.; Masuda, T.; Kawada, M.; Ishizuka, M.; Doki, Y.; Weinstein, I.B.; Imoto, M. Overexpression of cyclin DI contributes to malignant properties of esophageal tumor cells by increasing VEGF production and decreasing Fas expression. *Anticancer Res.* **2002**, *22*, 639–647.
46. Zheng, K.; Cubero, F.J.; Nevzorova, Y.A. c-MYC-Making Liver Sick: Role of c-MYC in Hepatic Cell Function, Homeostasis and Disease. *Genes* **2017**, *8*, 123. [CrossRef]
47. Akita, H.; Marquardt, J.U.; Durkin, M.E.; Kitade, M.; Seo, D.; Conner, E.A.; Andersen, J.B.; Factor, V.M.; Thorgeirsson, S.S. MYC activates stem-like cell potential in hepatocarcinoma by a p53-dependent mechanism. *Cancer Res.* **2014**, *74*, 5903–5913. [CrossRef]
48. Sharma, V.K.; Yang, X.; Kim, S.K.; Mafi, A.; Saiz-Sanchez, D.; Villanueva-Anguita, P.; Xiao, L.; Inoue, A.; Goddard, W.A., 3rd; Loh, Y.P. Novel interaction between neurotrophic factor-alpha1/carboxypeptidase E and serotonin receptor, 5-HTR1E, protects human neurons against oxidative/neuroexcitotoxic stress via beta-arrestin/ERK signaling. *Cell. Mol. Life Sci.* **2021**, *79*, 24. [CrossRef]
49. Bai, Z.; Feng, M.; Du, Y.; Cong, L.; Cheng, Y. Carboxypeptidase E down-regulation regulates transcriptional and epigenetic profiles in pancreatic cancer cell line: A network analysis. *Cancer Biomark.* **2020**, *29*, 79–88. [CrossRef]
50. Skalka, N.; Caspi, M.; Lahav-Ariel, L.; Loh, Y.P.; Hirschberg, K.; Rosin-Arbesfeld, R. Carboxypeptidase E (CPE) inhibits the secretion and activity of Wnt3a. *Oncogene* **2016**, *35*, 6416–6428. [CrossRef]
51. Xiao, L.; Yang, X.; Sharma, V.K.; Loh, Y.P. Cloning, gene regulation, and neuronal proliferation functions of novel N-terminal-truncated carboxypeptidase E/neurotrophic factor-alpha1 variants in embryonic mouse brain. *FASEB J.* **2019**, *33*, 808–820. [CrossRef] [PubMed]

Article

DNA Methylation Mediates EMT Gene Expression in Human Pancreatic Ductal Adenocarcinoma Cell Lines

Maria Urbanova [1,†], Verona Buocikova [1,†], Lenka Trnkova [1], Sabina Strapcova [2], Viera Horvathova Kajabova [1], Emma Barreto Melian [3], Maria Novisedlakova [4], Miroslav Tomas [1,5], Peter Dubovan [1,5], Julie Earl [3], Jozef Bizik [1], Eliska Svastova [2], Sona Ciernikova [1] and Bozena Smolkova [1,*]

1. Department of Molecular Oncology, Cancer Research Institute, Biomedical Research Center, Slovak Academy of Sciences, Dubravska Cesta 9, 845 05 Bratislava, Slovakia; maria.urbanova@savba.sk (M.U.); verona.buocikova@savba.sk (V.B.); lenka.trnkova@savba.sk (L.T.); viera.kajabova@savba.sk (V.H.K.); miroslav.tomas@nou.sk (M.T.); peter.dubovan@nou.sk (P.D.); jozef.bizik@savba.sk (J.B.); sona.ciernikova@savba.sk (S.C.)
2. Department of Tumor Biology, Institute of Virology, Biomedical Research Center, Slovak Academy of Sciences, Dubravska Cesta 9, 845 05 Bratislava, Slovakia; sabina.strapcova@savba.sk (S.S.); eliska.svastova@savba.sk (E.S.)
3. Molecular Epidemiology and Predictive Tumor Markers Group, Ramón y Cajal Health Research Institute (IRYCIS), Biomedical Research Network in Cancer (CIBERONC), Carretera Colmenar Km 9,100, 28034 Madrid, Spain; emma.barreto@salud.madrid.org (E.B.M.); julie.earl@live.co.uk (J.E.)
4. Oncology Outpatient Clinic, Hospital of the Hospitaller Order of Saint John of God, 814 65 Bratislava, Slovakia; mnovisedlakova@milosrdni.sk
5. Department of Surgical Oncology, National Cancer Institute, Slovak Medical University, Klenova 1, 833 10 Bratislava, Slovakia
* Correspondence: bozena.smolkova@savba.sk; Tel.: +421-2-3229-5138
† These authors share the first authorship.

Abstract: Due to abundant stroma and extracellular matrix, accompanied by lack of vascularization, pancreatic ductal adenocarcinoma (PDAC) is characterized by severe hypoxia. Epigenetic regulation is likely one of the mechanisms driving hypoxia-induced epithelial-to-mesenchymal transition (EMT), responsible for PDAC aggressiveness and dismal prognosis. To verify the role of DNA methylation in this process, we assessed gene expression and DNA methylation changes in four PDAC cell lines. BxPC-3, MIA PaCa-2, PANC-1, and SU.86.86 cells were exposed to conditioned media containing cytokines and inflammatory molecules in normoxic and hypoxic (1% O_2) conditions for 2 and 6 days. Cancer Inflammation and Immunity Crosstalk and Human Epithelial to Mesenchymal Transition RT^2 Profiler PCR Arrays were used to identify top deregulated inflammatory and EMT-related genes. Their mRNA expression and DNA methylation were quantified by qRT-PCR and pyrosequencing. BxPC-3 and SU.86.86 cell lines were the most sensitive to hypoxia and inflammation. Although the methylation of gene promoters correlated with gene expression negatively, it was not significantly influenced by experimental conditions. However, DNA methyltransferase inhibitor decitabine efficiently decreased DNA methylation up to 53% and reactivated all silenced genes. These results confirm the role of DNA methylation in EMT-related gene regulation and uncover possible new targets involved in PDAC progression.

Keywords: PDAC; inflammation; hypoxia; epithelial-to-mesenchymal transition; DNA methylation

1. Introduction

Pancreatic ductal adenocarcinoma (PDAC), representing more than 90% of all pancreatic cancers, is estimated to become the second leading cause of cancer-related deaths in developed countries by 2030 [1]. Patient prognosis is mainly affected by the time of disease diagnostics. However, only 11% of PDACs are detected early, with a 5-year survival rate of

39%. If cancer has spread to surrounding tissues or organs, a 5-year survival rate drops down to 13%, and for the 52% of patients diagnosed in the late stage, it decreases to only 3% [2]. High PDAC mortality is also a consequence of its aggressive nature with early local invasion and resistance to conventional treatment.

Accumulation of genetic, epigenetic, and morphological changes in pancreatic ductal cells is causal in disease initiation and development. The progression from hyperplasia through dysplasia to invasive PDAC is at the molecular level associated with telomere shortening and accumulation of mutations in *KRAS, ERBB2, CDKN2A* in low-grade, and *TP53, SMAD4*, and *BRCA2* in high-grade pre-invasive precursor lesions [3]. However, the mutational burden is not enough to comprehensively explain PDAC pathogenesis. Integration of genomic and epigenomic data demonstrates that mutational alteration in oncogenes, such as *KRAS*, induces downstream signaling leading to direct regulation of histone proteins as well as histone and DNA-modifying enzymes [4]. While genetics is critical for PDAC initiation and early progression, the acquisition of tumor heterogeneity is associated with specific epigenomic landscapes [5,6].

Besides cell-intrinsic (mutation background, epigenetic state), several extrinsic factors in the tumor microenvironment, such as inflammation, hypoxia with related oxidative stress, and acidosis, significantly contribute to PDAC aggressiveness [7,8]. The fibroinflammatory stroma of chronic pancreatitis resembles that of pancreatic cancer, and aberrant inflammatory signaling contributes to the malignant transformation of pancreatic cells [9,10]. On the other hand, hypoxia is one of the main players inducing metastatic cascade: tumor cell intravasation, migration, survival in the bloodstream, extravasation, and colonization [11]. The hypoxic PDAC microenvironment resides from poor vascularization and rapid proliferation of cancer cells. The presence of hypoxic areas in the tumors correlates with a worse prognosis [12]. Tumor cells develop efficient adaptive metabolic strategies in hypoxic conditions to satisfy their high energetic demands. Hypoxia-inducible factors (HIFs) are activating transcriptional factors (TFs), securing the physiological response of cancer cells to hypoxia by stimulation of genes involved in angiogenesis and glycolysis [13]. We and others have provided evidence that hypoxia is accompanied by HIF1 induction in various cancers, including PDAC [14–16]. Intratumoral hypoxia mediates epithelial to mesenchymal transition (EMT), whose major inducer is transforming growth factor-β (TGF-β) along with cytokines and growth factors secreted by the tumor microenvironment [17,18]. EMT results in loss of cell adhesion, abnormal apical-basal polarity, and cytoskeletal reorganization, which raises tumor cell motility, invasiveness, and stemness [19]. Mesenchymal phenotype increases resistance to apoptosis and elevates the production of extracellular matrix (ECM) components by activated pancreatic stellate cells. One of the main EMT features is the functional loss of E-cadherin expression [20]. Hypoxia-induced pathways critically contribute to the deregulation of EMT-TFs, including SNAI1, TWIST1, ZEB1, ZEB2, or SIP1 [21]. These TFs, promoting cell polarity loss by destroying tight junctions and degrading adhesion molecules, were detected to be overexpressed in PDAC [22]. The tumors' hypoxic environment can induce EMT by reducing the activity of ten-eleven translocation (TET) enzymes, which are essential in the process of cytosine demethylation, and bind the oxygen molecule as an essential cofactor [23].

Accumulating evidence reveals that hypoxia in cancers directly influences chromatin remodeling events like DNA methylation and histone modifications [24]. Epigenetic regulation is also implicated in dynamic changes underlying metastable or stable EMT transitions [25]. However, the study of epigenetic changes under hypoxic conditions is at the beginning in PDAC, with better-characterized microRNA and long non-coding RNA regulation, post-translational modifications of histones, and expression of epigenetic regulator proteins [26]. SNAI1 can recruit multiple chromatin-modifying enzymes, including LSD1, HDAC1, HDAC2, PRC2, and others to the E-cadherin promoter, inducing DNMT-mediated DNA methylation [27,28]. Earlier studies demonstrated that downregulation of E-cadherin in metastatic PDAC cells was guided by a SNAI1/HDAC1/HDAC2 repressor complex [29]. Importantly, PDAC models and human samples confirmed these findings. It is generally accepted that there is a global increase in DNA methylation after a period of hypoxia, which can be at least in part attributable to HIF-mediated expression of histone-modifying enzymes [30].

Given the limited options for PDAC treatment and the suggested role of DNA methylation in cancer treatment resistance, understanding epigenetic mechanisms underlying PDAC invasiveness and metastasis makes it possible to identify new therapeutic targets [31]. Herein, we examined the extent to which epigenetic regulation influences gene expression of EMT-related genes in PDAC. Particularly, the role of DNA methylation in the inflammation- and hypoxia-driven EMT model has been investigated in a subset of PDAC cell lines.

2. Results

Four PDAC cell lines, BxPC-3, MIA PaCa-2, and PANC-1, derived from the primary adenocarcinoma, and SU86.86 cells derived from liver metastasis, were used to assess EMT-related changes in gene expression and DNA methylation. Inflammatory conditions were modeled by indirect cell co-cultivation through a conditioned media (CM) containing a wide range of cytokines and inflammatory molecules produced by activated fibroblasts [32]. Cells were cultured in a monolayer for two and six days in either DMEM under normoxic conditions (Control), CM in normoxia (CM), DMEM in hypoxia (1% O_2, HY), or CM in hypoxia (CM + HY) (for details, see Material and Methods).

2.1. Inflammation and Hypoxia-Mediated Gene Expression Changes after 2-Day Exposure

To identify inflammation- and hypoxia-induced EMT-related gene expression changes, we used Cancer Inflammation and Immunity Crosstalk RT^2 Profiler and Human Epithelial to Mesenchymal Transition RT^2 Profiler PCR Arrays (PAHS-181Z and PAHS-090ZA, respectively). Each of them allowed us to analyze 84 genes or biological pathways, either mediating communication between tumor cells and the cellular mediators of inflammation and immunity or tumor metastasis, stem cell differentiation, and development. A two-fold change (FC) was set as a cut-off for upregulation and 0.5 for downregulation. An example of an inflammatory factor present in CM is CXCL12 (13.7% increase in CM over DMEM, unpublished data), a ligand for the C-X-C motif chemokine receptor 4 (CXCR4). Increased content of proinflammatory IL-1α in the CM (10.3%, unpublished data), which constitutively activates the NF-κB signaling pathway, could influence the expression of other inflammatory genes such as vascular endothelial growth factor A (*VEGFA*). However, only a few inflammatory genes showed more than two-fold change after cultivating cells in CM alone (Figure 1a). *VEGFA* upregulation by HY and CM + HY was found in all cell lines except for PANC-1. The highest upregulation of the C-C motif chemokine ligand 5 (*CCL5*) gene was induced by CM + HY. With the upregulation of 18 (Figure 1b) and downregulation of 14 genes (Figure 1c), the BxPC-3 cell line was the most sensitive to CM + HY exposure. Although 19 inflammatory genes were upregulated by more than two-fold in the MIA PaCa-2 cell line, the magnitude of these changes was lower, and only one was downregulated below 0.5-fold. The PANC-1 and SU.86.86 cell lines were more resistant to studied factors with upregulation of only a small number of the analyzed genes (7 and 8, respectively), while downregulation below 0.5-fold was observed only in 3 and 5 genes in these cell lines, respectively. In general, hypoxia was a more potent factor in inducing an inflammatory response in cells. The combination of CM + HY had the most pronounced effect on changes in inflammatory gene expression, with the *CXCR4* receptor gene being among the top upregulated in all cell lines. The top downregulated gene was *CCL11* by HY in BxPC-3 cells.

Extensive changes were found in the expression levels of EMT-related genes, although their magnitude was lower than for inflammatory genes (Figure 2a). In line with previous results, showing 17 and 22 upregulated and 10 and 13 downregulated genes by HY and CM + HY, respectively, the BxPC-3 cells were the most sensitive to studied factors (Figure 2b,c). Although the top-upregulated *VIM* gene showed an almost 100-fold change in BxPC-3 cells due to HY, no changes in *VIM* expression were found in the other cell lines. The top downregulated gene, *STEAP1*, with fold regulation value −27.0, was identified in the same cell line. CM-induced gene expression changes were milder, except for MIA PaCa-2 with 16 upregulated and 2 downregulated genes. However, only 2 genes were upregulated and 4 downregulated in this cell line by a combination of CM + HY. Interestingly, some of the genes upregulated in MIA PaCa-2 were downregulated in other cell lines, e.g., *KRT19*. The most resistant to all experimental conditions were PANC-1 cells, where CM + HY only upregulated 7 and downregulated 3 genes.

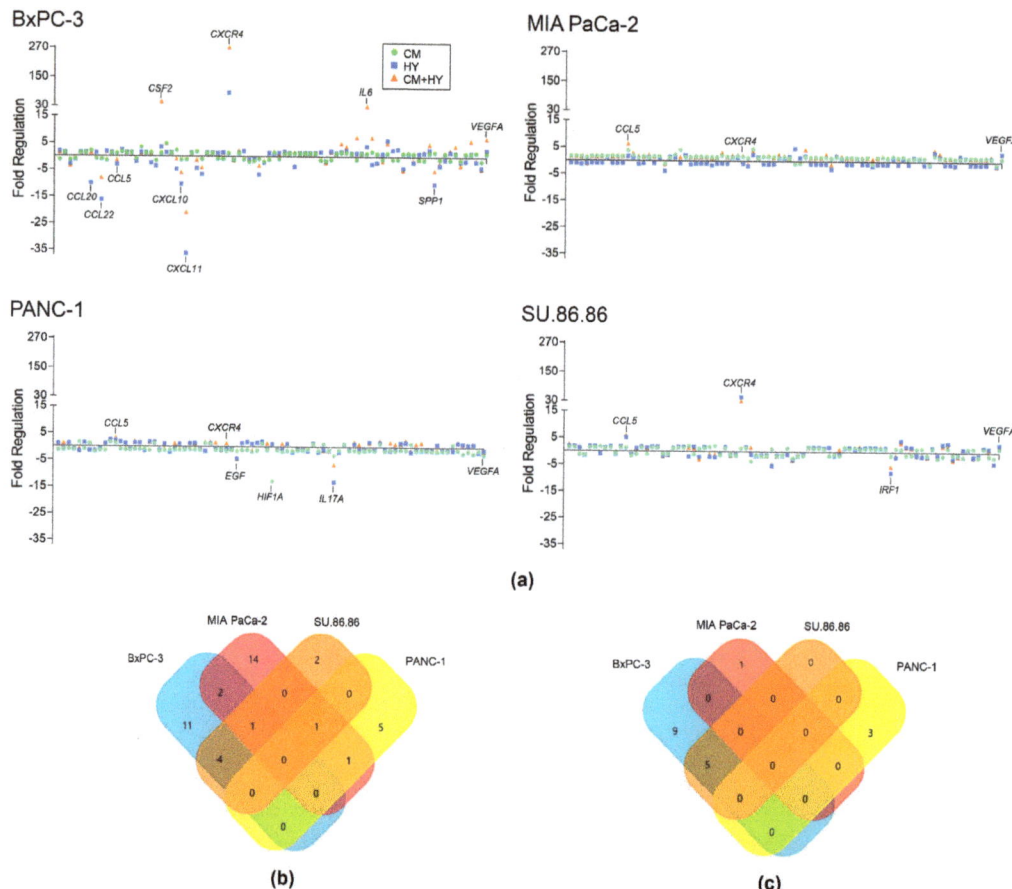

Figure 1. Inflammatory gene expression changes after 2-day cultivation of cells in inflammatory (CM), hypoxic (HY) conditions, and their combination (CM + HY) measured using Cancer Inflammation and Immunity Crosstalk RT^2 Profiler PCR Array (**a**). Gene expression changes are plotted as fold regulation values (−1/fold change for FC below 1); (**b**) Venn diagram showing overlapping genes with more than two-fold upregulation by CM + HY exposure; (**c**) Venn diagram showing overlapping genes with more than two-fold downregulation by CM + HY exposure. CM, conditioned media; HY, 1% hypoxia.

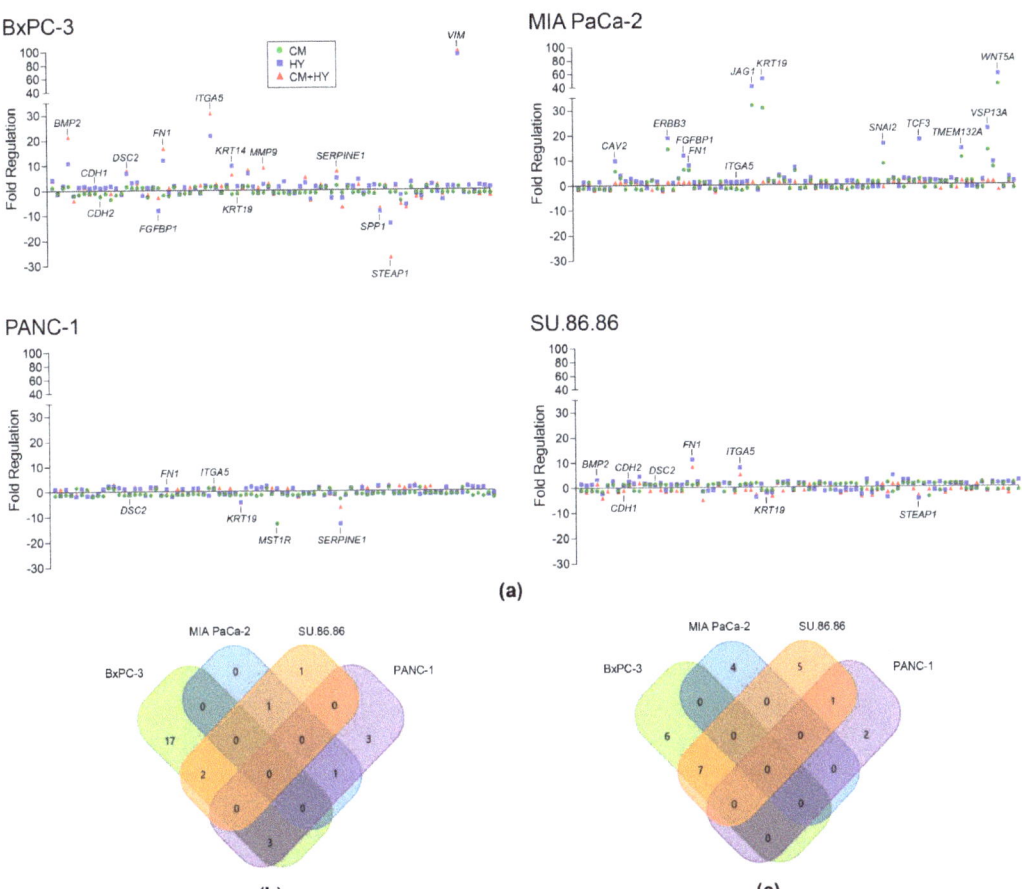

Figure 2. EMT gene expression changes after 2-days cultivation of cells in inflammatory (CM), hypoxic (HY) conditions and their combination (CM + HY) measured using Human Epithelial to Mesenchymal Transition RT^2 Profiler PCR Array (**a**) Gene expression changes are plotted as fold regulation values (−1/fold change for FC below 1); (**b**) Venn diagram showing overlapping genes with more than two-fold upregulation by CM + HY exposure; (**c**) Venn diagram showing overlapping genes with more than two-fold downregulation by CM + HY exposure. CM, conditioned media; HY, 1% hypoxia.

Based on these findings and published literature, three inflammatory genes (*CCL5, CXCR4, VEGFA*), five EMT-TFs (*SNAI1, SNAI2, ZEB1, ZEB2, TWIST1*), and 12 EMT-related genes (*CDH1, KRT19, OCLN, STEAP1, TSPAN13, CDH2, FN1, ITGA5, BMP2, NID2, SERPINE1,* and *DSC2*), were selected for validation/analysis by qRT-PCR. Genotyping assays and primer sequences are listed in Materials and Methods and Tables S1 and S2.

Gene expression changes after 2-day exposure to experimental conditions (CM, HY and CM + HY) are provided in Figure 3 and Table S3. In agreement with previous findings, *CXCR4* was upregulated by HY and CM + HY in all studied cell lines. A significant upregulation of *VEGFA* gene expression was observed due to CM and CM + HY in BxPC-3 cells and all studied combinations in SU.86.86 cells. MIA PaCa-2 and PANC-1 showed to be relatively resistant to all treatment conditions. In line with the data from the PCR array, the *CCL5* gene was downregulated in BxPC-3 cells, while its upregulation was observed in MIA PaCa-2, PANC-1, and SU.86.86 cell lines.

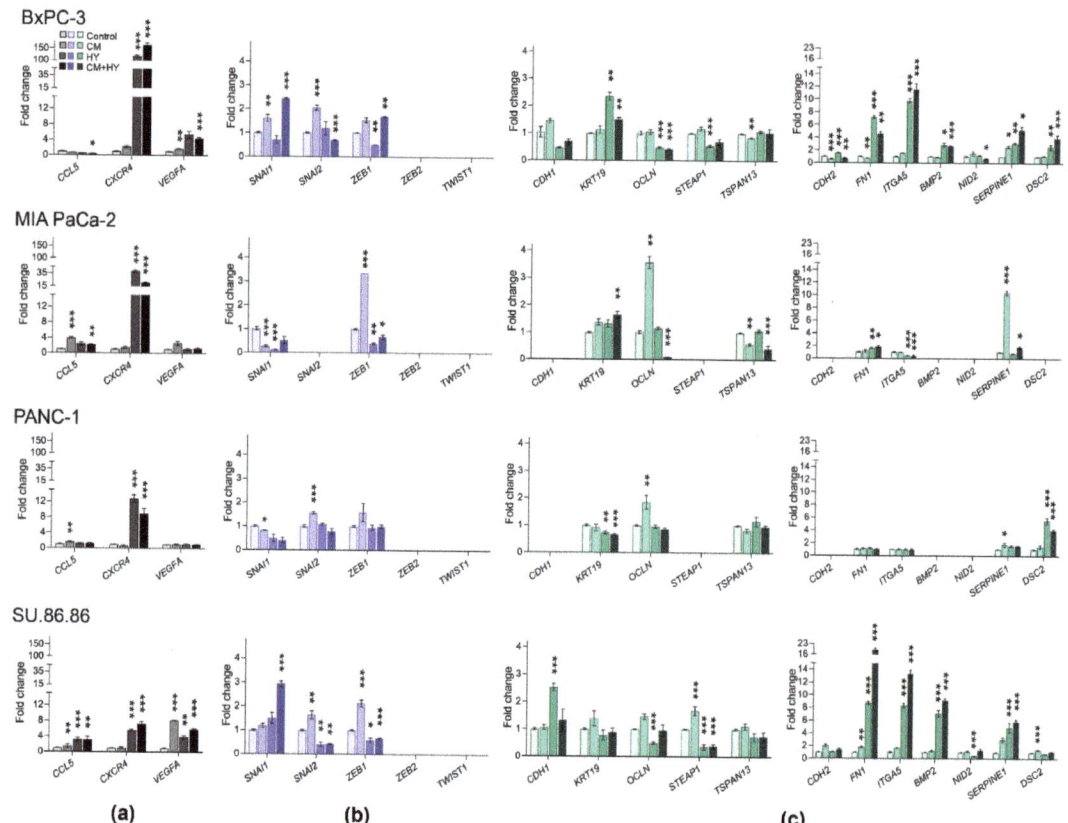

Figure 3. Changes in the expression of (**a**) inflammatory, (**b**) EMT-TFs, and (**c**) EMT-related genes after 2-day cell cultivation in inflammatory (CM), hypoxic (HY) conditions, and their combination (CM + HY), relative to Control. Inflammatory genes are highlighted by grey, EMT-TFs by blue, and EMT-related genes by green color; CM, conditioned media; HY, 1% hypoxia; * $p < 0.05$, ** $p < 0.01$, *** $p < 0.001$.

Gene expression of the EMT-TFs was affected moderately, with most changes below two-fold, except for *SNAI1* by CM + HY in BxPc-3 and SU.86.86 cells and *ZEB1* by CM in MIA PaCa-2 and SU.86.86. None of the analyzed cell lines expressed the *TWIST1* and *ZEB2* genes. Surprisingly, EMT-TFs were frequently downregulated after 2-day treatment.

CDH1 and *CDH2* genes were not expressed in the MIA PaCa-2 and PANC-1 cells. We confirmed the downregulation of several epithelial genes, mainly *OCLN* and *STEAP1*, in BxPc-3 and SU.86.86. The most significant upregulations of mesenchymal genes were found again in BxPC-3 and SU.86.86 cell lines, with the most significant changes in *FN1* and *ITGA5* due to HY and CM + HY exposure. *BMP2* was not expressed in MIA PaCa-2 and PANC-1, while its expression increased significantly due to HY and CM + HY in BxPC-3 and SU.86.86 cells. Gene expression changes in MIA PaCa-2 and PANC-1 cells were minor, mainly due to the relatively high number of silenced genes (*CDH1*, *STEAP1*, *CDH2*, *BMP2*, and *NID2*, while *DSC2* in MIA PaCa-2 only).

2.2. Global and Gene-Specific DNA Methylation in Individual Cell Lines

The LINE-1, which represents a surrogate marker of global methylation level and promoter DNA methylation of 15 EMT genes, including TFs, was assessed in all studied cell lines using the quantitative pyrosequencing method described in detail in Materials and Methods (Figure 4). Global DNA methylation varied between 46% in BxPC-3, 79% in MIA PaCa-2, 69% in PANC-1, and 60% in SU.86.86 cells. Low DNA methylation was found for EMT-TFs, with methylation levels below 10%. However, *SNAI1* and *SNAI2* in MIA PaCa-2 cells and *TWIST1* in all cell lines were highly methylated (between 53% and 95%). Importantly, the DNA methylation level strongly correlated with gene expression in most studied genes. High promoter methylation was found particularly in silenced genes, in MIA PaCa-2 and PANC-1 cells, *TWIST1* (95%, 79%), *STEAP1* (83%, 53%), *CDH2* (95%, 95%), *BMP2* (84%, 61%), *NID2* (88%, 84%), respectively and *DSC2* (80% in MIA PaCa-2). Nevertheless, DNA methylation of the *CDH1* gene was low (between 6% and 12%) despite inhibited gene expression in MIA PaCa-2 and PANC-1 cells.

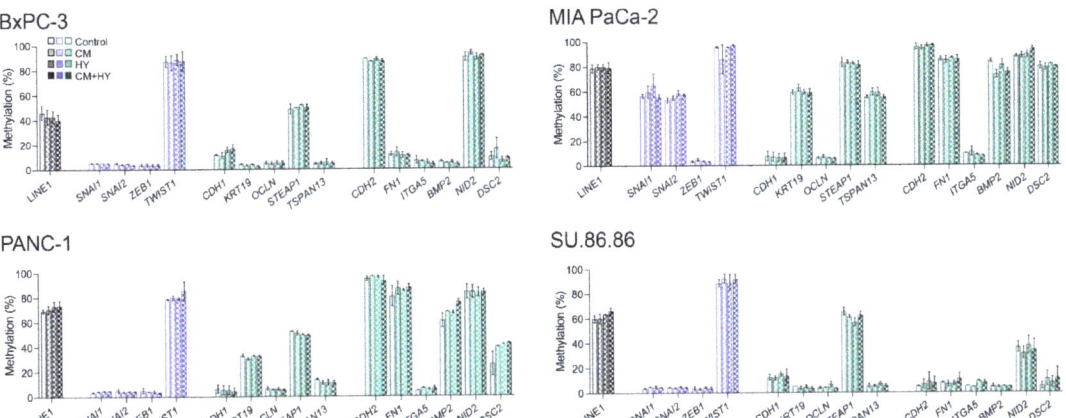

Figure 4. Global and promoter DNA methylation of individual genes and changes induced by 2-day exposure. EMT-TFs are highlighted by blue, EMT-related genes by green color; CM, conditioned media, HY, 1% hypoxia; no significant changes induced by a 2-day exposure to individual conditions were found.

In BxPC-3, only four genes, *TWIST1* (87%), *CDH2* (89%), *NID2* (90%), and *STEAP1* (49%), were highly methylated, while in SU.86.86 cells, there were only three genes, *TWIST1* (89%), *NID2* (36%), and *STEAP1* (65%). Experimental conditions did not significantly affect global or gene-specific DNA methylation after a 2-day exposure.

2.3. Prolonged Treatment-Induced EMT-Related Gene Expression and DNA Methylation Changes

Due to negative findings for DNA methylation changes after 2-days, we extended exposure time up to 6 days to rule out the possibility that the exposure time was too short for the methylation changes to take effect. During this time, the cells survived in the given experimental conditions without subculturing and significantly reduced viability (by more than 20%).

Gene expression changes after 6-day exposure to experimental conditions (CM, HY and CM + HY) are provided in Figure 5 and Table S4. Interestingly, in BxPC-3 and MIA PaCa-2 cells after 6-days, the extent of *CXCR4* upregulation by HY and CM + HY was lower than after 2-days. On the other hand, *CXCR4* expression increased from 8.8-fold to 25.6-fold in PANC-1 and *VEGFA* from 5.8-fold to 18.9-fold in SU.86.86 by CM + HY (Figures 3a and 5a). In addition, *CCL5* gene expression increased significantly due to CM in MIA PaCa-2 and all exposures in SU.86.86 cells. However, upregulation of *CCL5* was milder in comparison to other genes.

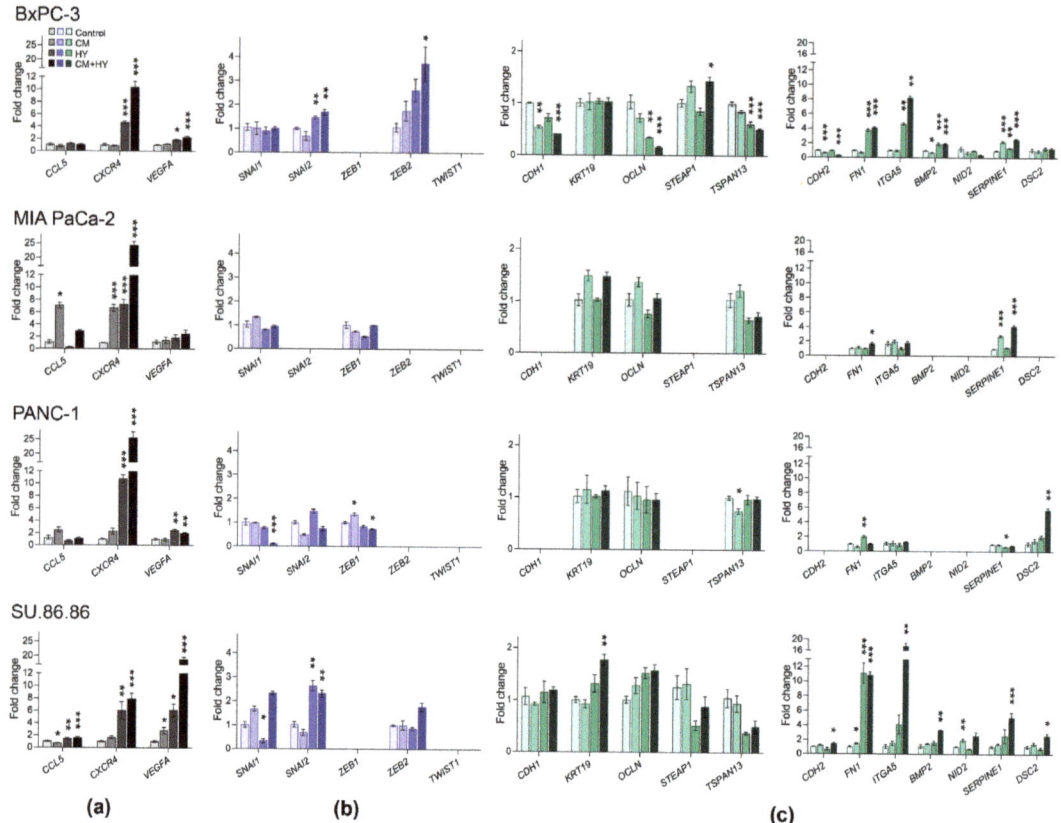

Figure 5. Changes in the expression of (**a**) inflammatory, (**b**) EMT-TFs, and (**c**) EMT-related genes after 6-day cell cultivation in inflammatory (CM), hypoxic (HY) conditions, and their combination (CM + HY), relative to Controls. Inflammatory genes are highlighted by grey, EMT-TFs by blue, and EMT-related genes by green color; CM, conditioned media, HY, 1% hypoxia; * $p < 0.05$, ** $p < 0.01$, *** $p < 0.001$.

Individual cell lines exhibited considerable differences in the expression of EMT genes (Figure 5b,c). All genes except *ZEB1* and highly methylated *TWIST1* were expressed in BxPC-3 and SU.86.86 cells. However, many genes, including *CDH1*, were not expressed in MIA PaCa-2 and PANC-1 cells.

A significant decrease of three epithelial genes, *CDH1*, *OCLN*, and *TSPAN13*, was identified in BxPC-3 cells. On the other hand, expression of four mesenchymal genes, *FN1*, *ITGA5*, *BMP2*, and *SERPINE1*, increased significantly, while *CDH2* was downregulated. In MIA PaCa-2 cells, upregulation of more than two-fold was identified in the *SERPINE1* gene only. In PANC-1 cells, downregulation of *SNAI1* was accompanied by upregulation of *DSC2*. Although expression of epithelial genes in SU.86.86 cells did not change more than two-fold, most mesenchymal genes were upregulated mainly by CM + HY, namely *FN1*, *ITGA5*, *BMP2*, *SERPINE1*, and *DSC2*.

Due to small DNA methylation changes after 2-day exposure, only LINE-1 and five representative genes with the most prominent expression changes were selected for analysis after 6-day exposure (Figure 6). Simultaneously, we assessed gene expression changes of three DNMTs and the *TET1* gene. *DNMT1* and *DNMT3B* decreased significantly in all cell lines except *DNMT1* in MIA PaCa-2. The *TET1* gene was not expressed in BxPC-3 cells; however, its expression increased significantly in MIA PaCa-2 by exposure to CM + HY while decreased by the same condition in PANC-1 cells. No changes were found in SU.86.86 cells.

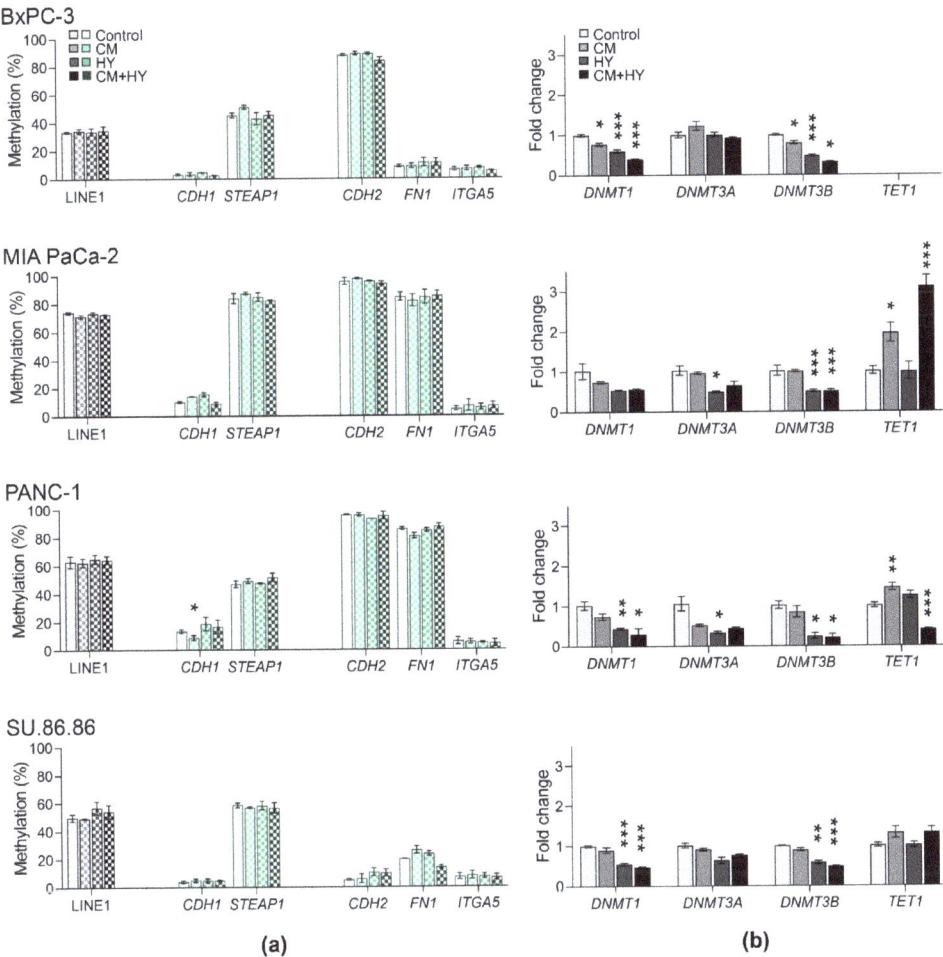

Figure 6. DNA methylation changes and gene expression after 6-day exposure; (**a**) global and gene-specific DNA methylation levels of selected genes; (**b**) expression of epigenetic effectors; CM, conditioned media, HY, 1% hypoxia; * $p < 0.05$, ** $p < 0.01$, *** $p < 0.001$.

The expression of hallmark EMT protein, E-cadherin, and DNMT1, considered maintenance DNMT, were assessed in all cell lines by western blot. This method confirmed changes found by qRT-PCR (Figure 7), showing that E-cadherin was expressed in BxPC-3 and SU.86.86 cells only. Its expression decreased significantly after 6-day exposure in the BxPC-3 cell line and SU.86.86 by CM. DNMT1 expression decreased significantly by CM + HY in BxPC-3, MIA PaCa-2, and SU.86.86 cells, while it increased by CM in PANC-1.

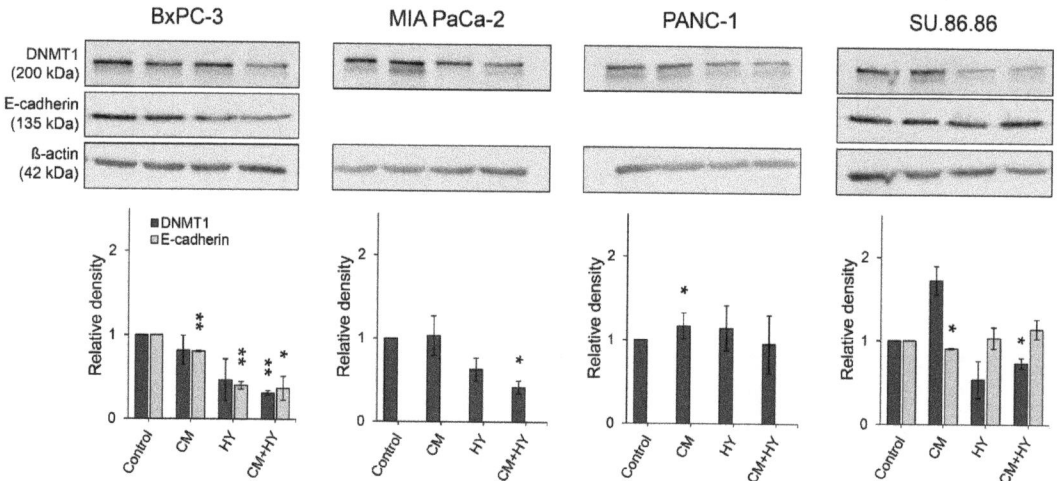

Figure 7. Western blot analysis and quantification by densitometry of DNMT1 and E-cadherin protein levels in the normoxic and hypoxic conditions enriched with conditioned media; CM, conditioned media, HY, 1% hypoxia; * $p < 0.05$, ** $p < 0.01$.

2.4. Gene Expression and DNA Methylation Changes Induced by Decitabine

To confirm that the expression of studied genes was mediated by DNA methylation, we used DNMT inhibitor decitabine (DAC) (Figure 8, Table S5). Non-cytotoxic DAC concentrations (cell viability over 80%) were selected based on the results of the luminescence assay (Figure 8a). Given the mode of action and low stability, DAC was added daily for 3 days to allow cell division. Due to the expected decrease of DNA methylation by DAC, only seven highly methylated genes were analyzed for DAC-induced DNA methylation changes, and genes with low promoter methylation were excluded from pyrosequencing analysis (Figure 8b). However, *TWIST1* and all EMT-related genes were assessed for gene expression changes (Figure 8c). DAC efficiently decreased DNA methylation in the majority of highly methylated genes. A significant decrease was found for *TWIST1*, *CDH2*, and *NID2* in BxPC-3; for all studied genes in MIA PaCa-2; *TWIST1*, *CDH2*, *FN1*, *NID2*, and *DSC2* in PANC-1 cells, and *TWIST1* in SU.86.86.

Gene expression of all studied genes except for *STEAP1* increased significantly after DAC treatment in BxPC-3 cells, with more than two-fold increase in *OCLN*, *CDH2*, *FN1*, *ITGA5*, *BMP2*, and *DSC2*. In MIA PaCa-2 five genes were upregulated, *KRT19*, *TSPAN13*, *FN1*, and *ITGA5*. In PANC-1 it was *TSPAN13* and *DSC2*. Finally, in SU.86.86 cell line *OCLN*, *CDH2*, *FN1*, *ITGA5*, *BMP2*, *NID2*, and *DSC2* genes were upregulated.

Importantly, DAC reactivated gene expression of all silenced genes (Figure 8d), including *TWIST1* in all cell lines, *CDH1* in MIA PaCa-2, and PANC-1. Moreover, *STEAP1*, *CDH2*, *BMP2*, *NID2*, and *DSC2* were reactivated in the MIA PaCa-2 cell line, and *CDH2*, *STEAP1*, *BMP2*, in PANC-1 cells. However, significant upregulation was also found in the genes with low methylation levels, whose methylation did not change significantly, e.g., *FN1*, *BMP2*, and *DSC2* in BxPC-3 cells, and *CDH2*, *FN1*, *BMP2*, and *DSC2* in SU.86.86 cells.

To evaluate the potential translational significance of our findings, we assessed the difference in the expression of analyzed EMT-related genes between PDAC and normal pancreatic tissues using The online Gene Expression Profiling Interactive Analysis (GEPIA) tool. GEPIA is a valuable and highly cited resource for gene expression analysis based on tumor and normal samples from The Cancer Genome Atlas (TCGA) and the Genotype-Tissue Expression (GTEx) databases (GEPIA (Gene Expression Profiling Interactive Analysis). Available online: http://gepia.cancer-pku.cn/ (accessed on 16 December 2021)) [33]. Based on the available data, mRNA expression of nearly all analyzed genes, except for *OCLN* and *TSPAN13*, was significantly upregulated in PDAC samples (Figure 9).

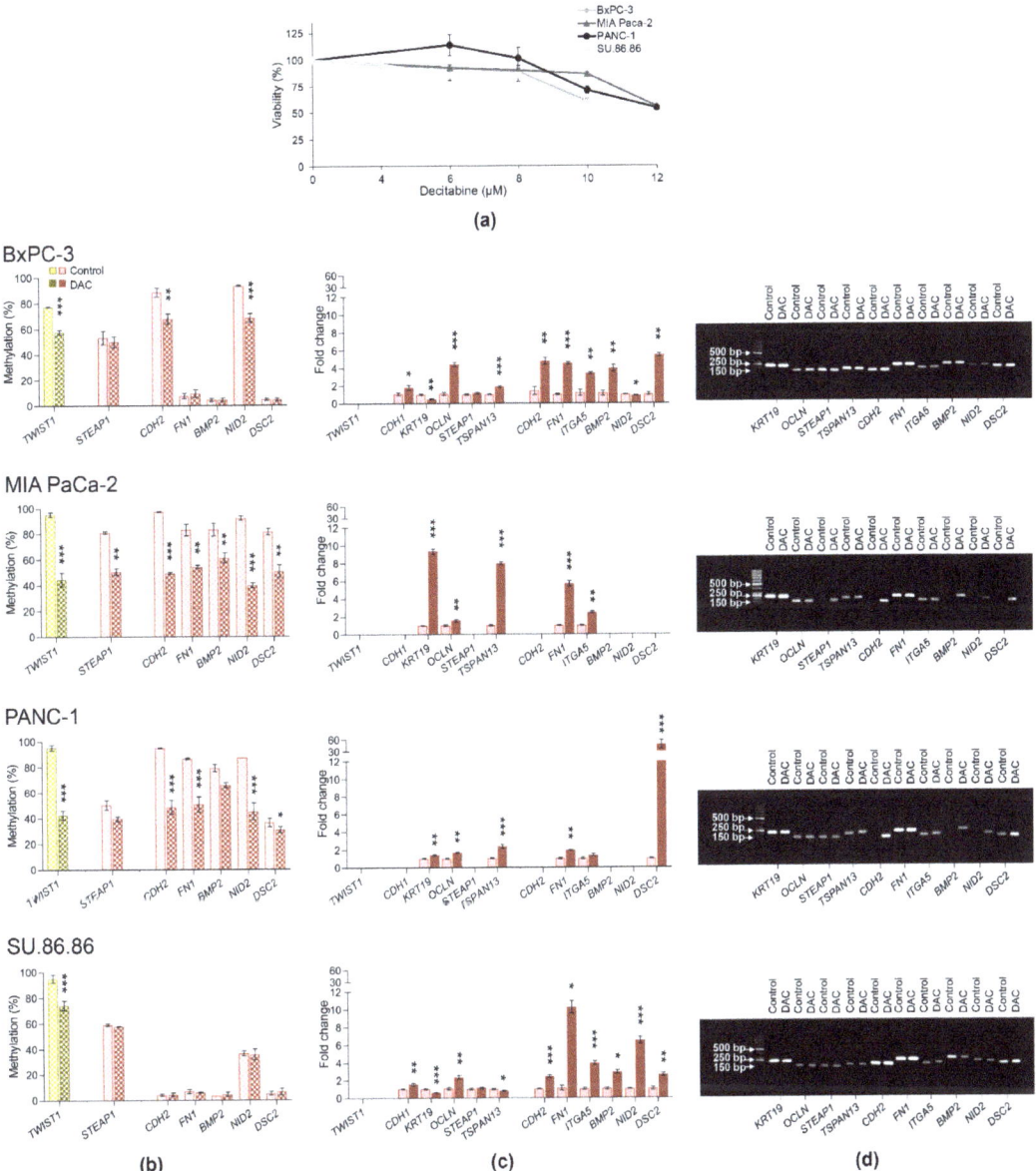

Figure 8. Changes in DNA methylation and gene expression induced by exposure to sub-cytotoxic decitabine (DAC) concentrations in PDAC cell lines. (**a**) Cell viability after DAC treatment; (**b**) DAC-induced DNA methylation changes in *TWIST1* (highlighted by yellow) and selected EMT-related genes (highlighted by red); (**c**) DAC-induced changes in the expression of *TWIST1* and EMT-related genes; (**d**) reactivation of gene expression; representative gels are shown for individual genes except for *TWIST1* and *CDH1*, * $p < 0.05$, ** $p < 0.01$, *** $p < 0.001$.

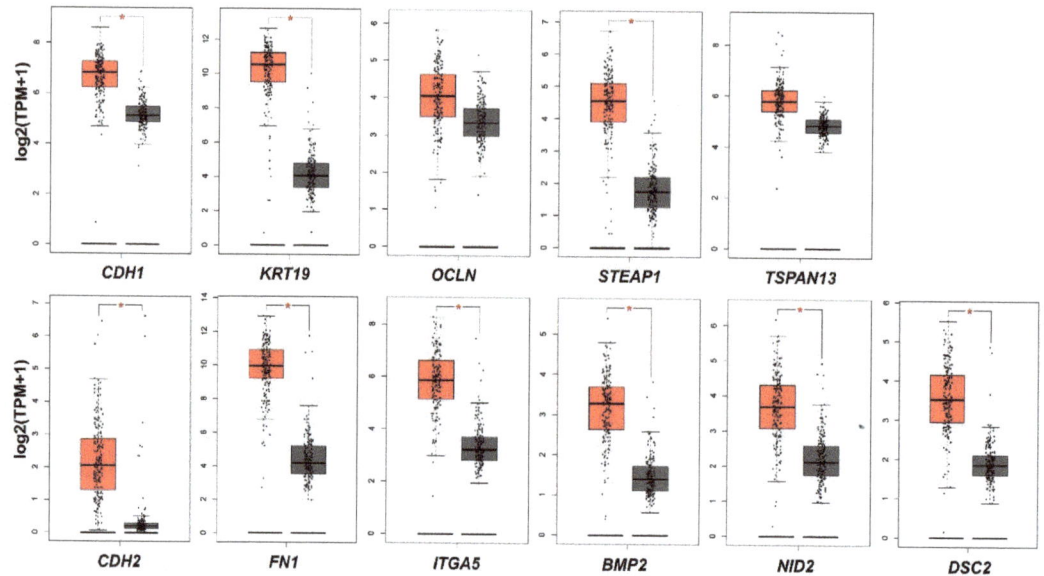

Figure 9. Comparison of studied EMT-related genes mRNA expression in PDAC and normal pancreatic tissues. * $p < 0.05$. The expression level is described as log2(TPM + 1). Red highlighted are PDAC tissues (n = 179), grey are normal pancreatic tissues (n = 171); TPM, transcript per million.

3. Discussion

Dense desmoplastic fibrotic stroma, the rapid proliferation of cancer cells, and poor vascularization contribute to the hypoxic microenvironment of PDAC [13]. Repression of E-cadherin and other genes involved in cell–cell and cell–basal membrane contacts are among the EMT features, leading to loss of epithelial characteristics, acquisition of a mesenchymal-like phenotype, and a worse prognosis. In addition to the EMT-TFs and cadherins, the role of other EMT-related genes has not been elucidated in PDAC.

In the present study, we focused on hypoxia- and inflammation-triggered gene expression changes of EMT genes and the role of DNA methylation in their regulation. Gene expression was modulated in a cell line-specific manner, with BxPC-3 cells manifesting the highest response to experimental conditions. BxPC-3 is the squamous or more basal-like human cell line, expressing the oncogenic ΔN form of TP63 (ΔNp63), present in human primary PDAC samples of this subtype. Interestingly, we found a high degree of similarity in gene expression and promoter DNA methylation patterns between BxPC-3 and metastatic SU.86.86 cells, the same as between MIA PaCa-2 and PANC-1 cells. Unique molecular features, including epithelial-mesenchymal phenotype and neuroendocrine differentiation attributed to MIA PaCa-2 and PANC-1 [34], together with divergent genetic profiles, may be responsible for a distinct response of the studied cell lines to experimental conditions [35].

Systemic and local chronic inflammation might enhance the risk of PDAC. The dynamic crosstalk between inflammatory and cancer cells is maintained by soluble mediators, cytokines, and chemokines, which are synthesized by the host tumor and stromal cells. They were shown to play an essential role in cellular proliferation, angiogenesis, metastasis, and immune evasion [36]. In agreement with the demonstrated role of hypoxia in inducing CXCR4 expression in cancer, we found *CXCR4* the most significantly upregulated gene by hypoxic conditions, independently of inflammatory stimuli. Accordingly, the expression of CXCR4 mediated the development of liver and lung metastasis in the pancreatic cancer animal model [37]. A positive correlation was documented between CXCR4 expression and PDAC progression, including hematogenous dissemination [38]. However, the relationship between the expression of CXCR4 in PDAC and clinicopathological parameters remains inconclusive. Although several studies described CXCR4 overexpression as a robust prognostic marker correlated with the risk of lymph node involvement and distant metastasis [39], recent findings from more than 3600 PDAC samples documented a higher CXCR4 expression in primary tumors than distant metastases [40]. CCL5 was one of 3 inflammatory cytokines deregulated in more than one cell line herein. The CCL5/ C-C motif chemokine receptor 5 (CCR5) axis gains increasing attention due to its involvement in tumor progression through multiple mechanisms, including immunosuppressive polarization, metabolic reprogramming, and ECM remodeling, facilitating migration and invasion of tumor cells [41]. The CCL5 has been identified as a key chemokine for Treg cells infiltration in PDAC. Moreover, besides elevated expression of CCL5 in poorly differentiated PDAC tissues compared to non-neoplastic and moderately differentiated, CCL5/CCR5 axis interaction was shown to promote migratory and invasiveness of PDAC BxPC-3, MIA PACa-2, and AsPC-1 cells [42]. Tumor proliferation is associated with the expression of pro-angiogenic factors, particularly VEGF. VEGF-A/VEGFR-2 signaling was shown to play a crucial role in the motility of pancreas cancer cells [43]. Accordingly, high expression of VEGFA was associated with a worse prognosis in PDAC [44].

Herein we found several EMT-related genes induced by hypoxia. This upregulation occurred only in cell lines and genes with low promoter DNA methylation. Although inflammation- and hypoxia-induced DNA methylation changes were negligible, differences in global and gene-specific DNA methylation between studied primary cell lines of the same origin (derived from pancreatic epithelial tissues) suggest an essential role of DNA methylation in PDAC tumorigenesis. However, in in vitro models, tumor cells acquire stable epigenetic marks after sustained cultivation of tumor cells under EMT-inducing conditions [45].

Furthermore, the regulatory function of DNA methylation in gene expression regulation was confirmed by the reactivation of silenced genes by DAC. This DNMT inhibitor is a deoxycytidine analog typically used to reactivate gene expression silenced by promoter methylation [46]. DAC incorporation into DNA leads to depletion of DNMT1 and passive demethylation. DAC induces gene expression changes also indirectly via demethylation of upstream genes, regulatory elements, or changes in histone modifications [47]. Although a significant decrease of DNA methylation accompanied reactivation of silenced genes, low DNA methylation levels of several upregulated genes, among them *CDH1*, suggest an indirect effect of DAC on their expression.

By default, in epithelial tissue-derived tumors, a reduction of epithelial genes and induction of mesenchymal phenotype is associated with EMT and higher tumor proliferation, motility, and metastasis. Among other reasons, high methylation levels of nearly all mesenchymal genes except for *ITGA5* in MIA PaCa-2 and PANC-1 cells can explain their resistance to experimental conditions. Herein, we discuss only genes differentially expressed in PDAC tissues compared to controls in TCGA dataset. Besides cadherins, whose role is well established in EMT and PDAC pathogenesis, we mainly focus on mesenchymal genes or those with a somewhat controversial role in EMT not associated yet with PDAC pathogenesis. The most upregulated *FN1* gene encodes the glycoprotein fibronectin found in the ECM, interacting with proteins such as collagen, fibrin, proteoglycans, and others [48]. Hypoxic conditions significantly increased *FN1* expression in BxPC-3 and SU.86.86 PDAC cell lines characterized by low promoter methylation. In agreement with previously published findings, FN1 induction by hypoxia directly correlated with the expression of its integrin receptor ITGA5 [49]. FN1 is primarily expressed in fibroblasts but can also be produced by other cell types, including cancer and endothelial cells [50]. Its expression is significantly increased in many solid tumors, including PDAC [51], promoting progression and metastasis [52]. High FN1 expression in PDAC tissues correlates with higher tumor weight, more advanced disease, and poorer prognosis after resection [53]. TGF-β stimulates FN1 expression and its transport to the extracellular space, where it participates in the EMT process. Knockdown of major TFs of the TGF-β pathway, SNAI1/2, and SMAD4, led to decreased FN1 expression, consequent EMT inhibition, and decreased tumor cell motility [54]. FN1 and ITGA5 also play an important role in tumor angiogenesis, although the mode of action has not been elucidated [55]. ITGA5 has been shown to potentiate the aggressiveness of cancer cells and their resistance to chemotherapy in animal models [56]. Increased methylation of the *ITGA5* gene has been associated with lower expression and increased invasiveness in breast tumors. However, its inactivation resulting in inhibition of cell division suggests diverse roles of ITGA5 [57]. The *STEAP1* belongs to the group of metalloreductases and is involved in tumor cell proliferation and suppresses apoptosis [58]. It is overexpressed in several types of human tumor tissues and cell lines, including tumors of the colon, pancreas, ovary, testis, and breast [59]. The role of this protein in cancer is controversial. While its expression inhibited metastasis in breast cancer, it was correlated with metastasis and EMT induction in lung adenocarcinoma [60,61]. In gastric tumors, the upregulation of *STEAP1* increased cell proliferation, migration, and invasion [62]. The *DSC2* gene is essential for desmosome formation in epithelial cells and is involved in epithelial morphogenesis, differentiation, wound healing, cell apoptosis, migration, and proliferation [63]. Low DSC2 expression has been reported to promote invasiveness and is involved in EMT in several types of epithelial tissue-derived tumors, including PDAC [64]. Highly differentiated PDAC tissues were also characterized by higher DSC2 expression compared to less differentiated ones, in which the complete absence of DSC2 was often observed [65]. The *NID2* gene encodes one of the basic components of the basement membrane and plays a key role in embryogenesis and the development of malignant tumors. In vitro experiments suggest that NID2 promotes invasiveness and migration in gastric carcinoma-derived tumor cells, where it was significantly overexpressed compared to healthy tissues [66]. Increased NID2 expression also correlated significantly with overall survival in gastric cancer patients [67]. Abnormal hypermethylation of the *NID2* promoter associated with suppression of its expression is known in aggressive types of breast tumors [68]. BMP2 is a growth factor that plays an important role in PDAC carcinogenesis [69]. It has been investigated as a potential prognostic marker in PDAC, but no significant correlation with survival or prognosis has been reported [70]. The BMP2 protein participates in the initiation and progression of several types of solid tumors, and its increased expression in the PDAC cell line PANC-1 has led to increased proliferation in both in vitro and in vivo models, presumably through impaired autocrine signaling [71]. BMP2 can also induce the EMT process and increase invasiveness in the PANC-1 cell line by activating the PI3K/Akt pathway [72]. The high level of BMP2 gene methylation in colorectal cancer is a negative prognostic marker typical for the third stage of the disease [73].

Hypoxia and inflammation play an essential role in the pathogenesis of PDAC, causing acidosis and the formation of reactive oxygen species and inducing genetic instability in pancreatic epithelial cells. Epigenomic landscapes explain the progression of PDAC into classical or more aggressive basal subtypes. Moreover, EMT plasticity suggests that the epigenetic landscapes are implicated in the dynamic events underlying mesenchymal and intermediate phenotypes responsible for tumor cell dissemination. This work shed light on the role of DNA methylation in the transcriptional regulation of several EMT genes. DNA methylation-mediated reactivation of silenced genes has a critical translational impact. However, further studies are warranted to investigate epigenetic drug efficacy in synergy with other anticancer therapies and possible off-target effects.

4. Materials and Methods

4.1. Pancreatic Cancer Cell Lines

In the present study, we used four epithelial PDAC cell lines, BxPC-3, MIA PaCa-2, PANC-1 derived from primary adenocarcinoma, and SU.86.86 derived from liver metastasis. The clinical course of the donor patients, site of derivation, histopathological appearance, and differentiation were described elsewhere [35]. These cells harbor different genetic backgrounds reflected in their phenotypic characteristics. BxPC-3 cells are KRAS negative, while MIA PaCa-2 possess G12C, PANC-1 G12D, and SU.86.86 G12D KRAS mutation, all have a homozygous deletion in exons 2 and 6 of p16 and variable mutations of *TP53*. Except for BxPC-3 with a homozygous deletion in exons 1–11, they do not carry *SMAD4* mutations. All cells were cultivated at 37 °C in a humidified atmosphere (5 % CO_2) and maintained in high-glucose (4.5 g/L) Dulbecco's modified Eagle medium (DMEM, PAA Laboratories GmbH, Pasching, Austria) supplemented with 10% fetal bovine serum (FBS, Biochrom AG, Berlin, Germany), 2 mM glutamine (PAA Laboratories GmbH), and 10 μg/mL gentamicin (Sandoz, Nürnberg, Germany). The cell cultures were regularly tested for mycoplasma contamination by PCR.

4.2. Cell Viability

For viability assay, the cells were seeded into 96-well plates at a density of 5.5×10^3 cells/well for BxPC-3, 1.9×10^3 cells/well for MIA PaCa-2, 3.0×10^3 cells/well for PANC-1, 4.8×10^3 cells/well for SU.86.86 and exposed to different concentrations of DAC (MedChem Express, Shanghai, China) (4–12 μM) added every 24 h in a total of 72 h. To assess the relative viability of cells, CellTiter-Glo® Luminescent Cell Viability Assay (Promega Corporation, Madison, WI, USA) and GloMax® Discover Microplate Reader (Promega Corporation, Madison, WI, USA) were used. Cell viability was determined as the luminescence intensity relative to untreated control cells (set to 100%). The results are presented as means ± SEM from at least two independent experiments in quadruplicates.

4.3. Cell Exposure

The pancreatic cells were indirectly co-cultured with contact-activated stromal fibroblasts to establish an experimental fibro-inflammatory in vitro model [74]. As previously described, activated fibroblasts were characterized by the production of inflammation-associated cytokines and growth factors, e.g., IL-1, IL-6, IL-8, IL-11, LIF, GM-CSF, and COX-2 related- prostaglandins [32]. All PDAC cell lines were cultivated with or without a conditioned medium (CM) for 2 and 6 days in normoxic or hypoxic conditions. Hypoxic experiments were carried out in the hypoxic workstation (Ruskinn Technologies, Bridgend, UK) in a 1% O_2, 2% H_2, 5% CO_2, 92% N_2 atmosphere at 37 °C.

For detection of the DAC-induced (DAC, MedChem Express, Shanghai, China) gene expression and DNA methylation changes, the cells were seeded on Petri dishes (60 mm) at a 250×10^3 cells/dish density. Subsequently, subcytotoxic concentrations of DAC (cell viability around 80%) were added every 24 h in a total of 72 h (for BxPC-3 and SU.86.86 6 μM DAC; for MIA PaCa-2 and PANC-1 8 μM DAC).

4.4. Expression Arrays

After exposure to individual experimental conditions, RNA was extracted from cell pellets using miRNeasy Mini Kit (Qiagen, Hilden, Germany). The RNA quality and quantity were assessed using NanoDrop® ND-1000 spectrophotometer (Thermo Fisher Scientific, Wilmington, DE, USA), and 2.5 μg of total RNA was reverse transcribed by RT^2 First Strand Kit (Qiagen, Hilden, Germany), following manufacturer instructions.

Cancer Inflammation and Immunity Crosstalk RT^2 Profiler PCR Array (PAHS-181Z; SABiosciences, Frederick, MD, USA) was used to analyze 84 genes or biological pathways involved in mediating communication between tumor cells and the cellular mediators of inflammation and immunity. In addition, 84 genes involved in tumor metastasis or stem cell differentiation and development were analyzed by Human Epithelial to Mesenchymal Transition RT^2 Profiler PCR Array (PAHS-090ZA; SABiosciences, Frederick, MD, USA). According to the manufacturer's protocol, real-time PCR was performed using RT^2 Profiler PCR Arrays containing pre-designed primer sets in combination with RT^2 SYBR Green/ROX PCR Master Mix (Qiagen, Hilden, Germany). PCR reaction was performed on Bio-Rad CFX96 real-time PCR detection system (Bio-Rad, Hercules, CA, USA) using a 3 step cycling program: 95 °C for 10 min, 45 cycles at 95 °C for 15 s and 60 °C for 60 s. Data analysis was performed using web-based RT^2 Profiler PCR Array Data Analysis version 3.5 (Gene globe data analysis. Available online: https://geneglobe.qiagen.com/us/analyze (accessed on 16 December 2021)). The expression levels of target genes were normalized relative to the values obtained for housekeepers (*ACTB*, *B2M*, *GAPDH*, *HPRT1*, and *RPLP0*) and quantified against controls. At least a two-fold change identified in two or more cell lines was considered for validation. To represent fold-change results in a biologically meaningful way, fold regulation values were calculated for FC below 1, as −1/fold change.

4.5. qRT-PCR Analysis

Total RNA from PDAC cell lines under individual culture conditions was isolated using the NucleoSpin® RNA kit (Machery-Nagel, Düren, Germany). The RNA quality and quantity were measured using NanoDrop® ND-1000 spectrophotometer (Thermo Fisher Scientific, Wilmington, DE, USA). Revert Aid TM H minus first-strand cDNA synthesis kit (Thermo Fisher Scientific, Loughborough, UK) was used for reverse transcription of total RNA (up to 4 µg from each sample).

qRT-PCR analyses were performed with TaqMan® assays (Thermo Fisher Scientific Loughborough, UK) or individually designed gene primers (Table S1). The following TaqMan gene expression assays, *CDH1* (Hs01023894_m1), *TWIST1* (Hs00361186_m1), *SNAI1* (Hs00195591_m1), *SNAI2* (Hs00161904_m1), *ZEB1* (Hs01566408_m1), *DNMT1* (Hs00945875_m1), *DNMT3A* (Hs01027166_m1), *DNMT3B* (Hs00171876_m1) and *TET1* (Hs00286756_m1) were employed, including *HPRT1* (Hs02800695_m1) used for normalization. The reaction mix contained 10 µL of 2× Taq-Man gene expression master mix (Thermo Fisher Scientific, Loughborough, UK), 1 µL of 20× TaqMan® Assay, 9 µL of 50 ng cDNA template, and ultrapure DNase/RNase-free water. Amplification was performed on a Bio-Rad CFX96 real-time PCR detection system (Bio-Rad, Hercules, CA, USA) using the cycling program: 50 °C for 2 min, 95 °C for 10 min and 40 cycles at 95 °C for 15 s followed by 56–63 °C for 60 s, depending on primers (amplification temperatures for individual primer pairs are listed in Table S1). All samples were analyzed in triplicates. qRT-PCR analysis of *ZEB2*, *FN1*, *SERPINE1*, *CDH2*, *KRT19*, *STEAP1*, *OCLN*, *DSC2*, *NID2*, *TSPAN13*, *BMP2*, *ITGA5*, *VEGFA*, *EGF*, *CXCR4*, and *CCL5* genes was performed with individually designed primers, using *HPRT1* for normalization (Table S1). The reaction mixture consisted of 7.5 µL of 2× GoTaq® qPCR Master Mix (Promega, Madison, WI, USA), 1 µL (0.67 µM) forward primer, 1 µL (0.67 µM) reverse primer, 4.5 µL ultrapure DNase/RNase-free water, and 50 ng cDNA. Amplification was carried out on a Bio-Rad CFX96 real-time PCR detection system (Bio-Rad, Hercules, CA, USA), all samples were analyzed in triplicates. Samples with ct values over 35 were considered unexpressed. Relative mRNA expression was calculated using the $2^{-\Delta\Delta Ct}$ method [75]. Statistical analysis was applied to the dCt values. FCs above 2.0 and below 0.5 with $p < 0.05$ were discussed only.

4.6. Western Blot

Samples from all studied cell lines exposed to experimental conditions for 6 days were used for protein isolation and Western blot analysis. For protein isolation, cells were lysed with RIPA buffer (Cell Signaling Technology, Danvers, MA, USA) supplemented with PhosSTOP™ (Roche, (Mannheim, Germany) and Complete™ Protease Inhibitor Cocktail (Roche, (Mannheim, Germany). Total protein concentration was determined by Pierce™ BCA Protein Assay Kit (Thermo Fisher Scientific, Waltham, MA, USA). A total amount of 40 µg of proteins per sample was used for analysis. Samples were diluted in 4× Laemmli Sample Buffer (Bio-Rad, Hercules, CA, USA) prior to the use and denatured by heating at 95 °C for 5 min. Proteins were separated by SDS-PAGE (7.5–10%) and transferred to nitrocellulose membrane (Whatman, Dassel, Germany). The membranes were blocked in 5% non-fat milk diluted in TBS (20 mM Tris, 150 mM NaCl) for 1 h and incubated overnight at 4 °C with primary antibodies against E-cadherin (Cell Signaling Technology, Danvers, MA, USA, cat. No. 14472) and DNMT1 (Cell Signaling Technology, Danvers, MA, USA, cat. No. 5032) diluted 1:1000 in 5% non-fat milk in TBST (20 mM Tris, 150 mM NaCl, 0.1 % Tween 20). Membranes were incubated with a primary antibody against β-actin (Sigma Aldrich, Taufkirchen, Germany, cat.no. A1978) diluted 1:4000 in 5% non-fat milk in TBST for 1 h at room temperature. Therefore, they were incubated with Goat anti-Rabbit IgG

(H + L) Highly Cross-Adsorbed Secondary Antibody, Alexa Fluor 680 or Goat anti-Mouse IgG (H + L) Highly Cross-Adsorbed Secondary Antibody, Alexa Fluor 680 (Thermo Fisher Scientific, Waltham, MA, USA) secondary antibodies diluted 1:10,000 in 5% non-fat milk in TBST for 1 h at room temperature. Proteins were visualized by Odyssey® Fc (LI-COR Biosciences, Lincoln, NE, USA) imaging system, and densitometry was performed using ImageJ/Fiji software. The results represent the ratio of protein to loading control (B-actin) relative to the control sample of two independent experiments.

4.7. DNA Methylation Analysis

Genomic DNA from studied PDAC cell lines ($1-2 \times 10^6$ cultured cells) was isolated using a FlexiGene DNA Kit (Qiagen, Hilden, Germany). DNA concentration and purity were measured using NanoDrop® ND-1000 spectrophotometer (Thermo Scientific, Wilmington, DE, USA). For sodium bisulfite treatment of extracted DNA (2 µg), EpiTect Bisulfite kit (Qiagen, Hilden, Germany) was used, following the provided protocol. EpiTect Bisulfite kit enables complete conversion of unmethylated cytosines to uracils, while methylated cytosines remain unaffected.

DNA methylation profiles of 15 top-ranked genes (*SNAI1, SNAI2, TWIST1, ZEB1, CDH1, FN1, CDH2, KRT19, STEAP1, OCLN, DSC2, NID2, TSPAN13, BMP2, ITGA5*) and methylation level of the long-interspersed nucleotide element 1 (LINE-1) were evaluated by the quantitative pyrosequencing method, carried out on a PyroMark Q24 platform, using PyroMark Gold Q24 Reagents (Qiagen GmbH, Hilden, Germany). Pyrosequencing assays for all genes were designed using the PyroMark assay design software (Qiagen GmbH, Hilden, Germany), primer sequences and PCR conditions are listed in Table S2. Designed assays were validated following the manufacturer's instructions. Methylation analyses were repeated twice. Between 2 and 7, CpGs were analyzed in each gene in the CpG islands of the promoter regions flanking the transcription start site. The results are presented as the percentage of average methylation in all CpG sites in each gene.

Global DNA methylation was analyzed with the PyroMark Q24 CpG LINE-1 kit (Qiagen, Hilden, Germany), allowing quantification of the methylation levels of three CpG sites in positions 331 to 318 of the LINE-1 sequence (GenBank accession number X58075). The PCR reactions were performed by the PyroMark PCR Kit (Qiagen, Hilden, Germany) following the manufacturer's instructions. Data analysis was performed by PyroMark Q24 2.0.6. software (Qiagen, Hilden, Germany).

4.8. Validation of mRNA Expression of Studied Genes between PDAC and Normal Tissue

The online tool GEPIA. Available online: http://gepia.cancer-pku.cn/ (accessed on 16 December 2021) [76] was used to validate the mRNA expression levels of the screened genes between PDAC and normal pancreatic tissues.

4.9. Statistical Analysis

Normality of distribution was tested by the Shapiro–Wilk test. Significant differences between normally distributed data were assessed by Student *t*-test or one-way analysis of variance (ANOVA) and Bonferroni or Tamhane post-hoc tests depending on assumed variances. Non-normally distributed data were evaluated using Mann–Whitney U-test or Kruskal–Wallis test followed by Dunn of Dunn–Bonferroni post-hoc methods. Data were analyzed using the SPSS software package version 23 (IBM SPSS, Inc., Chicago, IL, USA). Differences with $p < 0.05$ were considered statistically significant.

Supplementary Materials: The following supporting information can be downloaded at: https://www.mdpi.com/article/10.3390/ijms23042117/s1.

Author Contributions: Conceptualization, B.S. and S.C.; methodology, V.B., M.U., B.S., L.T. and S.S.; software, B.S.; validation, M.U., B.S. and E.B.M.; formal analysis, S.C. and M.N.; investigation, M.T. and P.D.; resources, S.C. and B.S.; data curation, B.S., M.U. and V.H.K.; writing—original draft preparation, V.B., B.S. and S.C.; writing—review and editing, V.H.K., E.S. and J.E.; visualization, V.B.

and B.S.; supervision, B.S. and J.B.; project administration, B.S. and S.C.; funding acquisition, S.C. and B.S. All authors have read and agreed to the published version of the manuscript.

Funding: This work was supported by VEGA 2/0052/18, APVV-20-0143, APVV-20-0480, H2020 GA 857381, and NExT-0711 grants.

Institutional Review Board Statement: Not applicable.

Informed Consent Statement: Not applicable.

Data Availability Statement: All data supporting the reported results can be found as Supplementary Files.

Acknowledgments: We would like to thank Alena Gabelova and Marina Cihova, for their help with the experiment design. We thank the Slovak Cancer Research Foundation for its continued support of our scientific activities. The graphical abstract was created with BioRender.com.

Conflicts of Interest: The authors declare no conflict of interest.

References

1. Rahib, L.; Wehner, M.R.; Matrisian, L.M.; Nead, K.T. Estimated Projection of US Cancer Incidence and Death to 2040. *JAMA Netw. Open* **2021**, *4*, e214708. [CrossRef] [PubMed]
2. Available online: https://www.cancer.net/cancer-types/pancreatic-cancer/statistics (accessed on 16 December 2021).
3. Maitra, A.; Adsay, N.V.; Argani, P.; Iacobuzio-Donahue, C.; De Marzo, A.; Cameron, J.L.; Yeo, C.J.; Hruban, R.H. Multicomponent analysis of the pancreatic adenocarcinoma progression model using a pancreatic intraepithelial neoplasia tissue microarray. *Mod. Pathol.* **2003**, *16*, 902–912. [CrossRef] [PubMed]
4. Liu, F.; Wang, L.; Perna, F.; Nimer, S.D. Beyond transcription factors: How oncogenic signalling reshapes the epigenetic landscape. *Nat. Rev. Cancer* **2016**, *16*, 359–372. [CrossRef] [PubMed]
5. Lomberk, G.; Blum, Y.; Nicolle, R.; Nair, A.; Gaonkar, K.S.; Marisa, L.; Mathison, A.; Sun, Z.; Yan, H.; Elarouci, N.; et al. Distinct epigenetic landscapes underlie the pathobiology of pancreatic cancer subtypes. *Nat. Commun.* **2018**, *9*, 1978. [CrossRef]
6. Lomberk, G.; Dusetti, N.; Iovanna, J.; Urrutia, R. Emerging epigenomic landscapes of pancreatic cancer in the era of precision medicine. *Nat. Commun.* **2019**, *10*, 3875. [CrossRef] [PubMed]
7. Strapcova, S.; Takacova, M.; Csaderova, L.; Martinelli, P.; Lukacikova, L.; Gal, V.; Kopacek, J.; Svastova, E. Clinical and Pre-Clinical Evidence of Carbonic Anhydrase IX in Pancreatic Cancer and Its High Expression in Pre-Cancerous Lesions. *Cancers* **2020**, *12*, 2005. [CrossRef] [PubMed]
8. Benej, M.; Svastova, E.; Banova, R.; Kopacek, J.; Gibadulinova, A.; Kery, M.; Arena, S.; Scaloni, A.; Vitale, M.; Zambrano, N.; et al. CA IX Stabilizes Intracellular pH to Maintain Metabolic Reprogramming and Proliferation in Hypoxia. *Front. Oncol.* **2020**, *10*, 1462. [CrossRef]
9. López-Novoa, J.M.; Nieto, M.A. Inflammation and EMT: An alliance towards organ fibrosis and cancer progression. *EMBO Mol. Med.* **2009**, *1*, 303–314. [CrossRef]
10. Wang, S.; Zheng, Y.; Yang, F.; Zhu, L.; Zhu, X.-Q.; Wang, Z.-F.; Wu, X.-L.; Zhou, C.-H.; Yan, J.-Y.; Hu, B.-Y.; et al. The molecular biology of pancreatic adenocarcinoma: Translational challenges and clinical perspectives. *Signal Transduct. Target. Ther.* **2021**, *6*, 249. [CrossRef]
11. Nguyen, D.X.; Bos, P.D.; Massagué, J. Metastasis: From dissemination to organ-specific colonization. *Nat. Rev. Cancer* **2009**, *9*, 274–284. [CrossRef]
12. Tao, J.; Yang, G.; Zhou, W.; Qiu, J.; Chen, G.; Luo, W.; Zhao, F.; You, L.; Zheng, L.; Zhang, T.; et al. Targeting hypoxic tumor microenvironment in pancreatic cancer. *J. Hematol. Oncol.* **2021**, *14*, 14. [CrossRef] [PubMed]
13. Yamasaki, A.; Yanai, K.; Onishi, H. Hypoxia and pancreatic ductal adenocarcinoma. *Cancer Lett.* **2020**, *484*, 9–15. [CrossRef] [PubMed]
14. Panisova, E.; Kery, M.; Sedlakova, O.; Brisson, L.; Debreova, M.; Sboarina, M.; Sonveaux, P.; Pastorekova, S.; Svastova, E. Lactate stimulates CA IX expression in normoxic cancer cells. *Oncotarget* **2017**, *8*, 77819–77835. [CrossRef] [PubMed]
15. Takacova, M.; Holotnakova, T.; Barathova, M.; Pastorekova, S.; Kopacek, J.; Pastorek, J. Src induces expression of carbonic anhydrase IX via hypoxia-inducible factor 1. *Oncol. Rep.* **2010**, *23*, 869–874.
16. Zhuang, H.; Wang, S.; Chen, B.; Zhang, Z.; Ma, Z.; Li, Z.; Liu, C.; Zhou, Z.; Gong, Y.; Huang, S.; et al. Prognostic Stratification Based on HIF-1 Signaling for Evaluating Hypoxic Status and Immune Infiltration in Pancreatic Ductal Adenocarcinomas. *Front. Immunol.* **2021**, *12*, 790661. [CrossRef]
17. Chen, S.; Chen, X.; Li, W.; Shan, T.; Lin, W.R.; Ma, J.; Cui, X.; Yang, W.; Cao, G.; Li, Y.; et al. Conversion of epithelial-to-mesenchymal transition to mesenchymal-to-epithelial transition is mediated by oxygen concentration in pancreatic cancer cells. *Oncol. Lett.* **2018**, *15*, 7144–7152. [CrossRef]
18. Miyazono, K.; Ehata, S.; Koinuma, D. Tumor-promoting functions of transforming growth factor-β in progression of cancer. *Ups J. Med. Sci.* **2012**, *117*, 143–152. [CrossRef]
19. Terashima, M.; Ishimura, A.; Wanna-Udom, S.; Suzuki, T. MEG8 long noncoding RNA contributes to epigenetic progression of the epithelial-mesenchymal transition of lung and pancreatic cancer cells. *J. Biol. Chem.* **2018**, *293*, 18016–18030. [CrossRef]

20. Zhang, Y.; Wei, J.; Wang, H.; Xue, X.; An, Y.; Tang, D.; Yuan, Z.; Wang, F.; Wu, J.; Zhang, J.; et al. Epithelial mesenchymal transition correlates with CD24+CD44+ and CD133+ cells in pancreatic cancer. *Oncol. Rep.* 2012, 27, 1599–1605. [CrossRef]
21. Schito, L.; Semenza, G.L. Hypoxia-Inducible Factors: Master Regulators of Cancer Progression. *Trends Cancer* 2016, 2, 758–770. [CrossRef]
22. Galván, J.A.; Zlobec, I.; Wartenberg, M.; Lugli, A.; Gloor, B.; Perren, A.; Karamitopoulou, E. Expression of E-cadherin repressors SNAIL, ZEB1 and ZEB2 by tumour and stromal cells influences tumour-budding phenotype and suggests heterogeneity of stromal cells in pancreatic cancer. *Br. J. Cancer* 2015, 112, 1944–1950. [CrossRef] [PubMed]
23. Kao, S.H.; Wu, K.J.; Lee, W.H. Hypoxia, Epithelial-Mesenchymal Transition, and TET-Mediated Epigenetic Changes. *J. Clin. Med.* 2016, 5, 24. [CrossRef] [PubMed]
24. Camuzi, D.; de Amorim, Í.S.S.; Ribeiro Pinto, L.F.; Oliveira Trivilin, L.; Mencalha, A.L.; Soares Lima, S.C. Regulation Is in the Air: The Relationship between Hypoxia and Epigenetics in Cancer. *Cells* 2019, 8, 300. [CrossRef] [PubMed]
25. Tam, W.L.; Weinberg, R.A. The epigenetics of epithelial-mesenchymal plasticity in cancer. *Nat. Med.* 2013, 19, 1438–1449. [CrossRef] [PubMed]
26. Geismann, C.; Arlt, A. Coming in the Air: Hypoxia Meets Epigenetics in Pancreatic Cancer. *Cells* 2020, 9, 353. [CrossRef] [PubMed]
27. Lin, Y.; Dong, C.; Zhou, B.P. Epigenetic regulation of EMT: The Snail story. *Curr. Pharm. Des.* 2014, 20, 1698–1705. [CrossRef] [PubMed]
28. Aghdassi, A.; Sendler, M.; Guenther, A.; Mayerle, J.; Behn, C.O.; Heidecke, C.D.; Friess, H.; Büchler, M.; Evert, M.; Lerch, M.M.; et al. Recruitment of histone deacetylases HDAC1 and HDAC2 by the transcriptional repressor ZEB1 downregulates E-cadherin expression in pancreatic cancer. *Gut* 2012, 61, 439–448. [CrossRef]
29. Von Burstin, J.; Eser, S.; Paul, M.C.; Seidler, B.; Brandl, M.; Messer, M.; von Werder, A.; Schmidt, A.; Mages, J.; Pagel, P.; et al. E-cadherin regulates metastasis of pancreatic cancer in vivo and is suppressed by a SNAIL/HDAC1/HDAC2 repressor complex. *Gastroenterology* 2009, 137, 361–371. [CrossRef]
30. Watson, J.A.; Watson, C.J.; McCann, A.; Baugh, J. Epigenetics, the epicenter of the hypoxic response. *Epigenetics* 2010, 5, 293–296. [CrossRef]
31. Romero-Garcia, S.; Prado-Garcia, H.; Carlos-Reyes, A. Role of DNA Methylation in the Resistance to Therapy in Solid Tumors. *Front. Oncol.* 2020, 10, 1152. [CrossRef]
32. Szabova, K.; Bizikova, I.; Mistrik, M.; Bizik, J. Inflammatory environment created by fibroblast aggregates induces growth arrest and phenotypic shift of human myeloma cells. *Neoplasma* 2015, 62, 938–948. [CrossRef] [PubMed]
33. Li, C.; Tang, Z.; Zhang, W.; Ye, Z.; Liu, F. GEPIA2021: Integrating multiple deconvolution-based analysis into GEPIA. *Nucleic Acids Res.* 2021, 49, W242–W246. [CrossRef] [PubMed]
34. Gradiz, R.; Silva, H.C.; Carvalho, L.; Botelho, M.F.; Mota-Pinto, A. MIA PaCa-2 and PANC-1 pancreas ductal adenocarcinoma cell lines with neuroendocrine differentiation and somatostatin receptors. *Sci. Rep.* 2016, 6, 21648. [CrossRef] [PubMed]
35. Deer, E.L.; González-Hernández, J.; Coursen, J.D.; Shea, J.E.; Ngatia, J.; Scaife, C.L.; Firpo, M.A.; Mulvihill, S.J. Phenotype and genotype of pancreatic cancer cell lines. *Pancreas* 2010, 39, 425–435. [CrossRef]
36. Opdenakker, G.; Van Damme, J. The countercurrent principle in invasion and metastasis of cancer cells. Recent insights on the roles of chemokines. *Int. J. Dev. Biol.* 2004, 48, 519–527. [CrossRef]
37. Saur, D.; Seidler, B.; Schneider, G.; Algül, H.; Beck, R.; Senekowitsch-Schmidtke, R.; Schwaiger, M.; Schmid, R.M. CXCR4 expression increases liver and lung metastasis in a mouse model of pancreatic cancer. *Gastroenterology* 2005, 129, 1237–1250. [CrossRef]
38. Wehler, T.; Wolfert, F.; Schimanski, C.C.; Gockel, I.; Herr, W.; Biesterfeld, S.; Seifert, J.K.; Adwan, H.; Berger, M.R.; Junginger, T.; et al. Strong expression of chemokine receptor CXCR4 by pancreatic cancer correlates with advanced disease. *Oncol. Rep.* 2006, 16, 1159–1164. [CrossRef]
39. Ding, Y.; Du, Y. Clinicopathological significance and prognostic role of chemokine receptor CXCR4 expression in pancreatic ductal adenocarcinoma, a meta-analysis and literature review. *Int. J. Surg.* 2019, 65, 32–38. [CrossRef]
40. Seeber, A.; Kocher, F.; Pircher, A.; Puccini, A.; Baca, Y.; Xiu, J.; Zimmer, K.; Haybaeck, J.; Spizzo, G.; Goldberg, R.M. High CXCR4 expression in pancreatic ductal adenocarcinoma as characterized by an inflammatory tumor phenotype with potential implications for an immunotherapeutic approach. *J. Clin. Oncol.* 2021, 39, 4021. [CrossRef]
41. Aldinucci, D.; Borghese, C.; Casagrande, N. The CCL5/CCR5 Axis in Cancer Progression. *Cancers* 2020, 12, 1765. [CrossRef]
42. Singh, S.K.; Mishra, M.K.; Eltoum, I.A.; Bae, S.; Lillard, J.W., Jr.; Singh, R. CCR5/CCL5 axis interaction promotes migratory and invasiveness of pancreatic cancer cells. *Sci. Rep.* 2018, 8, 1323. [CrossRef] [PubMed]
43. Doi, Y.; Yashiro, M.; Yamada, N.; Amano, R.; Noda, S.; Hirakawa, K. VEGF-A/VEGFR-2 signaling plays an important role for the motility of pancreas cancer cells. *Ann. Surg. Oncol.* 2012, 19, 2733–2743. [CrossRef] [PubMed]
44. Katsuta, E.; Qi, Q.; Peng, X.; Hochwald, S.N.; Yan, L.; Takabe, K. Pancreatic adenocarcinomas with mature blood vessels have better overall survival. *Sci. Rep.* 2019, 9, 1310. [CrossRef] [PubMed]
45. Dumont, N.; Wilson, M.B.; Crawford, Y.G.; Reynolds, P.A.; Sigaroudinia, M.; Tlsty, T.D. Sustained induction of epithelial to mesenchymal transition activates DNA methylation of genes silenced in basal-like breast cancers. *Proc. Natl. Acad. Sci. USA* 2008, 105, 14867–14872. [CrossRef]

46. Bohl, S.R.; Bullinger, L.; Rücker, F.G. Epigenetic therapy: Azacytidine and decitabine in acute myeloid leukemia. *Expert Rev. Hematol.* **2018**, *11*, 361–371. [CrossRef]
47. Seelan, R.S.; Mukhopadhyay, P.; Pisano, M.M.; Greene, R.M. Effects of 5-Aza-2′-deoxycytidine (decitabine) on gene expression. *Drug Metab. Rev.* **2018**, *50*, 193–207. [CrossRef]
48. Topalovski, M.; Brekken, R.A. Matrix control of pancreatic cancer: New insights into fibronectin signaling. *Cancer Lett.* **2016**, *381*, 252–258. [CrossRef]
49. Zhu, H.; Wang, G.; Zhu, H.; Xu, A. ITGA5 is a prognostic biomarker and correlated with immune infiltration in gastrointestinal tumors. *BMC Cancer* **2021**, *21*, 269. [CrossRef]
50. Pankov, R.; Yamada, K.M. Fibronectin at a glance. *J. Cell Sci.* **2002**, *115*, 3861–3863. [CrossRef]
51. Atay, S. Integrated transcriptome meta-analysis of pancreatic ductal adenocarcinoma and matched adjacent pancreatic tissues. *PeerJ* **2020**, *8*, e10141. [CrossRef]
52. Bendas, G.; Borsig, L. Cancer cell adhesion and metastasis: Selectins, integrins, and the inhibitory potential of heparins. *Int. J. Cell Biol.* **2012**, *2012*, 676731. [CrossRef] [PubMed]
53. Hu, D.; Ansari, D.; Zhou, Q.; Sasor, A.; Hilmersson, K.S.; Andersson, R. Stromal fibronectin expression in patients with resected pancreatic ductal adenocarcinoma. *World J. Surg. Oncol.* **2019**, *17*, 29. [CrossRef] [PubMed]
54. Olmeda, D.; Jordá, M.; Peinado, H.; Fabra, A.; Cano, A. Snail silencing effectively suppresses tumour growth and invasiveness. *Oncogene* **2007**, *26*, 1862–1874. [CrossRef]
55. Murphy, P.A.; Begum, S.; Hynes, R.O. Tumor angiogenesis in the absence of fibronectin or its cognate integrin receptors. *PLoS ONE* **2015**, *10*, e0120872. [CrossRef]
56. Kuninty, P.R.; Bansal, R.; De Geus, S.W.L.; Mardhian, D.F.; Schnittert, J.; van Baarlen, J.; Storm, G.; Bijlsma, M.F.; van Laarhoven, H.W.; Metselaar, J.M.; et al. ITGA5 inhibition in pancreatic stellate cells attenuates desmoplasia and potentiates efficacy of chemotherapy in pancreatic cancer. *Sci. Adv.* **2019**, *5*, eaax2770. [CrossRef]
57. Fang, Z.; Yao, W.; Xiong, Y.; Zhang, J.; Liu, L.; Li, J.; Zhang, C.; Wan, J. Functional elucidation and methylation-mediated downregulation of ITGA5 gene in breast cancer cell line MDA-MB-468. *J. Cell. Biochem.* **2010**, *110*, 1130–1141. [CrossRef] [PubMed]
58. Ohgami, R.S.; Campagna, D.R.; McDonald, A.; Fleming, M.D. The Steap proteins are metalloreductases. *Blood* **2006**, *108*, 1388–1394. [CrossRef]
59. Gomes, I.M.; Maia, C.J.; Santos, C.R. STEAP proteins: From structure to applications in cancer therapy. *Mol. Cancer Res.* **2012**, *10*, 573–587. [CrossRef]
60. Huo, S.-F.; Shang, W.-L.; Yu, M.; Ren, X.-P.; Wen, H.-X.; Chai, C.-Y.; Sun, L.; Hui, K.; Liu, L.-H.; Wei, S.-H. Steap1 facilitates metastasis and epithelial–mesenchymal transition of lung adenocarcinoma via the JAK2/STAT3 signaling pathway. *Biosci. Rep.* **2020**, *40*, BSR20193169. [CrossRef]
61. Xie, J.; Yang, Y.; Sun, J.; Jiao, Z.; Zhang, H.; Chen, J. STEAP1 inhibits breast cancer metastasis and is associated with epithelial–mesenchymal transition procession. *Clin. Breast Cancer* **2019**, *19*, e195–e207. [CrossRef]
62. Zhang, Z.; Hou, W.B.; Zhang, C.; Tan, Y.E.; Zhang, D.D.; An, W.; Pan, S.W.; Wu, W.D.; Chen, Q.C.; Xu, H.M. A research of STEAP1 regulated gastric cancer cell proliferation, migration and invasion in vitro and in vivos. *J. Cell. Mol. Med.* **2020**, *24*, 14217–14230. [CrossRef] [PubMed]
63. Nie, Z.; Merritt, A.; Rouhi-Parkouhi, M.; Tabernero, L.; Garrod, D. Membrane-impermeable Cross-linking Provides Evidence for Homophilic, Isoform-specific Binding of Desmosomal Cadherins in Epithelial Cells. *J. Biol. Chem.* **2011**, *286*, 2143–2154. [CrossRef] [PubMed]
64. Sun, C.; Wang, L.; Yang, X.-X.; Jiang, Y.-H.; Guo, X.-L. The aberrant expression or disruption of desmocollin2 in human diseases. *Int. J. Biol. Macromol.* **2019**, *131*, 378–386. [CrossRef] [PubMed]
65. Hamidov, Z.; Altendorf-Hofmann, A.; Chen, Y.; Settmacher, U.; Petersen, I.; Knösel, T. Reduced expression of desmocollin 2 is an independent prognostic biomarker for shorter patients survival in pancreatic ductal adenocarcinoma. *J. Clin. Pathol.* **2011**, *64*, 990–994. [CrossRef] [PubMed]
66. Yu, Z.-H.; Wang, Y.-M.; Jiang, Y.-Z.; Ma, S.-J.; Zhong, Q.; Wan, Y.-Y.; Wang, X.-W. NID2 can serve as a potential prognosis prediction biomarker and promotes the invasion and migration of gastric cancer. *Pathol. Res. Pract.* **2019**, *215*, 152553. [CrossRef] [PubMed]
67. Shan, Z.; Wang, W.; Tong, Y.; Zhang, J. Genome-Scale Analysis Identified NID2, SPARC, and MFAP2 as Prognosis Markers of Overall Survival in Gastric Cancer. *Med. Sci. Monit. Int. Med. J. Exp. Clin. Res.* **2021**, *27*, e929558-1. [CrossRef]
68. Strelnikov, V.V.; Kuznetsova, E.B.; Tanas, A.S.; Rudenko, V.V.; Kalinkin, A.I.; Poddubskaya, E.V.; Kekeeva, T.V.; Chesnokova, G.G.; Trotsenko, I.D.; Larin, S.S. Abnormal promoter DNA hypermethylation of the integrin, nidogen, and dystroglycan genes in breast cancer. *Sci. Rep.* **2021**, *11*, 2264. [CrossRef]
69. Kleeff, J.; Maruyama, H.; Ishiwata, T.; Sawhney, H.; Friess, H.; Büchler, M.W.; Korc, M. Bone morphogenetic protein 2 exerts diverse effects on cell growth in vitro and is expressed in human pancreatic cancer in vivo. *Gastroenterology* **1999**, *116*, 1202–1216. [CrossRef]
70. Rao, A.D.; Liu, Y.; von Eyben, R.; Hsu, C.C.; Hu, C.; Rosati, L.M.; Parekh, A.; Ng, K.; Hacker-Prietz, A.; Zheng, L. Multiplex proximity ligation assay to identify potential prognostic biomarkers for improved survival in locally advanced pancreatic cancer patients treated with stereotactic body radiation therapy. *Int. J. Radiat. Oncol. Biol. Phys.* **2018**, *100*, 486–489. [CrossRef]

71. Li, C.-S.; Tian, H.; Zou, M.; Zhao, K.-W.; Li, Y.; Lao, L.; Brochmann, E.J.; Duarte, M.E.L.; Daubs, M.D.; Zhou, Y.-H. Secreted phosphoprotein 24 kD (Spp24) inhibits growth of human pancreatic cancer cells caused by BMP-2. *Biochem. Biophys. Res. Commun.* **2015**, *466*, 167–172. [CrossRef]
72. Chen, X.; Liao, J.; Lu, Y.; Duan, X.; Sun, W. Activation of the PI3K/Akt pathway mediates bone morphogenetic protein 2-induced invasion of pancreatic cancer cells Panc-1. *Pathol. Oncol. Res.* **2011**, *17*, 257–261. [CrossRef] [PubMed]
73. Miura, T.; Ishiguro, M.; Ishikawa, T.; Okazaki, S.; Baba, H.; Kikuchi, A.; Yamauchi, S.; Matsuyama, T.; Uetake, H.; Kinugasa, Y. Methylation of bone morphogenetic protein 2 is associated with poor prognosis in colorectal cancer. *Oncol. Lett.* **2020**, *19*, 229–238. [CrossRef] [PubMed]
74. Kankuri, E.; Babusikova, O.; Hlubinova, K.; Salmenperä, P.; Boccaccio, C.; Lubitz, W.; Harjula, A.; Bizik, J. Fibroblast nemosis arrests growth and induces differentiation of human leukemia cells. *Int. J. Cancer* **2008**, *122*, 1243–1252. [CrossRef]
75. Livak, K.J.; Schmittgen, T.D. Analysis of relative gene expression data using real-time quantitative PCR and the 2(-Delta Delta C(T)) Method. *Methods* **2001**, *25*, 402–408. [CrossRef] [PubMed]
76. Tang, Z.; Li, C.; Kang, B.; Gao, G.; Li, C.; Zhang, Z. GEPIA: A web server for cancer and normal gene expression profiling and interactive analyses. *Nucleic Acids Res.* **2017**, *45*, W98–W102. [CrossRef] [PubMed]

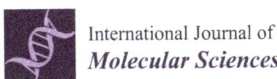

International Journal of Molecular Sciences

Article

Contribution of the STAT Family of Transcription Factors to the Expression of the Serotonin 2B (HTR2B) Receptor in Human Uveal Melanoma

Manel Benhassine [1], Gaëtan Le-Bel [1] and Sylvain L. Guérin [1,2,*]

1. Centre Universitaire d'Ophtalmologie-Recherche (CUO-Recherche), Axe Médecine Régénératrice, Hôpital du Saint-Sacrement, Centre de Recherche FRQS du CHU de Québec, Quebec City, QC G1S4L8, Canada; manal.benhassine.1@ulaval.ca (M.B.); gaetan.lebel17@gmail.com (G.L.-B.)
2. Département d'Ophtalmologie, Faculté de Médecine, Université Laval, Quebec City, QC G1V0A6, Canada
* Correspondence: sylvain.guerin@fmed.ulaval.ca; Tel.: +1-(418)-682-7565

Citation: Benhassine, M.; Le-Bel, G.; Guérin, S.L. Contribution of the STAT Family of Transcription Factors to the Expression of the Serotonin 2B (HTR2B) Receptor in Human Uveal Melanoma. *Int. J. Mol. Sci.* **2022**, *23*, 1564. https://doi.org/10.3390/ijms23031564

Academic Editors: Bozena Smolkova, Julie Earl and Agapi Kataki

Received: 20 December 2021
Accepted: 26 January 2022
Published: 29 January 2022

Publisher's Note: MDPI stays neutral with regard to jurisdictional claims in published maps and institutional affiliations.

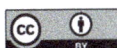

Copyright: © 2022 by the authors. Licensee MDPI, Basel, Switzerland. This article is an open access article distributed under the terms and conditions of the Creative Commons Attribution (CC BY) license (https://creativecommons.org/licenses/by/4.0/).

Abstract: Uveal melanoma (UM) remains the most common intraocular malignancy among diseases affecting the adult eye. The primary tumor disseminates to the liver in half of patients and leads to a 6 to 12-month survival rate, making UM a particularly aggressive type of cancer. Genomic analyses have led to the development of gene-expression profiles that can efficiently predict metastatic progression. Among these genes, that encoding the serotonin receptor 2B (HTR2B) represents the most discriminant from this molecular signature, its aberrant expression being the hallmark of UM metastatic progression. Recent evidence suggests that expression of HTR2B might be regulated through the Janus kinase/Signal Transducer and Activator of Transcription proteins (JAK/STAT) intracellular signalization pathway. However, little is actually known about the molecular mechanisms involved in the abnormally elevated expression of the *HTR2B* gene in metastatic UM and whether activated STAT proteins participates to this mechanism. In this study, we determined the pattern of STAT family members expressed in both primary tumors and UM cell-lines, and evaluated their contribution to *HTR2B* gene expression. Examination of the *HTR2B* promoter sequence revealed the presence of a STAT putative target site (5′-TTC (N)3 GAA3′) located 280 bp upstream of the mRNA start site that is completely identical to the high affinity binding site recognized by these TFs. Gene profiling on microarrays provided evidence that metastatic UM cell lines with high levels of HTR2B also express high levels of STAT proteins whereas low levels of these TFs are observed in non-metastatic UM cells with low levels of HTR2B, suggesting that STAT proteins contribute to *HTR2B* gene expression in UM cells. All UM cell lines tested were found to express their own pattern of STAT proteins in Western blot analyses. Furthermore, T142 and T143 UM cells responded to interleukins IL-4 and IL-6 by increasing the phosphorylation status of STAT1. Most of all, expression of HTR2B also considerably increased in response to both IL-4 and IL-6 therefore providing evidence that *HTR2B* gene expression is modulated by STAT proteins in UM cells. The binding of STAT proteins to the −280 HTR2B/STAT site was also demonstrated by electrophoretic mobility shift assay (EMSA) analyses and site-directed mutation of that STAT site also abolished both IL-4 and IL-6 responsiveness in in vitro transfection analyses. The results of this study therefore demonstrate that members from the STAT family of TFs positively contribute to the expression of HTR2B in uveal melanoma.

Keywords: HTR2B; STAT proteins; uveal melanoma; promoter; gene transcription

1. Introduction

Uveal melanoma (UM) is the most common intraocular malignancy in adults, with an incidence of four to six affected individuals per million in the United States [1]. Despite effective primary therapy, approximately 50% of patients will develop the metastatic disease [2]. Liver metastasis is a dreaded complication of this cancer as patients rarely survive more than five years following the initial detection of metastasis, with a death rate reaching 92% at two years [3]. Microarray analyses identified 12 genes, designated as the UM gene expression signature, that can distinguish between UM primary tumors that are at low or high risk of progressing towards the liver metastatic disease. The human gene encoding the 5-Hydroxytryptamine receptor 2B (*HTR2B*), also known as the serotonin receptor 2B, turns out to be the most discriminating among the class II genes for the identification of UM patients at high risk of evolving toward formation of liver metastases [4–6]. The serotonin receptors to which HTR2B belongs are gathered into a family of proteins that can be divided in seven subfamilies (HTR1-7). Interestingly, HTR2B has been described as an oncogene in hepatocellular carcinoma (HCC), prostate, small intestine and breast cancers [7–9], but as a tumor suppressor in ovarian cancer [10]. In addition to its function as a neurotransmitter, serotonin plays a role in its development, and most of its biological actions are transmitted within the cell through the activation of a few signal transduction pathways including the phospholipase C (PLC), the Receptor Tyrosin Kinase (RTK)/Phosphatidylinositol-4,5-bisphosphate-3-kinase (PI3K)/Extracellular signal-Regulated Kinase (ERK)/mammalian target of rapamycin (mTOR), the RAF/Mitogen activated protein Kinase Kinase (MEK)/ERK and the Janus kinase/Signal Transducer and Activator of Transcription proteins (JAK/STAT) pathways [10–15]. Although the serotonin-mediated activation of the JAK/STAT pathway has been shown to rely essentially on the 5-HT1A or 5-HT2A receptors [14,16–18], recent evidence also suggests that the HTR2B receptor might participate as well in the activation of this signal transduction pathway in uveal melanoma [19].

STAT proteins have the ability to transduce signals from the cell membrane into the nucleus, where they can alter the transcription of many responsive genes. Today, seven STAT genes have been identified in the human genome: *STAT1* to *STAT4*, *STAT5a*, *STAT5b* and *STAT6* [20]. STAT signaling is involved in many normal physiologic cell processes, including proliferation, differentiation, angiogenesis, immune system regulation and apoptosis. However, aberrant STAT regulation that may result from many possible irregularities can lead to various pathologic events, such as malignant cell transformation and metastasis [21]. It is noteworthy that some STAT proteins are currently even considered as oncogenes [22]. The aberrant activation of STAT proteins, most particularly STAT1, STAT3 and STAT5, has been suspected or proposed to significantly contribute to the progression of a variety of human tumors and cancer cell lines, including hematologic malignancies and solid tumors (reviewed in [23]).

Until very recently, STAT3 and STAT5 were probably the STAT family members with the most significant role in cancer development, in particular STAT3, as it clearly turned out to be the most thoroughly investigated STAT protein in cancer research. However, studies that relate cancer development to aberrant activation of STAT1 have blown-up over the last few years, the abnormal expression of STAT1 being now even used as a prognostic factor for patients with solid tumors [24]. By its capacity to control the immune system and promote tumor immune surveillance, STAT1 has been recognized as a tumor suppressor in breast cancer [25]. STAT2, STAT4 and STAT6 appear to have more limited roles in tumor biology. STAT proteins therefore play a major regulatory role in the maintenance and survival of cancer cells by allowing them to escape the host's anti-tumor responses. Cancer cells can then expand, metastasize and progress toward formation of solid tumors.

All STAT proteins have been reported to bind as dimers with varying affinities to the same palindromic DNA regulatory element (DRE: 5'-TTCN$_{2-4}$GAA-3') that is present in both hormone- and cytokine-responsive genes ([26]; also reviewed by [20,27]). Once they recognize promoter proximal DREs, STAT proteins then alter either positively (activation) or negatively (repression) the transcription of their target genes. STATs can also control enhancer activity, epigenetic status of associated genes, or instruct non-coding loci (e.g., miRNAs) by engaging more distal binding DREs.

The intercellular communication regulating developmental signaling is precisely controlled by both regulatory feedback loops that protect cells against signals that may be produced in the wrong time or place and which may lead to inappropriate developmental responses such as is frequently happening in cancer tissues. Such feedback loops can either be positive or negative depending on whether a gene increases or represses its own expression, respectively. It is believed that the most obvious use of negative feedback is to limit the duration of a signal that induces its own negative regulator so that when a threshold has been reached, this signal disappears. Cytokine signaling through the JAK/STAT signaling pathway well illustrates this mechanism. As many hormones, cytokines and growth factors receptors transduce their signals through this pathway, it is not surprising that regulatory feedback loops control their expression. For instance, expression of the glucocorticoid receptor (GR) has been shown to be under the regulatory influence of a negative feedback loop involving miR-29a [28]. Similarly, a negative feedback loop involving the transcription factor GATA2 also controls the transcription of the androgen receptor (ER) upon androgen deprivation in castration-resistant prostate cancers [29]. On the other hand, expression of the estrogen receptor (ER) has been demonstrated to be under the control of a positive feedback loop involving IL6 in oesophageal squamous cell carcinoma [30]. Therefore, in many instances, cancer cells appear to escape the cell's surveillance mechanism by altering the function of cellular targets within these regulatory feedback loops that are primed to respond to such signals.

Although studies that evaluated the relationship of STAT family members with cancer progression are particularly abundant, only a few examined activation of STAT proteins by serotonin in uveal melanoma [19,31]. In vascular smooth muscle cells, serotonin was found to activate JAK1, JAK2, and STAT1 through the HTR2A receptor [14]. However, blocking the signal transduction cascade mediated by the binding of serotonin to the HTR2B receptor using the selective serotonin receptor 2B antagonist PRX-08066 considerably reduced the phosphorylation of STAT2, STAT3, STAT6, and most remarkably that of both STAT5A and STAT5B, in three different UM cell lines [19] therefore demonstrating that HTR2B ligand recognition activates STAT proteins in UM. In the present study, we demonstrated that UM tumors and their derivative cell lines express different combinations of STAT genes and proteins. In addition, the *HTR2B* gene promoter was shown to bear multiple putative target sites for STAT proteins of which one (located at position −280 relative to the *HTR2B* mRNA start site) functionally binds members of the STAT family. Most of all, expression of HTR2B was found to positively respond to the STAT protein inducers IL-4 and IL-6, a mechanism ensured at least in part through the −280 STAT DRE, thereby further supporting the existence of an interleukin/JAK/STAT signalization pathway that may contribute to the metastatic properties of uveal melanoma.

2. Results

2.1. Multiple Putative DNA Target Sites for STAT Proteins Are Present in the Human HTR2B Gene Promoter and 5′-Flanking Sequences

In order to verify whether transcription of the *HTR2B* gene might be under the regulatory influence of STAT family members, we first searched for the presence of putative STAT DREs in both the promoter and 5′-flanking sequence of the *HTR2B* gene. A large segment of that gene extending up to approximately 2 Kbp upstream from the *HTR2B* mRNA start site was subjected to a search with the TFSEARCH program, a tool for the identification of putative DNA target sequences for nuclear-located transcription factors. We searched for putative STAT target sites that deviate from the consensus STAT DRE (5′-TTCN2–4GAA-3′) by no more than one nucleotide. Thirteen STAT target sites that fitted into this category could be identified along the entire promoter and 5′-flanking sequence of the *HTR2B* gene (Figure S1). Among them, three DREs that perfectly match the STAT consensus sequence could be identified at positions −982, −942 and −280 relative to the *HTR2B* mRNA start site (Figure S1B). The STAT DRE located at position −280 sounded particularly interesting in that most STAT proteins (especially STAT1 and STAT5) have an increased affinity for DREs in which both halves of the palindromic sequence are separated by a 3 nucleotides linker (as opposed to 2 and 4 nucleotides for the −982 and −942 DREs, respectively) [26]. On the other hand, STAT6 appears to clearly prefer a linker sequence comprising 4 nucleotides, as observed for the −942 DRE [26]. Therefore, we can conclude that multiple putative STAT binding sites are present in both the 5′-flanking and promoter sequence of the *HTR2B* gene.

2.2. Expression of STAT Genes Correlates with That of HTR2B in Uveal Melanoma

We have previously shown that the expression of the *HTR2B* gene at the transcriptional level correlates with the aggressiveness of the primary tumors from which UM cell lines are cultured [32]. We therefore searched our gene profiling on microarray datafiles to sort out which of the STAT genes are expressed by our UM cell lines and primary tumors, and attempted to correlate STAT genes expression with that of the *HTR2B* gene. Gene profiling analyses were conducted using total RNAs extracted from UM cell lines that express either low (T97, T108, T111, T128, T131, T132 and T143 cell lines) or high levels of *HTR2B* (T98, T142, T151 and T157 cell lines), or from primary tumors with either low (140, 149, 154 and 157 tumors) or high *HTR2B* levels (138, 139, 141, 142, 147 and 151 tumors) and used for microarray analyses. As shown on Figure 1A (and Figure S2), both UM cell lines (left) and primary tumors (right) that express high levels of *HTR2B* also express moderate to high levels of all STAT genes, with the only exception being *STAT4* (pooled data are presented; data for each individual cell line and tumor are shown on Supplementary Figure S1). On the other hand, a dramatic reduction in the expression of all STAT genes is observed in UM cell lines that have low *HTR2B* levels, whereas only *STAT1* expression is considerably reduced in low HTR2B tumors. Therefore, expression of *HTR2B* correlates perfectly with that of all STAT genes in UM cell lines whereas it is coordinated with that of STAT1 in the UM primary tumors.

We recently reported that cell passaging severely reduces the expression of genes encoding markers typical of UM, including those of the prognostic gene signature such as *HTR2B* [33]. We therefore examined whether the cell passage-dependent reduction in the expression of *HTR2B* also correlates with similar decreases in the expression of the STAT genes in T142 UM cells when compared to its primary tumor. As for *HTR2B*, expression of *STAT1*, *STAT2*, *STAT5A*, *STAT5B*, and *STAT6* genes, which were moderately to highly expressed in the primary tumor 142, was rapidly lost with cell passaging in the derivative T142 UM cell line (Figure 1B; similar results were also obtained with the 143 primary tumor and its derivative cell line T143 (data not shown)). These results suggest that expression of *HTR2B* correlates with that of STAT genes at the transcriptional level in uveal melanoma.

We next examined the pattern of STAT proteins expressed in UM cell lines cultured either from metastatic (T142) or non-metastatic (T97, T108 and T143) UM primary tumors. As shown in Figure 2, all STAT proteins are expressed at varying levels by all UM cell lines, irrespective of whether they have been cultured from metastatic tumors or not.

Data are also presented for the housekeeping gene β-2-microglobulin (B2M; control). Whereas STAT2, STAT3, STAT4 and STAT6 are more uniformly expressed between all four UM cell lines, high levels of STAT1 expression are observed in T108 cells, T97, T142 and T143 cells expressing, on the other hand, low to very low levels of this isoform. Interestingly, T97 apparently expresses no STAT5 whereas this isoform has a faster electrophoretic mobility in T108 UM cells. Furthermore, the metastatic T142 cell line expresses a STAT2 isoform with an apparent molecular mass higher than that observed in the remaining UM cells.

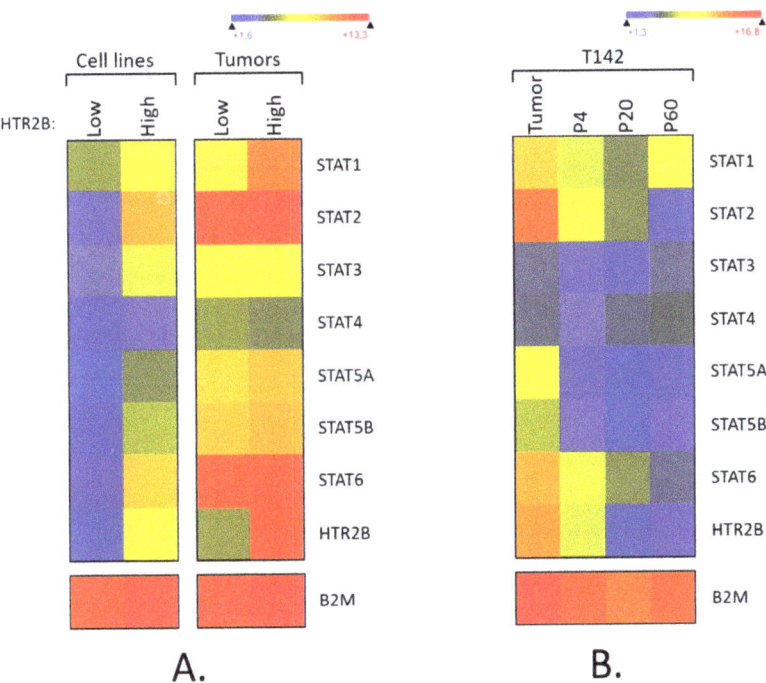

Figure 1. Expression of STAT genes in uveal melanoma. (**A**) Heatmap representation of all the STAT genes expressed by UM cell lines or the primary tumors from which they have been cultured. Data show the average of the individual transcriptome profile extracted from UM cell lines that express either low (T97, T108, T111, T128, T131, T132 and T143 cell lines) or high levels of *HTR2B* (T98, T142, T151 and T157 cell lines), or from primary tumors with either low (tumors 140, 149, 154 and 157) or high *HTR2B* levels (tumors 138, 139, 141, 142, 147 and 151). A dark blue color corresponds to a very low level of expression, whereas high levels appear in yellow/red. Moderate to high levels of all STAT genes except *STAT4* are observed in UM cell lines with high levels of *HTR2B* but not in UM cells with low expression of *HTR2B*. In UM primary tumors, only *STAT1* expression is considerably reduced in tumors with low *HTR2B* levels. (**B**) Heatmap representation of all STAT genes expressed by the UM primary tumor 142 (tumor) and its derivative cell line T142 cultured at passages P4, P20 and P60 as determined by DNA microarrays. As for *HTR2B*, expression of STAT genes, which is elevated in the primary tumor 142, is rapidly lost with cell passaging in the derivative T142 UM cell-line.

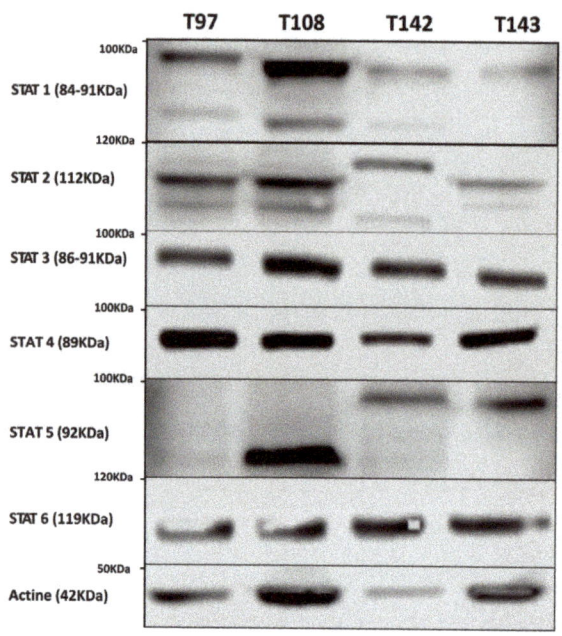
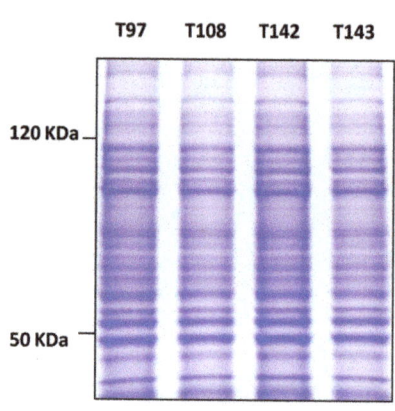

Figure 2. Western blot analysis of the STAT isoforms in UM cells. Total proteins isolated from the UM cell lines T97, T108, T142 and T143 were Western blotted using polyclonal antibodies directed against all STAT isoforms (STAT1 to STAT6). Actin was also blotted as a control. Coomassie blue staining (25 µg of each protein extract was used) is also shown beside the Western blots as a protein loading control. UM cell lines were found to express all STAT proteins to varying levels. In addition, the metastatic T142 cell line expresses a STAT2 isoform with an apparent molecular mass higher than that observed in the remaining UM cells.

2.3. Expression of HTR2B Responds to Stimulation by IL4 and IL6 in Uveal Melanoma

The previous experiments demonstrated that all UM cells express STAT proteins to different levels. However, this does not necessarily reflect the activation status of these transcription factors in unstimulated cells. We therefore verified both the total and phosphorylated STAT1, STAT3 and STAT5 proteins present in all our UM cell lines. These STAT family members were selected for this analysis as they are the most often involved in cancer development and also because they are expressed to relatively high levels in UM cells. As shown on Figure 3A, a large proportion of the STAT1, STAT3 and STAT5 proteins expressed by T97 and T108 is phosphorylated. On the other hand, T142 also expresses phospho-STAT3 but has no detectable phospho-STAT1 or phospho-STAT5. As for T142, T143 UM cells also had no detectable phospho-STAT1 nor phospho-STAT5 and only a weak level of phospho-STAT3. As T142 has a barely detectable level of total STAT1 and no activated STAT1, we therefore selected this UM cell line to verify whether it would respond to stimulation of STAT1 activation by interleukins 4 (IL-4) and 6 (IL-6). As expected, control T142 UM cells expressed no detectable level of total or phosphorylated STAT1 (Ctl; Figure 3B). However, the addition of either IL-4 or IL-6 dramatically increased expression of total STAT1 (Figure 3B,C). Furthermore, both these interleukins proved to be very efficient at activating STAT1, since as little as 100 pM considerably increased phosphorylation of this transcription factor in T142 cells relative to the unstimulated controls (Figure 3B).

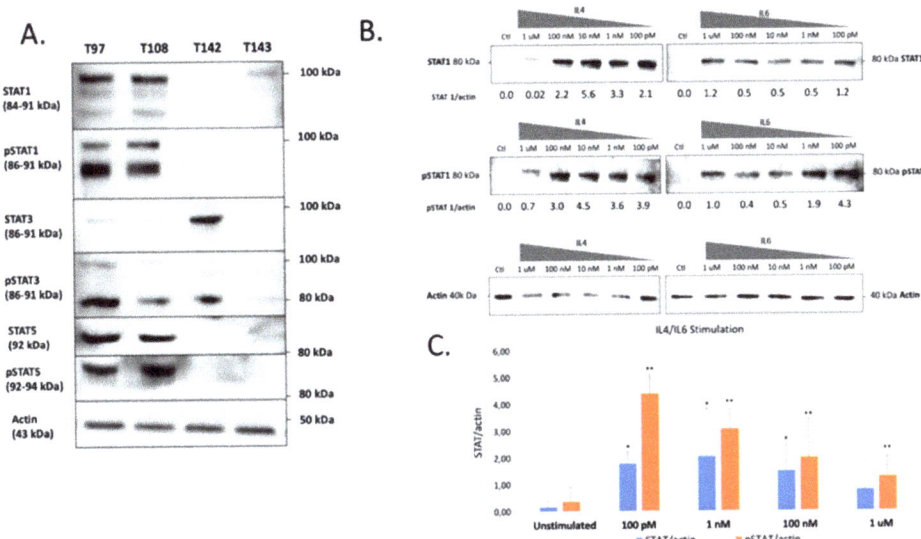

Figure 3. Western blot analysis of total and phosphorylated STAT1, STAT3 and STAT5 in UM cell lines. (**A**) Proteins from the UM cell lines T97, T108, T142 and T143 were Western blotted using antibodies that recognize only the phosphorylated (phospho-STAT1, phosphor-STAT3 and phosphor-STAT5) or total (comprising both inactive and phosphorylated) STAT1, STAT3 or STAT5 proteins (STAT1, STAT3 and STAT5). T97 and T108 UM cells express phosphorylated STAT1, STAT3 and STAT5 whereas T142 and T143 only express moderate and low levels of phospho-STAT3, respectively. The molecular mass of each STAT isoform is indicated in parenthesis. Actin is shown as a control. (**B**) Western blot analysis of either total (STAT1) or phosphorylated (pSTAT1) STAT1 in T142 UM cells that have been grown alone (Ctl) or in the presence of increasing doses (100 pM to 1 µM) of IL-4 and IL-6. The ratio of total (STAT1/actin) and phosphorylated (pSTAT1/actin) STAT1 over that of actin is also shown for both IL-4 and IL-6 stimulation. (**C**) Graph representation of the STAT/actin and pSTAT/actin ratios in either unstimulated or IL-4/IL-6 stimulated T142 UM cells. The addition of either IL-4 or IL-6 dramatically increased expression of total STAT1. Actin is shown as a control. * and **: Values considered to be statistically significant from those obtained for unstimulated total (STAT/actin) and phosphorylated (pSTAT/actin) STAT1, respectively (p value < 0.01).

That three DREs with a perfect match to the STAT consensus sequence could be found in the HTR2B gene promoter and 5′-flanking sequence does not warrant that they would resolve the appropriate activated STAT response in vitro. In order to verify whether expression of HTR2B indeed responds to activated STAT proteins, we cultured both T142 and T143 UM cells in the presence of varying concentrations (100 pM to 1 µM) of IL-4 and IL-6 and evaluated whether this would alter expression of HTR2B at the protein level. Consistent with the results shown on Figure 3, expression of HTR2B considerably increased in both T142 (4.7-fold increases in the HTR2B/actin ratio in the presence of IL-4 and IL-6 relative to negative controls, respectively) and T143 UM cells (7.7- and 11.5-fold increases in the HTR2B/actin ratio in the presence of IL-4 and IL-6 relative to controls, respectively) when as little as 100 pM of either IL-4 and IL-6 were added to the culture medium, relative to untreated cells (negative controls) (Figure 4). The HTR2B/actin ratio remained fairly stable as the concentration of both IL-4 and IL-6 is increased to 1 µM. We therefore conclude that expression of HTR2B increases in response to STAT-mediated interleukin signaling.

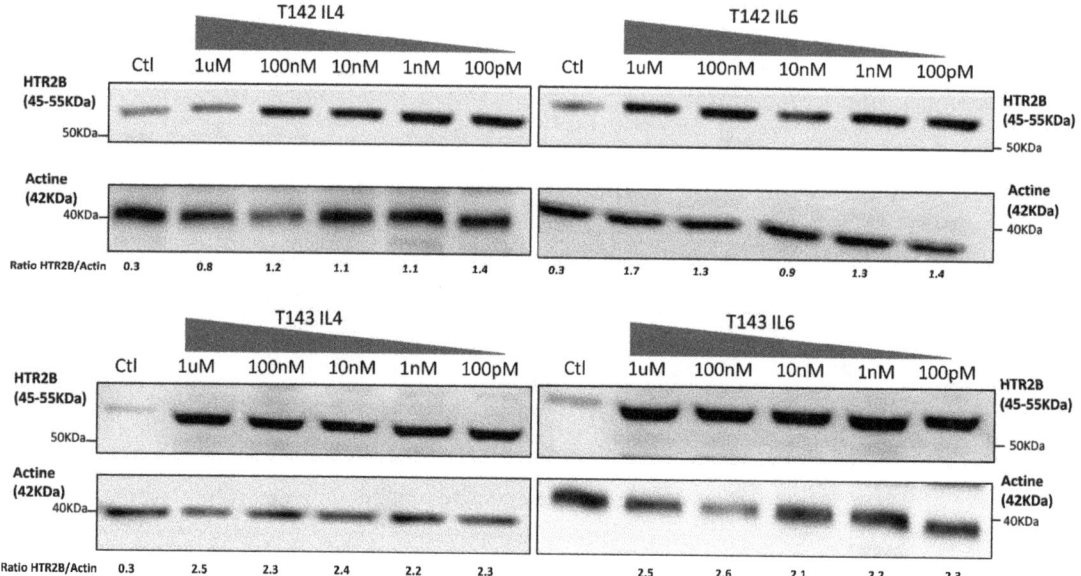

Figure 4. Expression of HTR2B in response to stimulation with IL-4 and IL-6. Expression of HTR2B was monitored by Western blot in both T142 and T143 UM cells cultured either alone (Ctl) or in the presence of increasing concentrations of IL4 and IL6 (100 pM to 1 µM). Values shown beneath each blot correspond to the ratio of the HTR2B signal over that of actin. Both IL-4 and IL-6 considerably increased expression of HTR2B in T142 and T143 UM cells relative to untreated cells (negative controls).

2.4. The −280 STAT Target Site Binds STAT Proteins and Contributes to HTR2B Promoter Activity In Vitro

As stated earlier, three distinct DNA regulatory elements that perfectly match the prototypical STAT target site have been identified in the HTR2B gene promoter (Supplementary Figure S1B). Because the −280 STAT DRE has its palyndromic repeats separated by a three nucleotides linker, a configuration that is also the most preferred for DNA binding of most STAT isoforms [26], it was selected to conduct the experiments in an electrophoretic mobility shift assay (EMSA). Therefore, 29 bp, double-stranded synthetic oligonucleotides bearing either the wild-type DNA sequence of the HTR2B −280 STAT site (WT), or a mutated STAT derivative in which the T, T and G residues at positions −284, −283 and −178 were changed for A, A and G, respectively (Table S1), were [^{32}P] 5′-end-labelled and used as labeled-probes in EMSAs. Incubation of increasing concentrations (5-, 15- and 20 µg) of nuclear proteins prepared from both T142 and T143 UM cells with the WT −280 STAT labeled probe yielded the formation of five distinct DNA-protein complexes (a to e) on a native polyacrylamide gel (Figure 5). Interestingly, substituting the wild-type probe for the mutated −280 STAT site (Mut) led to the complete disappearance of complex b (this is particularly evident using the T143 proteins) when the same amount of extracts from both T142 and T143 cells were used as the source of proteins, suggesting that formation of complex b results from the recognition of the WT labeled probe by STAT proteins. Furthermore, we also observed an increase in the DNA binding of complex d when extracts from T142 and T143 UM cells were used, respectively (Figure 5).

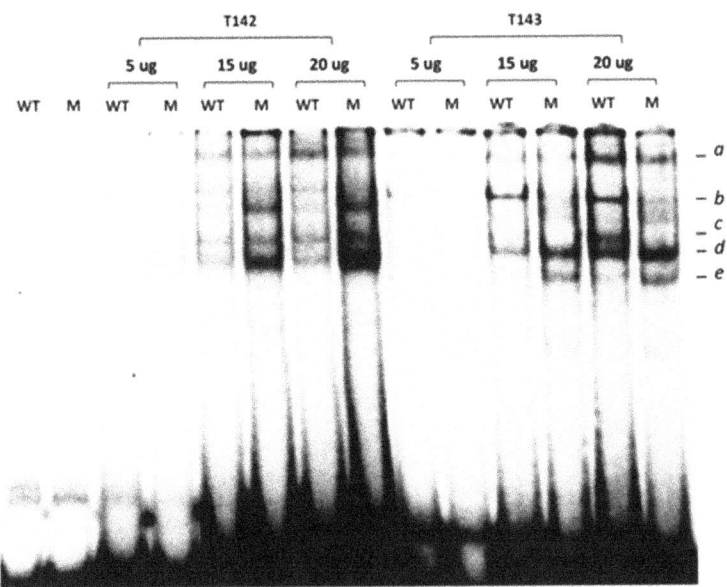

Figure 5. Gel shift analysis of the nuclear proteins binding to the *HTR2B* −280 STAT site. Nuclear proteins (5-, 15- or 20 μg) obtained from the UM cell lines T142 and T143 were incubated with a 5′ end-labeled, double-stranded oligonucleotide bearing either the wild-type sequence of the −280 STAT site identified in the *HTR2B* gene promoter (WT), or a derivative in which the −280 STAT site was mutated (M). Formation of DNA-protein complexes was then monitored by EMSA. The position of the multiple DNA-protein complexes formed is indicated (*a* to *e*), along with that of the free probe (U). Incubation of increasing concentrations of T142 and T143 nuclear proteins with the WT −280 STAT labeled probe yielded the formation of distinct DNA-protein complexes of which only complex *b* completely disappeared when the wild-type probe was substituted by the mutated −280 STAT site (Mut).

We recently cloned different segments from the HTR2B gene promoter and 5′-flanking sequences upstream from the chloramphenicol acetyl transferase (CAT) reporter gene in order to characterize the regulatory elements modulating expression of that gene in UM cells. This study led to the demonstration that HTR2B gene transcription was down-regulated by the presence of both a proximal and distal silencer element that proved functional only in non-metastatic UM cells in vitro [32]. As the −280 STAT target site identified in the present study is located right in the middle of the proximal silencer, we examined whether both IL-4 and IL-6 can impact on the activity directed by the HTR2B gene promoter and whether mutation of this STAT site would alter IL-4 and IL-6 responsiveness in vitro. Therefore, the −280 STAT site was mutated in a version of the HTR2B gene that includes 2 kb of the 5′ promoter and flanking sequence (in the HTR2B/-2000 construct) (Figure 6A). Because they are much easier to transfect than any other of our UM cell lines, the plasmids bearing both the wild-type −280 STAT site and its mutated derivative were transfected in T108 UM cells and the CAT activities were determined. The addition of 100 nM IL-4 and IL-6 significantly increased by 54% and 67% the CAT activity directed by HTR2B/-2000, respectively (in HTR2B/-2000(WT$_{STAT-280}$); Figure 6B). On the other hand, mutation of the −280 STAT site in HTR2B/-2000(MU$_{STAT-280}$) entirely abolished both IL-4 and IL-6 responsiveness in transfected T108 UM cells.

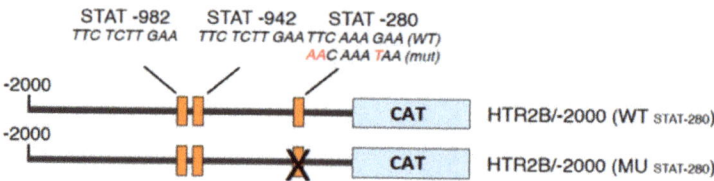

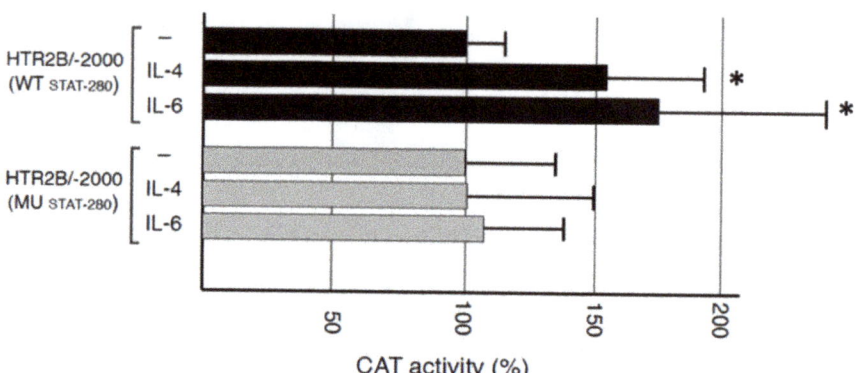

Figure 6. Responsiveness of the *HTR2B* gene promoter to IL-4 and IL-6 in transfected T108 cells: (**A**) Representation of the HTR2B/CAT recombinant plasmids used for transfection analyses. Numbers indicate the position relative to the *HTR2B* theoretical mRNA start site. The position of the three conserved STAT sites is indicated (STAT-982, STAT-942 and STAT-280) (**B**) CAT activities measured following transfection of the *HTR2B* constructs shown in panel B in the UM cell line T108. CAT activity is expressed relative to the level directed by the HTR2B/-2000 construct. *: Values considered to be statistically significant from those obtained with the HTR2B/-138 construct (p value < 0.01). Addition of IL-4 and IL-6 increased CAT activity encoded by the plasmid HTR2B/-2000(WT$_{STAT-280}$) but not when the −280 STAT site is mutated in HTR2B/-2000(MU$_{STAT-280}$).

3. Discussions

We recently investigated the molecular mechanisms that contribute to the increased expression of HTR2B in metastatic UM cells and demonstrated that both transcription factors Nuclear factor I (NFI) and Runt-related transcription factor 1 (RUNX1) interact with regulatory elements from the *HTR2B* gene to either activate (NFI) or repress (RUNX1) *HTR2B* expression in UM cells [32]. However, these TFs alone are insufficient to explain the elevated level of HTR2B protein observed in metastatic UM cells. The purpose of the present study was to investigate the potential contribution of proteins from the STAT transcription factors family to the expression of HTR2B in human UM cells. We demonstrated that all UM cell lines express their own combination of STAT isoforms and that some of them are obviously activated through phosphorylation. Furthermore, both IL-4 and IL-6 proved to be very efficient at activating STAT1 in metastatic T142 UM cells. Most of all, exposure to IL-4 and IL-6 dramatically increased the expression of HTR2B in both T142 and T143 UM cells. We could identify multiple putative target sites for STAT proteins within the promoter and 5′-flanking sequence of the *HTR2B* gene and demonstrated the binding of

STAT proteins to the DRE located at position −280. Mutation of this −280 STAT DRE totally abolished responsiveness of the *HTR2B* basal promoter toward IL-4 and IL-6, therefore establishing that transcription of the *HTR2B* gene is under the regulatory influence of STAT proteins in uveal melanoma.

We recently reported that the 292bp *HTR2B* promoter segment extending from positions −138 to −430, and therefore comprising the −280 proximal STAT DRE, shares a negative regulatory function typical of silencer elements [32]. That same DNA area was also shown to bind members of the NFI family of transcription factors, although the positive regulatory influence they exert through binding of this NFI site (located at position −210) was rather weak [32]. Therefore, STAT proteins that interact with the −280 site are also located close to other transcription factors, such as NFI, that also bind nearby the −280 STAT site. Besides this promoter proximal negative regulatory region, a more distal silencer element (located from positions −1297 to −710) was also shown to bind the positive transcription factor RUNX1 [32]. Direct interaction between STAT and RUNX proteins that mutually inhibits their transcriptional activity has been reported [34]. Furthermore, NFI-B2, a member from the NFI family of TFs, and STAT5 were found to bind nearby DNA target sites in the promoter of the whey acidic protein (WAP) to regulate its expression during pregnancy in the mouse mammary gland, although no direct physical interaction between both factors was demonstrated [35,36]. The fact that mutations that also prevent binding of STATs to the −280 STAT site did not prevent the formation of other DNA-protein complexes in EMSA (for instance, that of complexes *a*, *d* and *e*; Figure 6A) also suggests the presence of additional transcription factor binding sites located nearby, or overlapping with the −280 STAT target site. That an increased signal is observed for some of these DNA-protein complexes (such as for complex *d*) when the −280 STAT DRE is mutated is consistent with the possibility that it overlaps with the target sites recognized by these yet unknown factors. Unlike with the non-metastatic T97, T108 and T143 UM cell lines, both the *HTR2B* proximal and distal silencers are inactive in T142 metastatic cells. Therefore, STAT proteins most likely compete with the negative regulatory transcription factors that ensure the functionality of these silencer elements and a delicate balance between them must dictate the level to which the *HTR2B* gene is transcribed in non-metastatic UM cells. In metastatic T142 cells, this delicate balance is apparently shifted toward a regulatory function primarily ensured by positive regulatory TFs, including STAT proteins.

The increase in the molecular mass of STAT2 (a slight increase in that of STAT5 was also observed) in the metastatic T142 UM cell line relative to its apparent M_W in the non-metastatic T143 cell line is believed to result from post-translational modifications (PTMs) in T142 cells that are not occurring in T143 UM cells. Besides PTMs such as phosphorylation, ubiquitination, ISGylation, SUMOylation and acetylation, that do not significantly affect the molecular mass of the affected proteins, STATs have also been shown to be subjected to glycosylation, which, on the other hand, can cause substantial alterations in the electrophoretic mobility of the targeted proteins [37,38]. Indeed, wheat germ agglutinin affinity chromatography revealed that STAT1, STAT3, STAT5A, STAT5B and STAT6 are glucose-modified through the addition of O-linked N-acetylglucosamine (O-GlcNAc) residues on threonine or serine residues [39]. Serine/threonine phosphorylation of STAT1, STAT3 and STAT5 has been shown to contribute to the etiology of certain human cancers and immunodeficiencies [40]. In many cancers, STAT5 activation and its oncogenic gene expression is not only enhanced, but also kept persistent, whereas signaling involving activation of STAT5 is rather transient under physiological conditions. Interestingly, cancer-specific metabolic changes enhance glycosylation, which subsequently modulates STAT5 activity through enhanced tyrosine phosphorylation. Reducing the glycosylation status of the hyper-phosphorylated STAT5A variant, via glucose depletion or hypoxia, has been reported to restore transcription of oncogenic target genes back to their wild type level [41]. Glycosylation of proteins at threonine and/or serine residues, including transcription factors such as Sp1, SMAD4, DeltaLf (Delta-lactoferrin) and Nrf1 (Nuclear factor E2-related factor 1), to name a few, has been suggested to protect them from proteasomal degradation by masking nearby amino acids that are normally ubiquitinated [42–46], therefore increasing their steady-state stability. Therefore, and based on these observations, we can assume that the glycosylation status of both STAT2 and STAT5 might be related to the aggressiveness of the T142 UM cell line by ensuring an abnormally elevated intracellular signalization which also causes an increased expression of their target genes, such as HTR2B. Further experiments aimed at investigating the glycosylation status of STAT proteins in UM cells will surely prove particularly interesting as it may link this PTM to the UM metastatic properties.

Besides the −280 STAT site, our search for putative STAT target sites in the *HTR2B* promoter also revealed the presence of two other sequences with a perfect match to the STAT consensus target site at positions −982 and −942 relative to the *HTR2B* mRNA start site. The fact that mutation of the −280 proximal STAT site entirely abolished interleukin responsiveness in the context of the HTR2B/-2000 suggests that neither of these distant STAT sites can rescue the IL-4 and IL-6 responsiveness in T108 cells when the −280 STAT site is mutated. However, the apparent lack of functionality for both of these STAT distant sites might be context-dependent and a more in-depth characterization will be required before one can assume that neither are contributing to *hTR2B* gene expression in uveal melanoma.

The fact that both IL4 and IL6 not only contributed to the activation of STAT1 in T142 UM cells but also somehow restored its expression at the protein level (as very little STAT1 protein could be detected by Western blot in unstimulated UM cells) is particularly interesting, as it suggests *STAT1* gene transcription to be under the control of a positive feedback loop in T142 cells. Indeed, STAT1 has been shown to contribute to the transcription of its own gene through the presence of multiple STAT binding sites located within the *STAT1* gene proximal promoter, and mutation of these sites was found to disrupt reporter gene activity in response to leukemia inhibitory factor (LIF) [47]. Both the presence of an immune inflammatory phenotype and the tumor size correlates with a poor clinical prognosis in uveal melanoma. Interestingly, abnormally elevated levels of many cytokines, including IL-2, IL-4, IL-6 and IL-8, have been observed in the vitreous of eyes from patients with uveal melanoma [48–52]. IL-6 appears to be an important player in UM tumor progression, as increased expression in the level of this cytokine also correlates with an increased tumor prominence and the presence of both macrophage and T_{reg} infiltration of the primary tumor [48]. Among the tumor hallmarks of UM angiogenesis, the IL6-JAK-STAT3 pathway has been well-described to promote cancer progression as well as immunosuppression in an autocrine manner [53]. In the UM, activation of this signalization cascade also induces the trans-activation of the JunB subunit from the transcription factor AP-1, which, in turn, also promotes UM epithelial-mesenchymal transition and aggressiveness in UM [54].

Systemic therapies, including immunotherapy, have yielded poor results in the treatment of uveal melanoma [55]. Therefore, searching for new immune modulatory targets, incoming immunotherapy biomarkers and combined immune strategies with drugs offer a new therapeutic paradigm. Recent studies have shown an encouraging result in cutaneous melanoma (phase I clinical study) using these approaches [55]. However, despite the common origin from neural crest-derived cells, uveal and cutaneous melanomas have few overlapping genetic signatures. As a consequence, many therapies that have proven effective in cutaneous melanoma have little or no success in uveal melanoma. Immunotherapy with checkpoint inhibition showed promising results in the treatment of cutaneous melanoma, however, it did not appear to be equally effective with uveal melanoma. Moreover, angiogenesis seems to confer a worse prognosis to UM when compared to cutaneous melanoma [56]. Better insight into the molecular and genetic profile of uveal melanoma, such as the interest given in our study to the contribution of STAT family members to the expression of the serotonin receptor HTR2B, will facilitate the identification of new prognostic biomarkers and thus enable us to adapt the existing immunotherapy procedures in order to develop new forms of treatments specifically designed for uveal melanoma patients [57]. STAT family members have been involved in human cancer progression, development, survival, and resistance to treatment. This is especially the case for both STAT3 and STAT5 that are considered either as oncogenes or tumor suppressors, depending on the context and the delicate balance between the different counteracting transcription factors involved [23]. Immunotherapy approaches have been extensively investigated in recent years, and since these transcription factors are key members in the immune system response, it comes as no surprise that they are also embedded in the growing collection of potential new immune modulatory targets. Assessing the STAT signaling pathway and expression of its constituting mediators have been shown to predict sensitivity to immunotherapy and targeted STAT inhibition [23]. Knowing that STAT members are under the control of immune, interleukin/cytokine signals that differ from one patient to another may prove particularly informative as to whether any specific patient is a potential candidate for immunotherapy, depending on his STAT/interleukins/cytokines expression status.

In immunotherapy approaches, most attention is paid to the targeted inhibition of immune checkpoints using monoclonal antibodies, especially against PD-1 (programmed cell death protein 1), a cell-surface receptor that acts to restrain T cell-mediated immune responses when activated by its specific ligand PD-L1 (programmed death ligand 1) [58]. STAT1 and STAT3 are considered as potential biomarkers to define patients who are more likely to respond to immunotherapy, as both these family members induce the expression of PD-L1 [59–61]. Consequently, their baseline expression levels could be an indicator of PD-L1 manifestation in the tumor micro-environment, and thus help predict response to anti-PD-L1 immunotherapy [61]. According to recent developments, STAT1 emerged as a potential immunotherapy biomarker. Indeed, in their study, Zemek et al. compared the gene expression profiles of immune checkpoint inhibition responsive and non-responsive tumors in mice and validated their findings in cohorts of patients with cancer treated with immune checkpoint blocking antibodies [59]. They found that responsive tumors were characterized by an inflammatory gene expression signature consistent with an up-regulation of STAT1 signaling. This is particularly appealing in that their findings rendered possible the use of a biomarker-driven approach to patient management in order to properly establish whether a patient would benefit from treatment with sensitizing therapeutics before immune checkpoint blockade. In our study, the presence of a STAT2 protein with an abnormally elevated molecular mass combined to the presence of activated STAT3 distinguishes the T142 metastatic from the other non-metastatic UM cell lines and therefore militates toward a deeper involvement of both STAT2 and STAT3 in the aggressiveness of uveal melanoma. Analysis of the STAT2 and STAT3 expression and activation profiles in additional UM primary tumors and UM cell lines should prove particularly interesting to decipher whether both these mediators can be used as diagnostic markers for the identification of patients at risk of evolving toward liver metastatic disease.

In summary, we demonstrated that STAT proteins contribute to the transcription of the serotonin receptor HTR2B in uveal melanoma. The demonstration that STAT proteins can physically interact, or synergize with transcription factors such as NFI [35,36] that positively regulate transcription of the *HTR2B* gene, gives further support to the occurrence of an interleukin/JAK/STAT/NFI signalization cascade that likely contributes to the aggressiveness of uveal melanoma.

4. Materials and Methods

This study was conducted in agreement with the Helsinki declaration and was performed under the guidelines of the research ethics committee of the "CHU de Québec" (ethic code: F9-49776, protocol renewal approved on 4 September 2020).

4.1. Cell Culture

The UM cell lines T97, T98, T108, T111, T128, T131, T132, T142, T143, T151 and T157 were each cultured from the primary tumors of different patients diagnosed with this type of cancer and have already been previously described [33,62–64]. All cells were cultured in Dulbecco/Vogt modified Eagle's minimal essential medium (DMEM) Multicell (high glucose, with l-glut, without L-Pyruvate; Wisent, Québec, QC, Canada) supplemented with

10% fetal bovine serum (FBS) High quality (Wisent, Québec, QC, Canada) and 0.002% v/v gentamicin (Life Technologies (distributed by Thermo Fisher Scientific Inc., Rockford, IL, USA) at 37 °C under 5% CO_2.

4.2. Plasmid Construct, Oligonucleotides and Site-Directed Mutagenesis

Construction of the HTR2B/-2000 plasmid bearing the HTR2B promoter segment from −2000 to +96 relative to the theoretical mRNA start site has been described previously [32]. The putative STAT target site identified at position −280 upstream of the HTR2B theoretical mRNA start site was mutated into the HTR2B/-2000 construct (to yield HTR2B/-2000($MU_{STAT-280}$)) using the Quick Change Lightning Multi Site-Directed Mutagenesis Kit from Agilent Technologies (Santa Clara, CA, USA) according to manufacturer's instructions (see Supplementary Table S1 for DNA sequence of the mutated primers used). The DNA insert from each recombinant plasmid was sequenced by chain-termination dideoxy sequencing (SANGER Sequencing platform, CHU de Québec-Université Laval Research Center, CHUL, Québec, Canada) to confirm the mutations.

The double-stranded oligonucleotides used either as labeled probe or unlabeled competitors in the EMSAs were chemically synthesized using a Biosearch 8700 apparatus (Integrated DNA Technologies, Inc., Coralville, WA, USA). Their DNA sequences are listed in Supplementary Table S1.

4.3. Transient Transfections and CAT Assays

The HTR2B/-2000 plasmids bearing the wild-type −280 STAT target site (HTR2B/-2000($WT_{STAT-280}$)) and its derivative bearing mutations in the −280 STAT site (HTR2B/-2000($MU_{STAT-280}$)) were transiently transfected into sub-confluent (80% coverage of the culture plate) T108 UM cells. Six-wells tissue-culture plates were used along with the K2® Transfection System following the manufacturer's instructions (BIONTEX, München, Germany). Each tissue-culture well received 1.5 g of the test plasmid and 0.5 g of the hGH-encoding plasmid PXGH5. All cells were harvested 48 h following transfection and CAT activities were determined and normalized to the hGH secreted in the medium as previously described [32]. Values shown are the mean of three separate transfections, each done in triplicate.

4.4. Preparation of Nuclear Extracts and EMSA

All tissue-cultured UM cells were grown to mid-confluence (70% coverage of the culture flasks) prior to preparation of nuclear extracts and their use in EMSAs following previously described procedures [65,66]. EMSAs were carried out by incubating 5×10^4 cpm of the ^{32}P-end-labelled, double-stranded oligonucleotide bearing the DNA sequence of the HTR2B −280 STAT site with the amount of nuclear proteins specified in the legend of each figure, in the presence of 2 μg of poly(dI:dC) (Amersham Biosciences, Piscataway, NJ, USA) and 50 mM KCl in buffer D [10 mM Hepes pH 7.9, 10% v/v glycerol, 0.1 mM EDTA, 0.5 mM DTT (dithiothreitol; Sigma-Aldrich Canada, Oakville, ON, Canada) and 0.25 mM phenylmethylsulfonyl fluoride (PMSF; Sigma-Aldrich Canada)]. DNA–protein complexes were next separated by gel electrophoresis through 8% non-denaturing polyacrylamide gels run against a Tris-glycine buffer (50 mM Tris, 2.5 mM EDTA, 0.4 M glycine) at 4 °C. The position of the DNA–protein complexes was then revealed upon autoradiography of the dried gels at −80 °C.

4.5. Western Blots

Western blots were conducted as described [32,62–64,67] using antibodies directed against the following proteins: Total STAT1 (D1K9Y (polyclonal), 1/300; Cell Signaling Technology), Total STAT2 (D9J7L (polyclonal), 1/300; Cell Signaling Technology, Danvers, MA, USA), Total STAT3 (sc-8019 (monoclonal), 1/100; Santa Cruz Biotechnology, Dallas, TX, USA), Total STAT4 (sc-398228 (monoclonal), 1/100; Santa Cruz Biotechnology), Total STAT5 (sc-74442 (monoclonal), 1/100; Santa Cruz Biotechnology), Total STAT6 (sc-374021 (monoclonal), 1/100; Santa Cruz Biotechnology), HTR2B (HPA-012867 (monoclonal), 1/100; Millipore Sigma), Phospho STAT1 (sc-8394 (monoclonal), 1/100; Santa Cruz Biotechnology), Phospho STAT3 (sc-8059 (monoclonal), 1/100; Santa Cruz Biotechnology), Phospho STAT5 (sc-81524 (monoclonal), 1/100; Santa Cruz Biotechnology), and a peroxidase-conjugated AffiniPure Goat secondary antibody against mouse IgG (1:2500 dilution; Jackson ImmunoResearch Laboratories, West Grove, PA, USA).

4.6. Gene Expression Profiling

Isolation of total RNA and microarray analysis, which all comply with the Minimum Information About a Microarray Experiment (MIAME) requirements, were conducted as recently reported [67]. All data generated from the arrays were also analyzed by robust multi-array analysis (RMA) for background correction of the raw values. They were then transformed in Log2 base and quantile normalized before a linear model was fitted to the normalized data to obtain an expression measure for each probe set on each array. Heat maps were generated using the ArrayStar V4.1 (DNASTAR, Madison, WI, USA) software. All microarray data presented in this study comply with the Minimum Information About a Microarray Experiment (MIAME) requirements. Data have been deposited in NCBIs Gene Expression Omnibus (GEO, available online: http://www.ncbi.nlm.nih.gov/geo/) and are accessible through GEO Series accession number GSE GSE86915 (last accessed date: 25 January 2022).

4.7. Statistical Analyses

A Student's *t*-test was performed for comparison of the groups in transfection analyses. Differences were considered to be statistically significant at $p < 0.05$. All data are also expressed as mean $\pm$ SD.

Supplementary Materials: The following supporting information can be downloaded at: https://www.mdpi.com/article/10.3390/ijms23031564/s1.

Author Contributions: Conceptualization, S.L.G.; Data curation, M.B. and G.L.-B.; Formal analysis, M.B. and G.L.-B.; Funding acquisition, S.L.G.; Investigation, S.L.G.; Methodology, M.B. and G.L.-B.; Project administration, S.L.G.; Supervision, S.L.G.; Validation, S.L.G.; Writing—original draft, M.B.; Writing—review & editing, S.L.G. All authors have read and agreed to the published version of the manuscript.

Funding: This work was supported by a grant from the Cancer Research Society (CRS) to S.L.G. (grant #24004). The Québec Ocular tissue bank and the Uveal Melanoma Infrastructure are financially supported by the Réseau de recherche en santé de la vision from the Fonds de recherche du Québec—Santé (FRQS).

Institutional Review Board Statement: This study was conducted according to the guidelines of the Declaration of Helsinki, and approved by the Institutional Review Board (or Ethics Committee) of "CHU de Québec" (ethic code: F9-49776, protocol renewal approved on 1 September 2020).

Informed Consent Statement: Not applicable.

Data Availability Statement: All microarray data presented in this study can be accessed at NCBI Gene Expression Omnibus (GEO# GSE86915; https://www.ncbi.nlm.nih.gov/geo/query/acc.cgi?acc=GSE86915) (last accessed date: 19 December 2022).

Acknowledgments: The authors would like to thank Solange Landreville (CUO-Recherche, CHU de Québec) for providing some of the UM microarray annotation files whose data were used in this study. The Banque d'yeux Nationale is partly supported by the Réseau de Recherche en Santé de la Vision from the FRQS. M.B. is supported by a studentship from the FRQS.

Conflicts of Interest: The authors declare that they have no conflict of interest.

Abbreviations

EMSA   Electrophoretic mobility shift assay

References

1. Yang, J.; Manson, D.K.; Marr, B.P.; Carvajal, R.D. Treatment of uveal melanoma: Where are we now? *Ther. Adv. Med. Oncol.* **2018**, *10*, 1758834018757175. [CrossRef] [PubMed]
2. Carvajal, R.D.; Schwartz, G.K.; Tezel, T.; Marr, B.; Francis, J.H.; Nathan, P.D. Metastatic disease from uveal melanoma: Treatment options and future prospects. *Br. J. Ophthalmol.* **2017**, *101*, 38–44. [CrossRef] [PubMed]
3. Diener-West, M.; Reynolds, S.M.; Agugliaro, D.J.; Caldwell, R.; Cumming, K.; Earle, J.D.; Hawkins, B.S.; Hayman, J.A.; Jaiyesimi, I.; Jampol, L.M.; et al. Development of Metastatic Disease after Enrollment in the COMS Trials for Treatment of Choroidal Melanoma. *Arch. Ophthalmol.* **2005**, *123*, 1639–1643. [CrossRef]
4. Onken, M.D.; Worley, L.A.; Ehlers, J.P.; Harbour, J.W. Gene expression profiling in uveal melanoma reveals two molecular classes and predicts metastatic death. *Cancer Res.* **2004**, *64*, 7205–7209. [CrossRef] [PubMed]
5. Onken, M.D.; Worley, L.A.; Tuscan, M.D.; Harbour, J.W. An accurate, clinically feasible multi-gene expression assay for predicting metastasis in uveal melanoma. *J. Mol. Diagn.* **2010**, *12*, 461–468. [CrossRef] [PubMed]
6. Zhang, Y.; Yang, Y.; Chen, L.; Zhang, J. Expression analysis of genes and pathways associated with liver metastases of the uveal melanoma. *BMC Med. Genet.* **2014**, *15*, 29. [CrossRef]
7. Dizeyi, N.; Bjartell, A.; Hedlund, P.; Taskén, K.A.; Gadaleanu, V.; Abrahamsson, P.-A. Expression of Serotonin Receptors 2B and 4 in Human Prostate Cancer Tissue and Effects of Their Antagonists on Prostate Cancer Cell Lines. *Eur. Urol.* **2005**, *47*, 895–900. [CrossRef]
8. Svejda, B.; Kidd, M.; Giovinazzo, F.; Eltawil, K.; Gustafsson, B.I.; Pfragner, R.; Modlin, I.M. The 5-HT2B receptor plays a key regulatory role in both neuroendocrine tumor cell proliferation and the modulation of the fibroblast component of the neoplastic microenvironment. *Cancer* **2010**, *116*, 2902–2912. [CrossRef]
9. Soll, C.; Jang, J.H.; Riener, M.-O.; Moritz, W.; Wild, P.J.; Graf, R.; Clavien, P.-A. Serotonin promotes tumor growth in human hepatocellular cancer. *Hepatology* **2010**, *51*, 1244–1254. [CrossRef]
10. Henriksen, R.; Dizeyi, N.; Abrahamsson, P.-A. Expression of serotonin receptors 5-HT1A, 5-HT1B, 5-HT2B and 5-HT4 in ovary and in ovarian tumours. *Anticancer. Res.* **2012**, *32*, 1361–1366.
11. Harbour, J.W.; Onken, M.D.; Roberson, E.D.; Duan, S.; Cao, L.; Worley, L.A.; Council, M.L.; Matatall, K.A.; Helms, C.; Bowcock, A.M. Frequent mutation of BAP1 in metastasizing uveal melanomas. *Science* **2010**, *330*, 1410–1413. [CrossRef] [PubMed]
12. Raymond, J.R.; Mukhin, Y.V.; Gelasco, A.; Turner, J.; Collinsworth, G.; Gettys, T.W.; Grewal, J.S.; Garnovskaya, M.N. Multiplicity of mechanisms of serotonin receptor signal transduction. *Pharmacol. Ther.* **2001**, *92*, 179–212. [CrossRef]
13. van Raamsdonk, C.D.; Bezrookove, V.; Green, G.; Bauer, J.; Gaugler, L.; O'Brien, J.M.; Simpson, E.M.; Barsh, G.S.; Bastian, B.C. Frequent somatic mutations of GNAQ in uveal melanoma and blue naevi. *Nature* **2009**, *457*, 599–602. [CrossRef] [PubMed]
14. Banes, A.K.L.; Shaw, S.M.; Tawfik, A.; Patel, B.P.; Ogbi, S.; Fulton, D.; Marrero, M.B. Activation of the JAK/STAT pathway in vascular smooth muscle by serotonin. *Am. J. Physiol. Cell Physiol.* **2005**, *288*, C805–C812. [CrossRef] [PubMed]
15. Naito, K.; Tanaka, C.; Mitsuhashi, M.; Moteki, H.; Kimura, M.; Natsume, H.; Ogihara, M. Signal Transduction Mechanism for Serotonin 5-HT2B Receptor-Mediated DNA Synthesis and Proliferation in Primary Cultures of Adult Rat Hepatocytes. *Biol. Pharm. Bull.* **2016**, *39*, 121–129. [CrossRef] [PubMed]
16. Watanabe, T.; Pakala, R.; Katagiri, T.; Benedict, C.R. Serotonin potentiates angiotensin II—induced vascular smooth muscle cell proliferation. *Atherosclerosis* **2001**, *159*, 269–279. [CrossRef]
17. Donegan, J.J.; Patton, M.S.; Chavera, T.S.; Berg, K.A.; Morilak, D.A.; Girotti, M. Interleukin-6 Attenuates Serotonin 2A Receptor Signaling by Activating the JAK-STAT Pathway. *Mol. Pharmacol.* **2015**, *87*, 492–500. [CrossRef]
18. Coelho, W.S.; Sola-Penna, M. Serotonin regulates 6-phosphofructo-1-kinase activity in a PLC–PKC–CaMK II- and Janus kinase-dependent signaling pathway. *Mol. Cell. Biochem.* **2013**, *372*, 211–220. [CrossRef]
19. Weidmann, C.; Berube, J.; Piquet, L.; de La Fouchardiere, A.; Landreville, S. Expression of the serotonin receptor 2B in uveal melanoma and effects of an antagonist on cell lines. *Clin. Exp. Metastasis* **2018**, *35*, 123–134. [CrossRef]
20. Darnell, J.E., Jr. STATs and Gene Regulation. *Science* **1997**, *277*, 1630–1635. [CrossRef]
21. Bowman, T.; Garcia, R.; Turkson, J.; Jove, R. STATs in oncogenesis. *Oncogene* **2000**, *19*, 2474–2488. [CrossRef] [PubMed]
22. Calò, V.; Migliavacca, M.; Bazan, V.; Macaluso, M.; Buscemi, M.; Gebbia, N.; Russo, A. STAT proteins: From normal control of cellular events to tumorigenesis. *J. Cell. Physiol.* **2003**, *197*, 157–168. [CrossRef] [PubMed]
23. Verhoeven, Y.; Tilborghs, S.; Jacobs, J.; de Waele, J.; Quatannens, D.; Deben, C.; Prenen, H.; Pauwels, P.; Trinh, X.B.; Wouters, A.; et al. The potential and controversy of targeting STAT family members in cancer. *Semin. Cancer Biol.* **2020**, *60*, 41–56. [CrossRef] [PubMed]
24. Zhang, J.; Wang, F.; Liu, F.; Xu, G. Predicting STAT1 as a prognostic marker in patients with solid cancer. *Ther. Adv. Med. Oncol.* **2020**, *12*, 1758835920917558. [CrossRef] [PubMed]
25. Koromilas, A.E.; Sexl, V. The tumor suppressor function of STAT1 in breast cancer. *JAK-STAT* **2013**, *2*, e23353. [CrossRef]
26. Ehret, G.B.; Reichenbach, P.; Schindler, U.; Horvath, C.M.; Fritz, S.; Nabholz, M.; Bucher, P. DNA Binding Specificity of Different STAT Proteins: Comparison of In Vitro Specificity with Natural Target Sites. *J. Biol. Chem.* **2001**, *276*, 6675–6688. [CrossRef]

27. Schindler, C.; Darnell, J.E., Jr. Transcriptional responses to polypeptide ligands: The JAK-STAT pathway. *Annu. Rev. Biochem.* **1995**, *64*, 621–651. [CrossRef]
28. Glantschnig, C.; Koenen, M.; Gil-Lozano, M.; Karbiener, M.; Pickrahn, I.; Williams-Dautovich, J.; Patel, R.; Cummins, C.L.; Giroud, M.; Hartleben, G.; et al. A miR-29a-driven negative feedback loop regulates peripheral glucocorticoid receptor signaling. *FASEB J.* **2019**, *33*, 5924–5941. [CrossRef]
29. He, B.; Lanz, R.B.; Fiskus, W.; Geng, C.; Yi, P.; Hartig, S.M.; Rajapakshe, K.; Shou, J.; Wei, L.; Shah, S.S.; et al. GATA2 facilitates steroid receptor coactivator recruitment to the androgen receptor complex. *Proc. Natl. Acad. Sci. USA* **2014**, *111*, 18261–18266. [CrossRef]
30. Dong, H.; Xu, J.; Li, W.; Gan, J.; Lin, W.; Ke, J.; Jiang, J.; Du, L.; Chen, Y.; Zhong, X.; et al. Reciprocal androgen receptor/interleukin-6 crosstalk drives oesophageal carcinoma progression and contributes to patient prognosis. *J. Pathol.* **2017**, *241*, 448–462. [CrossRef]
31. Booth, L.; Roberts, J.L.; Sander, C.; Lalani, A.S.; Kirkwood, J.M.; Hancock, J.F.; Poklepovic, A.; Dent, P. Neratinib and entinostat combine to rapidly reduce the expression of K-RAS, N-RAS, Gαq and Gα11 and kill uveal melanoma cells. *Cancer Biol. Ther.* **2019**, *20*, 700–710. [CrossRef] [PubMed]
32. Benhassine, M.; Guérin, S.L. Transcription of the Human 5-Hydroxytryptamine Receptor 2B (HTR2B) Gene Is under the Regulatory Influence of the Transcription Factors NFI and RUNX1 in Human Uveal Melanoma. *Int. J. Mol. Sci.* **2018**, *19*, 3272. [CrossRef] [PubMed]
33. Mouriaux, F.; Zaniolo, K.; Bergeron, M.-A.; Weidmann, C.; de la Fouchardiere, A.; Fournier, F.; Droit, A.; Morcos, M.W.; Landreville, S.; Guérin, S.L. Effects of Long-term Serial Passaging on the Characteristics and Properties of Cell Lines Derived from Uveal Melanoma Primary Tumors. *Investig. Opthalmology Vis. Sci.* **2016**, *57*, 5288–5301. [CrossRef]
34. Ogawa, S.; Satake, M.; Ikuta, K. Physical and Functional Interactions between STAT5 and Runx Transcription Factors. *J. Biochem.* **2008**, *143*, 695–709. [CrossRef]
35. Mukhopadhyay, S.S.; Wyszomierski, S.L.; Gronostajski, R.M.; Rosen, J.M. Differential Interactions of Specific Nuclear Factor I Isoforms with the Glucocorticoid Receptor and STAT5 in the Cooperative Regulation of WAP Gene Transcription. *Mol. Cell. Biol.* **2001**, *21*, 6859–6869. [CrossRef] [PubMed]
36. Robinson, G.W.; Kang, K.; Yoo, K.H.; Tang, Y.; Zhu, B.-M.; Yamaji, D.; Colditz, V.; Jang, S.J.; Gronostajski, R.M.; Hennighausen, L. Coregulation of Genetic Programs by the Transcription Factors NFIB and STAT5. *Mol. Endocrinol.* **2014**, *28*, 758–767. [CrossRef] [PubMed]
37. Rauth, M.; Freund, P.; Orlova, A.; Grünert, S.; Tasic, N.; Han, X.; Ruan, H.-B.; Neubauer, H.A.; Moriggl, R. Cell Metabolism Control Through O-GlcNAcylation of STAT5: A Full or Empty Fuel Tank Makes a Big Difference for Cancer Cell Growth and Survival. *Int. J. Mol. Sci.* **2019**, *20*, 1028. [CrossRef] [PubMed]
38. Jitschin, R.; Böttcher, M.; Saul, D.; Lukassen, S.; Bruns, H.; Loschinski, R.; Ekici, A.B.; Reis, A.; Mackensen, A.; Mougiakakos, D. Inflammation-induced glycolytic switch controls suppressivity of mesenchymal stem cells via STAT1 glycosylation. *Leukemia* **2019**, *33*, 1783–1796. [CrossRef]
39. Gewinner, C.; Hart, G.; Zachara, N.; Cole, R.; Beisenherz-Huss, C.; Groner, B. The Coactivator of Transcription CREB-binding Protein Interacts Preferentially with the Glycosylated Form of Stat5. *J. Biol. Chem.* **2004**, *279*, 3563–3572. [CrossRef]
40. Friedbichler, K.; Hoelbl, A.; Li, G.; Bunting, K.D.; Sexl, V.; Gouilleux, F.; Moriggl, R. Serine phosphorylation of the Stat5a C-terminus is a driving force for transformation. *Front. Biosci.* **2011**, *16*, 3043–3056. [CrossRef]
41. Freund, P.; Kerenyi, M.A.; Hager, M.; Wagner, T.; Wingelhofer, B.; Pham, H.T.T.; Elabd, M.; Han, X.; Valent, P.; Gouilleux, F.; et al. O-GlcNAcylation of STAT5 controls tyrosine phosphorylation and oncogenic transcription in STAT5-dependent malignancies. *Leukemia* **2017**, *31*, 2132–2142. [CrossRef]
42. Kim, Y.J.; Kang, M.J.; Kim, E.; Kweon, T.H.; Park, Y.S.; Ji, S.; Yang, W.H.; Yi, E.C.; Cho, J.W. O-GlcNAc stabilizes SMAD4 by inhibiting GSK-3β-mediated proteasomal degradation. *Sci. Rep.* **2020**, *10*, 19908. [CrossRef]
43. Han, J.W.; Valdez, J.L.; Ho, D.V.; Lee, C.S.; Kim, H.M.; Wang, X.; Huang, L.; Chan, J.Y. Nuclear factor-erythroid-2 related transcription factor-1 (Nrf1) is regulated by O-GlcNAc transferase. *Free Radic. Biol. Med.* **2017**, *110*, 196–205. [CrossRef]
44. Hardivillé, S.; Hoedt, E.; Mariller, C.; Benaïssa, M.; Pierce, A. O-GlcNAcylation/Phosphorylation Cycling at Ser10 Controls Both Transcriptional Activity and Stability of Δ-Lactoferrin. *J. Biol. Chem.* **2010**, *285*, 19205–19218. [CrossRef]
45. Su, K.; Roos, M.D.; Yang, X.; Han, I.; Paterson, A.J.; Kudlow, J.E. An N-terminal Region of Sp1 Targets Its Proteasome-dependent Degradation in Vitro. *J. Biol. Chem.* **1999**, *274*, 15194–15202. [CrossRef]
46. Zhu, Y.; Liu, T.-W.; Cecioni, S.; Eskandari, R.; Zandberg, W.F.; Vocadlo, D.J. O-GlcNAc occurs cotranslationally to stabilize nascent polypeptide chains. *Nat. Chem. Biol.* **2015**, *11*, 319–325. [CrossRef]
47. He, F.; Ge, W.; Martinowich, K.; Becker-Catania, S.; Coskun, V.; Zhu, W.; Wu, H.; Castro, D.; Guillemot, F.; Fan, G.; et al. A positive autoregulatory loop of Jak-STAT signaling controls the onset of astrogliogenesis. *Nat. Neurosci.* **2005**, *8*, 616–625. [CrossRef]
48. Nagarkatti-Gude, N.; Bronkhorst, I.H.G.; van Duinen, S.G.; Luyten, G.P.M.; Jager, M.J. Cytokines and Chemokines in the Vitreous Fluid of Eyes with Uveal Melanoma. *Investig. Opthalmology Vis. Sci.* **2012**, *53*, 6748–6755. [CrossRef]
49. Chen, M.-X.; Liu, Y.-M.; Li, Y.; Yang, X.; Wei, W.-B. Elevated VEGF-A & PLGF concentration in aqueous humor of patients with uveal melanoma following Iodine-125 plaque radiotherapy. *Int. J. Ophthalmol.* **2020**, *13*, 599–605. [CrossRef]

50. Lee, C.S.; Jun, I.H.; Kim, T.-I.; Byeon, S.H.; Koh, H.J.; Lee, S.C. Expression of 12 cytokines in aqueous humour of uveal melanoma before and after combined Ruthenium-106 brachytherapy and transpupillary thermotherapy. *Acta Ophthalmol.* **2012**, *90*, e314–e320. [CrossRef]
51. Cheng, Y.; Feng, J.; Zhu, X.; Liang, J. Cytokines concentrations in aqueous humor of eyes with uveal melanoma. *Medicine* **2019**, *98*, e14030. [CrossRef]
52. Midena, E.; Parrozzani, R.; Midena, G.; Trainiti, S.; Marchione, G.; Cosmo, E.; Londei, D.; Frizziero, L. In vivo intraocular biomarkers: Changes of aqueous humor cytokines and chemokines in patients affected by uveal melanoma. *Medicine* **2020**, *99*, e22091. [CrossRef]
53. Johnson, D.E.; O'Keefe, R.A.; Grandis, J.R. Targeting the IL-6/JAK/STAT3 signalling axis in cancer. *Nat. Rev. Clin. Oncol.* **2018**, *15*, 234–248. [CrossRef]
54. Gong, C.; Shen, J.; Fang, Z.; Qiao, L.; Feng, R.; Lin, X.; Li, S. Abnormally expressed JunB transactivated by IL-6/STAT3 signaling promotes uveal melanoma aggressiveness via epithelial–mesenchymal transition. *Biosci. Rep.* **2018**, *38*. [CrossRef]
55. Castet, F.; Garcia-Mulero, S.; Sanz-Pamplona, R.; Cuellar, A.; Casanovas, O.; Caminal, J.M.; Piulats, J.M. Uveal Melanoma, Angiogenesis and Immunotherapy, Is There Any Hope? *Cancers* **2019**, *11*, 834. [CrossRef]
56. Smit, K.N.; Jager, M.J.; de Klein, A.; Kili, E. Uveal melanoma: Towards a molecular understanding. *Prog. Retin. Eye Res.* **2020**, *75*, 100800. [CrossRef]
57. Kaštelan, S.; Antunica, A.G.; Oresković, L.B.; Pelčić, G.; Kasun, E.; Hat, K. Immunotherapy for Uveal Melanoma-Current Knowledge and Perspectives. *Curr. Med. Chem.* **2020**, *27*, 1350–1366. [CrossRef]
58. Chemnitz, J.M.; Parry, R.V.; Nichols, K.E.; June, C.H.; Riley, J.L. SHP-1 and SHP-2 Associate with Immunoreceptor Tyrosine-Based Switch Motif of Programmed Death 1 upon Primary Human T Cell Stimulation, but Only Receptor Ligation Prevents T Cell Activation. *J. Immunol.* **2004**, *173*, 945–954. [CrossRef]
59. Attili, I.; Karachaliou, N.; Bonanno, L.; Berenguer, J.; Bracht, J.; Codony-Servat, J.; Codony-Servat, C.; Ito, M.; Rosell, R. STAT3 as a potential immunotherapy biomarker in oncogene-addicted non-small cell lung cancer. *Ther. Adv. Med. Oncol.* **2018**, *10*, 1758835918763744. [CrossRef]
60. Zemek, R.M.; de Jong, E.; Chin, W.L.; Schuster, I.S.; Fear, V.S.; Casey, T.H.; Forbes, C.; Dart, S.J.; Leslie, C.; Zaitouny, A.; et al. Sensitization to immune checkpoint blockade through activation of a STAT1/NK axis in the tumor microenvironment. *Sci. Transl. Med.* **2019**, *11*, eaav7816. [CrossRef]
61. Nakayama, Y.; Mimura, K.; Tamaki, T.; Shiraishi, K.; Kua, L.-F.; Koh, V.; Ohmori, M.; Kimura, A.; Inoue, S.; Okayama, H.; et al. Phospho-STAT1 expression as a potential biomarker for anti-PD-1/anti-PD-L1 immunotherapy for breast cancer. *Int. J. Oncol.* **2019**, *54*, 2030–2038. [CrossRef]
62. Duval, C.; Zaniolo, K.; Leclerc, S.; Salesse, C.; Guérin, S.L. Characterization of the human $\alpha 9$ integrin subunit gene: Promoter analysis and transcriptional regulation in ocular cells. *Exp. Eye Res.* **2015**, *135*, 146–163. [CrossRef]
63. Landreville, S.; Agapova, O.A.; Kneass, Z.T.; Salesse, C.; Harbour, J.W. ABCB1 identifies a subpopulation of uveal melanoma cells with high metastatic propensity. *Pigment Cell Melanoma Res.* **2011**, *24*, 430–437. [CrossRef]
64. Molloy-Simard, V.; St-Laurent, J.-F.; Vigneault, F.; Gaudreault, M.; Dargis, N.; Guérin, M.-C.; Leclerc, S.; Morcos, M.; Black, D.; Molgat, Y.; et al. Altered Expression of the Poly(ADP-Ribosyl)ation Enzymes in Uveal Melanoma and Regulation of PARG Gene Expression by the Transcription Factor ERM. *Investig. Opthalmology Vis. Sci.* **2012**, *53*, 6219–6231. [CrossRef]
65. Roy, R.J.; Gosselin, P.; Guérin, S.L. A short protocol for micro-purification of nuclear proteins from whole animal tissue. *Biotechniques* **1991**, *11*, 770–777.
66. Gaudreault, M.; Gingras, M.-E.; Lessard, M.; Leclerc, S.; Guérin, S.L. Electrophoretic Mobility Shift Assays for the Analysis of DNA-Protein Interactions. In *DNA-Protein Interactions*; Methods in Molecular Biology; Humana Press: Totowa, NJ, USA, 2009; Volume 543, pp. 15–35. [CrossRef]
67. Couture, C.; Zaniolo, K.; Carrier, P.; Lake, J.; Patenaude, J.; Germain, L.; Guérin, S.L. The tissue-engineered human cornea as a model to study expression of matrix metalloproteinases during corneal wound healing. *Biomaterials* **2016**, *78*, 86–101. [CrossRef]

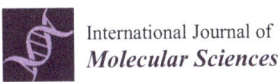

Article

miR-205-5p Downregulation and *ZEB1* Upregulation Characterize the Disseminated Tumor Cells in Patients with Invasive Ductal Breast Cancer

Lenka Kalinkova [1,†], Nataliia Nikolaieva [1,†], Bozena Smolkova [2], Sona Ciernikova [1], Karol Kajo [1,3], Vladimir Bella [4], Viera Horvathova Kajabova [2], Helena Kosnacova [1], Gabriel Minarik [5] and Ivana Fridrichova [1,*]

1. Department of Genetics, Cancer Research Institute, Biomedical Research Center of the Slovak Academy of Sciences, 84505 Bratislava, Slovakia; lenka.kalinkova@savba.sk (L.K.); nataliia.nikolaieva@savba.sk (N.N.); sona.ciernikova@savba.sk (S.C.); karol.kajo@ousa.sk (K.K.); helena.svobodova@savba.sk (H.K.)
2. Department of Molecular Oncology, Cancer Research Institute, Biomedical Research Center of the Slovak Academy of Sciences, 84505 Bratislava, Slovakia; bozena.smolkova@savba.sk (B.S.); viera.kajabova@savba.sk (V.H.K.)
3. Department of Pathology, St. Elisabeth Cancer Institute, 81250 Bratislava, Slovakia
4. Department of Senology, St. Elisabeth Cancer Institute, 81250 Bratislava, Slovakia; vladimir.bella@ousa.sk
5. Institute of Molecular Biomedicine, Faculty of Medicine, Comenius University, 81108 Bratislava, Slovakia; gabriel.minarik@gmail.com
*   Correspondence: ivana.fridrichova@savba.sk; Tel.: +421-02-32295188
†   These authors contributed equally to this work.

Abstract: Background: Dissemination of breast cancer (BC) cells through the hematogenous or lymphogenous vessels leads to metastatic disease in one-third of BC patients. Therefore, we investigated the new prognostic features for invasion and metastasis. Methods: We evaluated the expression of miRNAs and epithelial-to-mesenchymal transition (EMT) genes in relation to *CDH1*/E-cadherin changes in samples from 31 patients with invasive ductal BC including tumor centrum (TU-C), tumor invasive front (TU-IF), lymph node metastasis (LNM), and CD45-depleted blood (CD45-DB). Expression of miRNA and mRNA was quantified by RT-PCR arrays and associations with clinico-pathological characteristics were statistically evaluated by univariate and multivariate analysis. Results: We did not verify *CDH1* regulating associations previously described in cell lines. However, we did detect extremely high *ZEB1* expression in LNMs from patients with distant metastasis, but without regulation by miR-205-5p. Considering the ZEB1 functions, this overexpression indicates enhancement of metastatic potential of lymphogenously disseminated BC cells. In CD45-DB samples, downregulated miR-205-5p was found in those expressing epithelial and/or mesenchymal markers (CTC+) that could contribute to insusceptibility and survival of hematogenously disseminated BC cells mediated by increased expression of several targets including *ZEB1*. Conclusions: miR-205-5p and potentially *ZEB1* gene are promising candidates for markers of metastatic potential in ductal BC.

Keywords: invasive ductal breast cancer; *CDH1* gene; EMT genes; miRNA and mRNA expression; E-cadherin

1. Introduction

The International Agency for Research on Cancer's GLOBOCAN 2018 reported the global burden of cancer across 20 world regions and revealed almost 2.1 million new breast cancer (BC) patients and 0.63 million associated deaths. That means a 24.2% incidence and 15% mortality rate in female cancer patients [1]. Among BC patients, metastatic disease has been reported in the range from 7% to 35% [2–4]. Metastatic breast cancer is generally considered incurable and regardless of some improvement in overall survival only 13% of BC patients with primary stage IV survive 10 years after diagnosis [5]. Cancer cells spread from the tumor mass either via blood or via lymphatic circulation after the intensive neo-vascularization and neo-lymphangiogenesis, respectively [6]. Detached cancer cells enter blood vessels directly, but those traveling through the lymphatic vasculature either form metastases in lymph nodes or they pass into the blood circulation through the thoracic duct [7]. However, the factors determining the method of cancer cell dissemination depend mainly on the cancer type and features of the tumor microenvironment [8].

In BC, lymphovascular invasion inside and around the tumor tissue indicate the mechanisms of cancer spread and metastases in lymph nodes are considered as the key prognostic marker of tumor spread and aggressiveness [9–11]. On the other hand, many studies performed in the last decade have investigated the role of circulating tumor cells (CTCs) in haematogenous dissemination of cancer and their clinical utility in prognosis is under examination in ongoing clinical trials. Detection and count of CTCs are used as independent prognostic factors for primary and metastatic BC contributing to the monitoring and treatment stratification of BC patients [12–14]. Various technologies for CTC detection and isolation have been developed (including the validated CellSearch® system) and most of them have utilized the epithelial characters for CTC enrichment [15,16]. In BC, heterogeneous CTC subpopulations were found, counting cells with epithelial characters co-existing with those with epithelial-to-mesenchymal transition (EMT) features; however, EMT CTCs have been identified more frequently in metastatic BC patients and are associated with poor prognosis [17–20].

Mesenchymal cell phenotype is associated with an increased migratory capacity, invasiveness, apoptosis, and resistance; therefore, EMT is considered an essential event in BC haematogenous dissemination [20,21]. On the other hand, TGF-1-induced EMT was recently described to promote the chemotaxis-mediated migration of BC cells through the lymphatic vessels [22]. The main feature of EMT induction is the loss of cell–cell adherent junctions via inhibition of E-cadherin encoded by the *CDH1* gene. Key EMT inducers, which act as direct *CDH1* repressors, belong to three distinct families; the Snail family (SNAIL1, SNAIL2/SLUG, and SNAIL3/SMUC), the Zeb family (ZEB1/2), and the b-HLH family (TWIST1/2). Their encoding genes inhibit E-cadherin expression via binding to the E-box elements in the promoter region of the *CDH1* gene [23,24].

Genetic and epigenetic mechanisms of E-cadherin downregulation were previously described. Several *CDH1* somatic or germline mutations and loss of heterozygosity were found almost exclusively in invasive lobular BC [25,26]. In addition, epigenetic modulation by *CDH1* promoter methylation [27,28] or by miRNA post-transcription regulation have been documented [29].

In BC cells, MYC/MYCN-activated miR-9 was found to be a direct regulator of the *CDH1* gene, and increased miR-9 levels were associated with metastatic status and local recurrence in BC patients [30,31]. The miR-221 a member of the miR-221/222 cluster directly targeted the open reading frame of *CDH1* and a higher miR-221 expression, significantly upregulated by SNAIL2/SLUG, was observed in metastatic BC cells and BC patients with LNMs and distant metastases [32–34]. Moreover, the miR-221/222 cluster decreased expression of E-cadherin indirectly via targeting of transcription repressor *TRPS1*, the direct regulator of *ZEB2* transcription, resulting in abundance of *ZEB2* and promotion of EMT [35].

Several *CDH1* repressors and therefore EMT inducers were found to be regulated by members of a well-investigated miR-200 cluster including miR-200b/200a/429 and miR-200c/141. Decreased expression of all members of the miR-200 cluster followed by upregulation of *SNAI1*, *SNAI2*, *ZEB1*, and *ZEB2* genes was observed in EMT in vitro models of breast basal cell lines and BC patients, more markedly in those with metaplastic tumors. Moreover, the inactivation of miR-200c/141 expression could be caused by hypermethylation of its promoter [36]. Among them, miR-200c targeted *ZEB1* and the other two *TKS5* and *MYLK* genes acting in invadopodia formation. Co-expression of these three genes and low expression of miR-200c in several BC lines as well as in BC patients are associated with EMT activation, higher invasion and invadopodia creation [37,38]. In a recent study, miR-200c targeted *ZEB2* and the role of this repressor in metastasis was found in triple-negative BC (TNBC) cells and tissues [39]. Furthermore, both *ZEB1* and *ZEB2* were directly regulated by miR-205 and decreased levels of miR-205 initiated EMT and were associated with a metastatic phenotype of BC patients [40,41].

Other BC in vitro studies showed that expression levels of miR-203 and miR-200 cluster were decreasing in a time-dependent manner during SNAI1-induced EMT. The miR-203-reduced *SNAI1* endogenous levels generated a double-negative miR-203/SNAI1 feedback loop and together with the miR200/ZEB1 feedback loop, the plasticity of the epithelial cell during differentiation and tumorigenesis was controlled [42]. The miR-203 also directly regulated *SNAI2* gene and this miRNA was upregulated and downregulated in non-metastatic and metastatic cell lines, respectively, compared to non-tumorigenic cells. Moreover, decreasing levels of miR-203 in metastatic cells were associated with promoter hypermethylation [43]. Downregulation of miR-124 was found in TNBC cell lines and patient tissues. It was documented that miR-124 directly targeted the *ZEB2* gene and contributed to EMT and metastasis suppression [44]. Other authors showed that miR-124 also directly targeted the *SNAI2/SLUG* gene, which allowed E-cadherin expression and inhibition of cell invasion and metastasis. In BCs, the significantly reduced miR-124 levels negatively correlated with histological grade [45].

Compared to the above-mentioned EMT-associated transcription factors, the miRNA regulation of *TWIST1* expression in BC has been less frequently investigated. The *TWIST1* gene was directly targeted by miR-720 and significant downregulation of miR-720 followed by increasing *TWIST1* levels were observed predominantly in metastatic BC [46].

Generally, in BCs and many other epithelial cancers, the attenuation of E-cadherin adhesion is considered the main event in invasion and metastasis. Regarding the prognostic value, high levels of E-cadherin were found to be a good prognostic marker in most cancers. In a previous study, the variable trend of decreasing E-cadherin expression was observed from ductal BCs in situ, from ductal BCs without LNMs to those with LNMs, but increased E-cadherin levels were found in LNM tissues compared to primary tumors [47]. However, a more recent study showed that high E-cadherin correlated with shorter survival in invasive ductal BCs in contrast to the lobular subtype of BC, and reduced or lost E-cadherin expression was inversely associated with tumor stage, indicating more complex and possible divergent functions of this protein in BCs [48]. This hypothesis is supported by results from mouse experimental models, where the loss of E-cadherin improved cancer cell invasion, but reduced cell proliferation and survival, the number of CTCs in systemic circulation, and dissemination of cancer cells in distant organs. The authors indicated that E-cadherin could contribute to metastasis through apoptosis inhibition [49].

In this study, we investigated epigenetic changes associated with regulation of the E-cadherin encoding *CDH1* gene to contribute to a better understanding of the specific functions of E-cadherin and associated miRNAs and genes in invasive ductal BCs. We analyzed the expression of *CDH1*, five well-known EMT genes, and seven regulating miRNAs (Figure 1) in tumor centrum (TU-C), tumor invasive front (TU-IF), and in lymph node metastasis (LNM) and CTC-enriched blood fraction samples (by CD45 depletion) to identify aberrantly expressed miRNAs and genes, and understand their associations with clinical parameters of invasive and metastatic processes including LNM, CTC, lymphovascular invasion (LVI), and distant metastasis (MTS). Our results did not confirm *CDH1* regulating associations previously described in cell line models. However, we detected extremely high *ZEB1* expression in LMN samples from patients with MTS, which was not regulated by miR-205-5p. Due to *ZEB1* functions, its overexpression indicates enhancement of metastatic potential of disseminated BC cells spread through the lymphatic vessels. In CD45-depleted blood (CD45-DB) fractions, the downregulated miR-205-5p was found in samples expressing epithelial and/or mesenchymal markers (CTC+) that could contribute to reduced susceptibility and increased survival of hematogenously disseminated BC cells mediated by increased expression of several target genes including *ZEB1*. Both, miR-205-5p and potentially *ZEB1* are promising candidates as markers for metastatic potential of disseminated ductal BC cells.

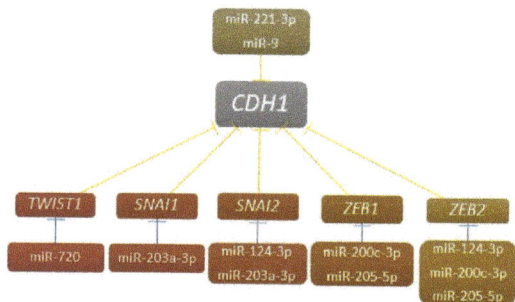

Figure 1. Diagram of associations in inhibition of *CDH1* expression adapted from results of in vitro studies.

2. Results

2.1. miRNA and mRNA Expressions vs. Controls

In the group of 31 patients with invasive ductal breast cancer, we evaluated the expressions of seven miRNAs regulating *CDH1* and EMT repressors (miR-9-5p, miR-124-3p, miR-200c-3p, miR-203a-3p, miR-205-5p, miR-221-3p, and miR-720) and mRNA expression for *CDH1* and associated EMT genes (*TWIST1*, *SNAI1*, *SNAI2*, *ZEB1*, and *ZEB2*). The analyses were performed in TU-C, TU-IF and LNM samples, and in CD45-DB fractions enriched by CTCs with and without identified epithelial and/or mesenchymal markers (CTC+ and CTC-, respectively). The controls for all patients' tissue samples and depleted fractions were non-neoplastic breast specimens (C-breast) and CD45-depleted fractions from healthy women (C-blood). In TU-C, significant upregulation was detected for miR-9-5p (fold change, FC 7.915, $p = 0.042$) and miR-203a-3p (FC 2.356, $p = 0.042$) and downregulation for *CDH1* (fold change, FC 0.123, $p = 0.002$), *SNAI2* (FC 0.16, $p = 0.021$) and *ZEB2* (FC 0.125, $p < 0.001$) genes compared to controls. Similarly, TU-IFs were downregulated for *CDH1* (FC 0.108, $p = 0.001$), *SNAI2* (FC 0.102, $p = 0.002$) and *ZEB2* (FC 0.086, $p < 0.001$) genes and LNM samples were downregulated for miR-205-5p (FC 0.21, $p = 0.012$), and upregulated for *ZEB1* (FC 22.08, $p = 0.043$) and *ZEB2* (FC 0.122, $p = 0.003$). In CTC-depleted bloods, miR-124-3p (FC 9.766, $p = 0.036$) was upregulated and in CTC+ samples, miR-221-3p (FC 0.289, $p = 0.017$) and *ZEB2* (FC 0.395, $p = 0.037$) were downregulated compared to controls (Figure 2, Table 1).

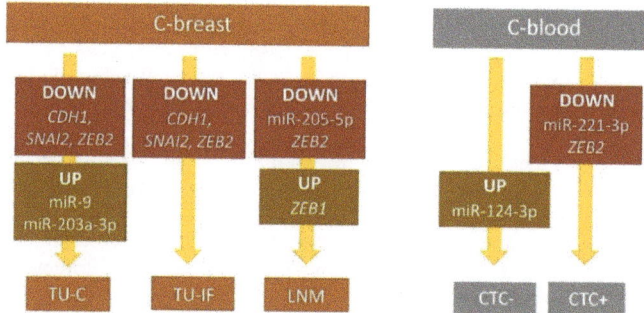

Figure 2. Significantly different expressions of miRNAs and mRNA of *CDH1* and EMT genes in tumor centrum (TU-C), tumor invasive front (TU-IF) and lymph node metastasis (LNM), and in CD45-DB fractions enriched by CTCs compared to adequate controls (C-breast, non-neoplastic breast tissues and C-blood, CD45-depleted fractions from healthy women).

Table 1. Comparison of miRNA and mRNA of CDH1 and EMT gene expressions between controls and different types of BC patients' specimens and between each other's samples.

miRNAs/ Genes	TU-C vs. C-Breast			TU-IF vs. C-Breast			LNM vs. C-Breast		
	FC	p-Value	95% CI	FC	p-Value	95% CI	FC	p-Value	95% CI
miR-9-5p	7.915	**0.042**	0.012–41.946	0.838	0.790	0.004–263.197	0.551	0.422	0.004–180.863
miR-124-3p	1.789	0.553	0.001–4.238	1.632	0.557	0.002–1.277	0.649	0.634	0.002–624.915
miR-200c-3p	1.686	0.382	0.054–45.865	2.137	0.092	0.215–59.281	1.821	0.271	0.156–48.471
miR-203a-3p	2.356	**0.042**	0.077–79.574	1.556	0.294	0.042–38.469	1.287	0.593	0.039–29.094
miR-205-5p	0.512	0.251	0.009–36.730	0.350	0.054	0.002–10.925	0.210	**0.012**	0.002–8.057
miR-221-3p	1.335	0.423	0.081–17.503	1.365	0.290	0.168–13.709	1.096	0.802	0.091–19.943
miR-720	1.152	0.735	0.050–33.593	1.398	0.245	0.130–15.221	1.033	0.939	0.042–22.785
CDH1	0.123	**0.002**	0.004–2.366	0.108	**0.001**	0.004–2.015	0.630	0.754	0.005–461.981
TWIST1	0.449	0.765	0.000–19.953	0.320	0.097	0.000–29.212	2.866	0.717	0.000–84,067.528
SNAI1	0.711	0.586	0.027–23.260	0.706	0.658	0.020–55.154	1.460	0.740	0.024–246.709
SNAI2	0.161	**0.021**	0.003–13.083	0.102	**0.002**	0.001–9.663	0.302	0.168	0.001–140.598
ZEB1	0.482	0.117	0.032–9.616	0.474	0.052	0.064–6.320	22.08	**0.043**	0.083–522,995.072
ZEB2	0.125	**<0.001**	0.002–3.578	0.086	**<0.001**	0.001–3.209	0.122	**0.003**	0.001–13.175

	CTC− vs. C-Blood			CTC+ vs. C-Blood			CTC+ vs. CTC−		
	FC	p-Value	95% CI	FC	p-Value	95% CI	FC	p-Value	95% CI
miR-9-5p	0.428	0.366	0.001–157.642	0.374	0.223	0.002–39.997	0.873	0.880	0.004–373.287
miR-124-3p	9.766	**0.036**	0.007–15,744.196	5.914	0.150	0.007–12,237.005	0.606	0.696	0.000–6364.879
miR-200c-3p	0.398	0.171	0.005–43.795	0.299	0.052	0.008–10.359	0.751	0.645	0.012–25.075
miR-203a-3p	1.176	0.643	0.000–745.653	0.148	0.089	0.000–16.253	0.125	0.064	0.000–174.337
miR-205-5p	10.792	0.082	0.004–167,893.014	0.443	0.370	0.002–138.141	0.041	**0.010**	0.000–69.820
miR-221-3p	0.771	0.634	0.023–36.002	0.289	**0.017**	0.016–6.790	0.374	0.077	0.005–14.906
miR-720	0.667	0.451	0.020–37.507	0.534	0.339	0.004–18.729	0.801	0.712	0.006–25.216
CDH1	1.031	0.918	0.071–29.950	0.948	0.912	0.132–17.345	0.919	0.782	0.024–7.315
TWIST1	0.518	0.362	0.006–18.831	0.685	0.606	0.010–25.111	1.321	0.543	0.052–21.295
SNAI1	0.456	0.136	0.016–6.304	0.424	0.125	0.013–7.586	0.931	0.658	0.072–9.000
ZEB1	0.683	0.206	0.032–12.101	1.121	0.751	0.029–23.244	1.641	0.410	0.085–19.595
ZEB2	0.451	0.066	0.022–6.546	0.395	**0.037**	0.024–2.350	0.876	0.824	0.135–3.364

	TU-IF vs. TU C			LNM vs. TU C			LNM vs. TU IF		
	FC	p-Value	95% CI	FC	p-Value	95% CI	FC	p-Value	95% CI
miR-9-5p	0.106	**0.001**	0.000–48.840	0.070	**<0.001**	0.000–28.042	0.658	0.437	0.005–113.159
miR-124-3p	0.912	0.898	0.000–1595.729	0.363	0.215	0.000–775.000	0.398	0.201	0.001–451.409
miR-200c-3p	1.267	0.531	0.089–30.484	1.080	0.892	0.069–25.098	0.852	0.556	0.064–9.123
miR-203a-3p	0.661	0.199	0.016–16.564	0.546	0.103	0.01–11.711	0.827	0.614	0.018–32.217
miR-205-5p	0.684	0.612	0.003–68.594	0.409	0.100	0.002–48.151	0.598	0.318	0.005–112.073
miR-221-3p	1.022	0.934	0.079–19.973	0.821	0.540	0.043–18.746	0.803	0.452	0.054–13.541
miR-720	1.213	0.481	0.040–22.891	0.897	0.766	0.015–29.349	0.739	0.325	0.021–11.792
CDH1	0.882	0.662	0.048–16.349	5.135	**0.048**	0.081–4310.936	5.819	**0.034**	0.087–4172.813
TWIST1	0.712	0.148	0.025–31.480	6.378	0.158	0.017–88,008.904	8.96	0.102	0.019–132,814.422
SNAI1	0.994	0.986	0.043–54.895	2.055	0.208	0.052–259.574	2.067	0.224	0.019–316.497
SNAI2	0.635	0.198	0.005–16.977	1.875	0.258	0.022–238.470	2.955	0.070	0.025–644.682
ZEB1	0.982	0.947	0.111–15.056	45.794	**0.015**	0.139–1,074,172.923	46.615	**0.014**	0.225–1,274,282.570
ZEB2	0.69	0.191	0.029–8.390	0.979	0.962	0.027–58.004	1.419	0.415	0.034–76.961

Abbreviations: C-breast, non-neoplastic breast tissue controls; TU-C, tumor centrum; TU-IF, tumor invasive front; LNM, lymph node metastasis; C-blood, CD45-DB fractions from healthy women; CTC− and CTC+, CD45-DB fractions from patients without and with identified epithelial and mesenchymal markers, respectively. Significant results are highlighted in bold.

2.2. miRNA and mRNA Expressions in Different Types of Samples

Expression of two miRNAs, and *CDH1* and *ZEB1* genes was found to be statistically different between BC samples. In both TU-IF and LMN, miR-9-5p was downregulated and in LNM, *CDH1* and *ZEB1* were upregulated compared to TU-C. Similarly, upregulated *CDH1* and *ZEB1* genes were found in LNM against expressions in TU-IF. CTC+ samples presented miR-205-5p downregulation compared to CTC- (Table 1, Figure 3).

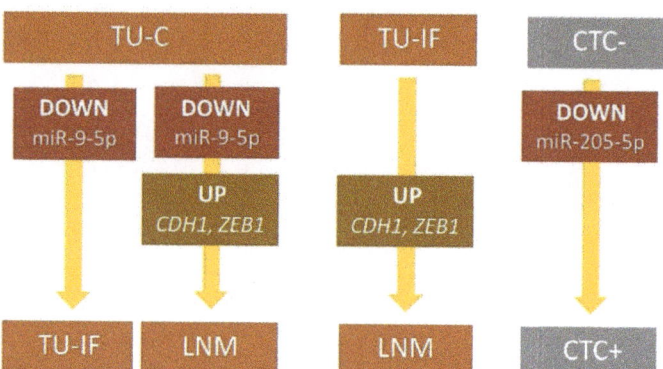

Figure 3. Expression of miRNAs, and *CDH1* and EMT genes between different types of BC patients' samples, namely in tumor centrum (TU-C), tumor invasive front (TU-IF) and lymph node metastasis (LNM), and in CD45-depleted blood (CD45-DB) fractions without and with identified epithelial and/or mesenchymal markers (CTC- and CTC+).

To evaluate the inhibitory function of miRNAs we analyzed the correlation between expressions of miRNAs, and *CDH1* and EMT genes, and between *CDH1* and each of EMT genes (Table 2 and Table S1). Negative correlation was found between miR-221-3p and *TWIST1* gene in TU-Cs (correlation coefficient (r), $r = -0.470$, $p = 0.015$), and miR-9 and *SNAI1* gene in LNMs ($r = -0.607$, $p = 0.013$). In CD45-DB fractions the negative correlations were observed more frequently, in CTC- samples between miR-124-3p and *TWIST1* ($r = -0.883$, $p = 0.020$), and miR-221-3p and *ZEB2* ($r = -0.543$, $p = 0.024$). In CTC+ specimens, miR-9, miR-205-5p and miR-720 negatively correlated with both *SNAI1* and *ZEB1* (r ranged from -0.853 to -0.588 and p-value from 0.001 to 0.044), miR-221-3p with *ZEB1* ($r = -0.610$, $p = 0.035$) (Table 2). No negative correlations were detected between expressions of *CDH1* and any of EMT genes in tumor, LNM and CTC samples (Table S1).

In this study, several associations between miRNAs and genes indicating regulation events previously documented by in vitro results were shown. In TU-Cs, upregulated miR-9 and downregulated *CDH1*, and upregulated miR-203a-3p, and downregulated *SNAI2* were found compared to controls. LNM samples presented downregulation of miR-205-5p with upregulation of the *ZEB1* gene (Table 1). However, in none of these associations were significant negative correlations between miRNA and mRNA expressions of *CDH1* and EMT genes observed.

Table 2. Significant correlations between miRNA and mRNA of *CDH1*, and EMT gene expressions in BC samples.

Sample	miRNA	Gene	Correlation Coefficient (r)	p-Value
C-breast	miR-124-3p	SNAI1	0.964	0.036
TU-C	miR-203a-3p	CDH1	0.409	0.031
		ZEB1	0.479	0.018
		ZEB2	0.406	0.036
	miR-205-5p	SNAI1	0.383	0.048
	miR-221-3p	TWIST1	−0.470	0.015
	miR-200c-3p	SNAI1	0.387	0.046
TU-IF		TWIST1	0.417	0.034
	miR-720	SNAI1	0.527	0.005
		SNAI2	0.383	0.040
LNM	miR-9	SNAI1	−0.607	0.013
	miR-221-3p	TWIST1	0.726	0.011
		ZEB1	0.581	0.048
C-blood	miR-9	ZEB1	0.610	0.046
		ZEB2	0.627	0.039
	miR-200c-3p	ZEB1	0.616	0.043
		ZEB2	0.682	0.021
	miR-203a-3p	TWIST1	0.967	0.007
		SNAI1	0.797	0.032
		ZEB1	0.800	0.010
		ZEB2	0.900	0.001
		TWIST1	0.885	0.019
	miR-221-3p	SNAI1	0.784	0.021
		ZEB1	0.785	0.004
		ZEB2	0.936	<0.000
		TWIST1	0.869	0.025
	miR-720	ZEB1	0.743	0.009
		ZEB2	0.736	0.010
CTC-	miR-124-3p	TWIST1	−0.883	0.020
	miR-221-3p	ZEB2	−0.543	0.024
	miR-9	SNAI1	−0.835	0.001
		ZEB1	−0.853	0.001
CTC+	miR-205-5p	SNAI1	−0.653	0.021
		ZEB1	−0.588	0.044
	miR-221-3p	ZEB1	−0.610	0.035
	miR-720	SNAI1	−0.616	0.033
		ZEB1	−0.623	0.031

Abbreviations: C-breast, non-neoplastic breast tissue controls; TU-C, tumor centrum, TU-IF, tumor invasive front; LNM, lymph node metastasis; C-blood, CD45-DB fractions from healthy women; CTC- and CTC+, CD45-DB fractions from patients without and with identified epithelial and mesenchymal markers, respectively. Negative correlations are highlighted in bold.

2.3. Association between miRNA and mRNA Expression and Clinico-Pathological Parameters

Using univariate statistical analysis, we found spectrum of associations between up- or downregulated expressions of miRNAs and *CDH1* and EMT genes and relevant clinico-pathological characteristics for each group of samples (Table 3). In TU-C, downregulated levels of miR-124-3p and miR-203a-3p were detected in patients with MTS and TNM staging III and IV compared to those without MTS and lower TNM, respectively. Furthermore, miR-200c-3p was downregulated in HER2 positive BCs and reduced *CDH1*, *SNAI1*, and *ZEB2* expression was identified in ER+ and /or PR+ tumors. TU-IF samples showed downregulation for miR-200c-3p in ER+ tumors, decreased expression for *TWIST1* in ER+ BCs and several combinations of downregulated EMT genes, namely *SNAI2* and *ZEB1* associated with lymph node metastasis (LNM) positive phenotype and higher TNM, respectively; *SNAI2* and *ZEB2* with distant metastasis (MTS) presence and *SNAI2*, and both, *ZEB1* and *ZEB2* with LVI. Decreased *ZEB2* was also associated with tumors sized ≤20 mm. In LNM tissues, upregulation of miR-124-3p, SNAI1 and ZEB1 was associated with ER+, higher TNM and MTS+ in the primary tumor, respectively. In CD45-DB samples, downregulation of SNAI1 and upregulation of miR-9 were found in patients with HER2+ tumors, and upregulation of CDH1 in grade 3 cancers, respectively. miR-205-5p were found upregulated in patients with LNM+ and higher TNM but significantly downregulated in patients with CTC+ phenotype (Figure 4). FCs and p-values for these associations are summarized in Table 3.

Immunohistochemical analyses in TU-C samples showed that 17 and 5 patients presented strong homogenous expression (3+) and heterogeneous strong and moderate expression (3+ and 2+) of E-cadherin in different portions in individual patients, respectively. These samples were considered as those with high E-cadherin expression. In nine patients with low E-cadherin expression, strictly heterogeneous phenotype with different portion of strong, moderate, poor, and no expression (3+/2+/1+, 3+/2+/1+/0 and 2+/1+) was observed. The associations between CDH1 gene expression in high and low E-cadherin expression were tested by univariate statistical analysis. An increasing trend in CDH1 expression in E-cadherin high compared to low expression was found; however, without upregulation and statistically significant difference in CDH1 expression between E-cadherin high and low groups (FC 1.134, p = 0.777).

Table 3. Significant up- and downregulation of miRNA and mRNA of CDH1, and EMT gene expression in BC patients with different clinico-pathological parameters.

Sample	Clinical Characteristics	miRNAs/Genes	FC	p-Value	95% CI
TU-C	MTS+ vs. MTS-	miR-124-3p	0.075	0.049	0.000–35.995
	HER2+ vs. HER2-	miR-200c-3p	0.440	0.018	0.030–12.772
	TNM III and IV vs. TNM I and II	miR-203a-3p	0.316	0.008	0.009–4.922
	ER+ vs. ER-	SNAI1	0.465	0.007	0.049–7.093
		ZEB2	0.486	0.017	0.113–5.252
	PR+ vs. PR-	CDH1	0.366	0.025	0.028–3.448
		SNAI1	0.336	0.008	0.049–6.071
TU-IF	≤20 mm vs. >20 mm	ZEB2	0.343	0.011	0.024–4.821
	LNM+ vs. LNM-	SNAI2	0.326	0.023	0.002–9.962
		ZEB1	0.497	0.035	0.079–4.408
	MTS+ vs. MTS-	SNAI2	0.432	0.041	0.034–94.834
		ZEB2	0.344	0.030	0.006–7.949
	TNM III and IV vs. TNM I and II	SNAI2	0.246	0.007	0.002–4.248
		ZEB1	0.438	0.007	0.059–2.126
	LVI+ vs. LVI-	SNAI2	0.294	0.015	0.002–6.602
		ZEB1	0.482	0.034	0.079–3.844
		ZEB2	0.350	0.026	0.024–3.722
	ER+ vs. ER-	miR-200c-3p	3.795	0.048	0.684–24.343
		TWIST1	0.420	0.049	0.011–15.353
LNM	MTS + vs. MTS-	ZEB1	824.73	0.018	0.283–1,584,361.881
	TNM III and IV vs. TNM I and II	SNAI1	5.959	0.025	0.227–432.565
	ER+ vs. ER-	miR-124-3p	6.819	0.018	0.091–887.828
CD45-DB	CTC+ vs. CTC-	miR-205-5p	0.041	0.010	0.000–69.820
	LNM+ vs. LNM-	miR-205-5p	22.961	0.035	0.012–400,412.929
	TNM III and IV vs. TNM I and II	miR-205-5p	39.056	0.006	0.039–692,990.143
	HER2+ vs. HER2-	miR-9	10.321	0.027	0.088–1098.021
		SNAI1	0.439	0.041	0.061–9.288
	Grade 3 vs. Grade 1 and 2	CDH1	1.468	0.033	0.151–11.647

Abbreviations: FC, fold change; CI, confidence interval; TU-C, tumor centrum, TU-IF, tumor invasive front; LNM, lymph node metastasis; CD45-DB, CD45-depleted blood; CTC, circulating tumor cell; MTS, metastatic; TNM, TNM staging system (T, tumor; N, lymph node; M, metastasis); LN, lymph node; LVI, lymphovascular invasion; ER, estrogen receptor; PR, progesterone receptor; HER2, human epidermal growth factor receptor 2.

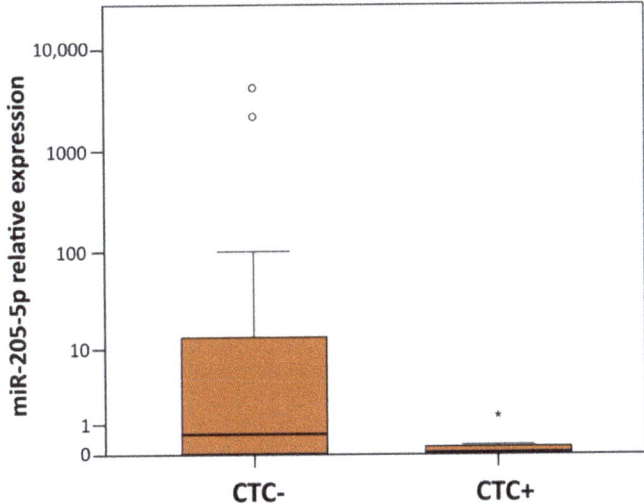

Figure 4. Individual expression levels of miR-205-5p in CD45-depleted peripheral blood of CTC negative (CTC-) and positive (CTC+) BC patients. The median is depicted by a horizontal line within each bar. The length of the boxes is the interquartile range (IQR) that represents values between the 75th and 25th percentiles of individual fold change values. Values more than 3 IQRs from the end of the box are labeled as extreme (*). Values more than 1.5 IQRs but less than 3 IQRs from the end of the box are labeled as outliers (O). Abbreviations: BC, breast cancer; CTC, circulating tumor cells.

Multivariate analysis was used to test for risk factors influencing hematogenous and lymphogenous dissemination, namely CTC, LNM, and LVI positivity, and the presence of distant MTS. Variables that were significant in univariate analysis were used in multivariate analysis.

Firstly, logistic regression was applied to predict the potential influence of miR-205-5p expression on the dissemination of tumor cells characterized by CTC positivity. In multivariate models, the clinical parameters of age, tumor size, histological grade, and HER2 status were included to control for potential confounders. The multivariate model correctly classified 88.9% of CTC negative and 91.7% of CTC positive patients, respectively, with an overall success rate of 90.0%. The presence of CTC positivity was negatively correlated with miR-205-5p expression in CD45-DB fractions (Table 4). Multivariate models for LNM, LVI, and MTS risk prediction were not significant.

Table 4. Risk estimation of miR-205-5p expression and clinical status for the presence of CTC in CD45-DB of BC patients (logistic regression adjusted for age).

Risk Factor	Variables	p-Value	OR	95% CI
CTCs presence	Age	0.061	0.893	0.792–1.005
	High grade (G3)	0.075	46.197	0.683–3124.868
	miR-205-5p *	0.028	4.326	1.170–15.995
	Tumor size > 20 mm	0.047	96.081	1.066–8661.849
	HER2 positivity [§]	0.036	2153.786	1.628–2,849,343.631
	Constant	0.126	0.000	

* ΔCt values in CD45-DB samples; [§] cut-off 10%. Abbreviations: CI, Confidence interval; CTCs, circulating tumor cells; HER2, Human epidermal growth factor receptor 2; OR, Odds ratio. Model summary: −2 Log likelihood 18.870; R squared (Cox & Snell) 0.512; R squared (Nagelkerke) 0.692. Input variables to model: age, histological grade, miR-205-5p expression, tumor size, and HER2 status.

3. Discussion

Based on the generally accepted knowledge of the key role of E-cadherin (encoded by *CDH1* gene) in cancer cell spread, we investigated the influence of aberrant expression of several EMT genes and their regulating miRNAs, in addition to miRNAs which directly targeted *CDH1* gene expression on ductal BC development in several stages of disease.

Our results showed decreasing levels of *CDH1* expression in both TU-C and TU-IF compared to C-breast, but without a statistically significant difference between the two. LMN samples were characterized by a similar expression of *CDH1* gene as in C-breast, but its upregulation compared to TU-C and TU-IF indicates a possible role of *CDH1* gene in lymphogenous cancer spread. On the other hand, similar *CDH1* expression was found in CTC- and CTC+ samples compared to C-blood.

In our patients, immunohistochemical E-cadherin expression was carefully evaluated in TU-C. In all tumors, full E-cadherin expression (3+) was found in 17 samples; however, 14 presented locally decreased levels of E-cadherin. Among them, increasing *CDH1* levels were observed in those with high E-cadherin (3+ and 3+/2+ phenotype) compared to low levels (3+/2+/1+, 3+/2+/1+/0 and 2+/1+), but without a statistically significant difference. The reason we were not able to show *CDH1*/E-cadherin association could the variability of immunohistochemistry results in ductal BCs. In technical terms, it may be that qualitative analyses of *CDH1* expression and semiquantitative E-cadherin immunohistochemistry cannot be performed in the same region of tumor. However, the association between expression of *CDH1* and E-cadherin has been documented by other authors [50] and the upregulated *CDH1* levels in LNM tissues identified in our study could correspond with the previously published increase in E-cadherin expression in LNM tissues [47].

In this study, the relatively complicated scheme of *CDH1* regulation by miRNAs and EMT genes was used to investigate possible regulators of *CDH1* in several types of samples from invasive ductal BC patients. All evaluated associations were previously identified in vitro [30,33,38,40,42–46]. Among them, only upregulated miR-9 with downregulated *CDH1* associating with invasive phenotype and upregulated miR-203a-3p with downregulated *SNAI2* gene indicating inactive EMT process were detected in TU-C. Our results were in accordance with other studies showing upregulation of miR-203a-3p in cell lines and primary BCs. According to the findings, a negative association between downregulated miR-203a-3p and upregulated SNAI2 was observed in metastatic cells [43,51,52]. LNM samples presented downregulated levels of miR-205-5p with upregulation of the *ZEB1* gene, indicating the important role of *ZEB1* in invasion. However, a negative correlation between the expression of these miRNAs and associated genes was not detected. On the other hand, we found several negative correlations that were not investigated in vitro. They could designate the new regulating connection as in the case of miR-9 and *SNAI1* expression observed in both, LNM and CTC+ samples. The other possibility is that these findings show only the independent co-existence observed in particular stages of BCs in relation to their functions (Table 2).

Similarly to LNM tissues, CTC+ samples showed miR-205-5p downregulation, and a negative correlation between miR-205-5p and *ZEB1* expression was detected.

The ZEB1 transcription factor is regulated by multiple signaling pathways and molecules as TGF-β, β-catenin and miRNAs, and it alone regulates a high number of genes, as was found in TNBCs [53,54]. In addition to EMT promotion, *ZEB1* overexpression contributes to maintenance of stem-like features, immune evasion, and epigenetic reprogramming [55]. Moreover, *ZEB1* initiates chemoresistance but inhibits the apical–basal polarity of cancer cells and antiestrogen sensitivity [53]. All these functions could contribute to the insusceptibility and survival of disseminated BC cells located in LNM samples due to elevated levels of the *ZEB1* gene found in our study.

To evaluate the association between aberrant expression of *CDH1*, and regulation of miRNAs and EMT genes and selected clinico–pathological parameters, we found a varying combination of changes in individual types of patient's samples. Patients with ER+ tumors showed downregulation of *SNAI1* and *TWIST1* in TU-C and TU-IF, respectively. Similarly, downregulation on protein and mRNA levels were observed in primary BCs by other authors, respectively [56,57]. In our study, upregulation of miR-200c-3p and miR-124-3p in TU-IF and LNM samples was observed in ER+ patients compared to ER-, respectively. The identical finding for miR-200c-3p was described also in other studies [58,59]. Differences in PR status were observed only in TU-C where PR+ samples were characterized by downregulated *CDH1* and *SNAI1* genes. Other authors identified a similar association between decreased SNAI1 protein and the PR+ phenotype [60]. In addition, HER2+ against HER2- tumors showed downregulation miR-200c-3p, and upregulation of miR-9 and downregulation of *SNAI1* were found in TU-C and CD45-DB fractions, respectively. In patients with advanced BCs in advanced stage (TNM III and IV), downregulated miR-203a-3p, and *SNAI2* with *ZEB1* were detected in TU-C and TU-IF, and upregulation of *SNAI1* and miR-205-5p was found in samples with disseminated cancer cells, LNM and CD45-DB fractions, respectively. Finally, in TU-F, tumors >20 mm presented downregulated *ZEB2* and in CD45-DB fractions, upregulation of *CDH1* in Grade 3 tumors compared to patients with smaller and highly or moderately differentiated BCs, respectively.

For evaluation of the influence of expression change on hematogenous or lymphogenous dissemination, the presence of LVI, LNM, CTC, and MTS were crucial parameters that were consequently used for the creation of multivariate models. In patients with LVI+, downregulation of *SNAI2*, *ZEB1*, and *ZEB2* was observed in TU-IF. The presence of LNM was associated with downregulation of *SNAI2* and *ZEB1* in TU-IF and upregulation of miR-205-5p in the CD45-DB fraction. Patients with distant metastasis showed downregulated miR-124-3p in TU-C, and *SNAI2* and *ZEB2* in TU-IF. Consistent with these findings, in vitro and in vivo studies showed that miR-124-3p inhibit the metastasis process [61,62]. The markedly upregulated levels of *ZEB1* in LMN tissues from patients with MTS could indicate its previously hypothesized role in metastasis [63]. The presence of CTC was associated with downregulation of miR-205-5p in the CD45-DB fractions that was verified in the multivariate risk model for CTC risk prediction (Table 4).

Regardless of the many questions remaining about the role of miR-205-5p in normal breast physiology, tumor-suppressor activities of this miRNA were documented in many studies. Decreasing levels of miR-205-5p were observed from less aggressive BC subtypes and ER+/PR+ tumors to more aggressive cases as TNBCs and those with high metastatic capabilities, poor response to therapy and patient survival [41,64]. To date, more than 20 genes targeted by miR-205-5p associating with processes and pathways involved in breast tumorigenesis were identified [64,65]. Decreased levels of miR-205-5p expression in CTC+ samples allow higher expression of the *ZEB1* gene, which could contribute to better condition and protection of cancer cells by several processes as previously discussed. Expression of other target genes *ITGA5* and *NOTCH2* could improve the stemness and metastatic potential of hematogenously disseminated cancer cells [66,67]. Moreover, after the reduction in miR-205-5p, CTCs could acquire chemoresistance features resulting from overexpression of *VEGF-A* and *FGF2*, leading to increased apoptosis upon chemotherapy treatment [68].

To our knowledge, miRNA expression analyses in CD45-DBs have been published very rarely. We found only one in silico study, in which specific differentially expressed miRNAs were identified, miR-99a and miR-151-3p for ductal BCs in situ, miR-145 and miR-210 for invasive BCs, and miR-361-5p and miR-205 for metastatic BCs [41]. Our study therefore brings original results. On the other hand, gene expression profiles were investigated in CTC samples by several research groups. In these studies, the gene expression profiles in CTCs obtained from patients with metastatic BCs were different compared to primary tumors that can be utilized for characterization of CTCs, and evaluation of prognosis and therapeutic prediction. However, expression profiles of mesenchymal CTCs were omitted for EpCAM separation of CTC-enriched fractions [69–72]. In our study, CTC+ samples were characterized by epithelial and/or mesenchymal features; therefore, we consider our results to be more objective.

Generally, the positive expression of E-cadherin is used to discriminate between ductal and lobular subtypes of BC. However, detailed examination reveals different levels of E-cadherin inhibition in the many regions of invasive ductal tumor tissues. In this BC subtype, genetic changes in the E-cadherin encoding gene *CDH1* are very rare; therefore, we investigated the influence of aberrant expression of *CDH1* and regulating miRNA and EMT genes on invasive and metastatic features in samples which represent several stages of BC cell dissemination. In this study, we showed a variable spectrum of upregulated or downregulated expressions of the *CDH1* gene and associated miRNAs and EMT genes and did not verify any regulating relationships, which were previously described in cell line studies, except an association between miR-205-5p and *ZEB1* expressions in the CTC+ fraction. However, we did observe extremely high *ZEB1* expression in LMN samples obtained from patients with distant metastases that was not explained by miR-205-5p decreasing. This finding indicates that *ZEB1* overexpression could enhance the metastatic potential of cancer cells disseminated through the lymphatic circulation. In CD45-DB fractions, the samples with the identified presence of CTCs showed downregulation of miR-205-5p expression that could contribute to maintaining the stemness and initiation of such protective features as immune evasion and chemoresistance through the increased expression of several target genes including *ZEB1*. Together, we identified miR-205-5p and *ZEB1* as potential markers for metastatic behavior of disseminated BC cells originating from a ductal tumor; however, their clinical relevance needs to be widely investigated.

4. Materials and Methods

4.1. Patients

We analyzed patient's RNA samples isolated from CD45-DB fractions and FFPE specimens from the central region and invasive front of tumor and lymph node metastases. The controls were non-neoplastic breast tissues and CD45-DB fractions of age-matched women. At the Department of Senology and Department of Pathology, St. Elisabeth Cancer Institute, Bratislava, 69 patients suspected of an invasive type of breast cancer were preselected and blood samples were collected. After the evaluation of post-operation tumor samples, 31 patients with invasive ductal BC were included in this study. 13 non-neoplastic breast tissues and 12 CD45-DB from heathy women at matched age were used as controls. This study was approved by St. Elizabeth Cancer Institute Review Board in Bratislava and written informed consent was obtained from all patients and controls. The age of patients ranged from 42 to 86 years, (median 65 years), controls were aged between 52 and 79 years (median 67 years) and between 54 and 66 years (median 59 years) in breast tissue and CD45-DB samples, respectively. No statistical differences in age were found between patients and controls. The clinical and histopathological characteristics and immunohistochemical data (tumor size, histological grade, LN and MTS status, TNM stage, LVI, hormone receptor (ER, PR) and HER2 status, Ki-67 and E-cadherin expression) were obtained from patients records and tumors were defined according to TNM classification (Table 5). No patient underwent preoperative radiotherapy or chemotherapy before specimen collection, and control women had no signs or symptoms of cancer or other serious diseases.

Table 5. Clinical characteristics.

Variables		n	%
All		31	100.0
Age	≤50	3	9.68
	>50	28	90.32
Histological grade	1 and 2	14	45.16
	3	17	54.84
Tumor size (mm)	≤20	12	38.71
	>20	19	61.29
LNM status [a]	0	9	29.03
	≥1	22	70.97
MTS status	Negative	24	77.42
	Positive	7	22.58
TNM stage	I. and II.	13	41.94
	III. and IV.	18	58.06
CTC occurrence [b]	Negative	18	58.06
	Positive	13	41.94
LVI	Negative	7	22.58
	Positive	24	77.42
ER status [c]	Negative	5	16.13
	Positive	26	83.87
PR status [c]	Negative	11	35.48
	Positive	20	64.52
HER2 status [d]	Negative	23	74.19
	Positive	8	25.81
Ki-67 proliferative index [e]	Low	4	12.90
	High	27	87.10
E-cadherin expression [f]	High	22	70.97
	Low	9	29.03

Abbreviations: LNM, lymph node metastasis; MTS, metastatic; LVI, lymphovascular invasion; ER, estrogen receptor; PR, progesterone receptor; HER2, human epidermal growth factor receptor 2. [a] LNM status was categorized according to the number of metastatic LNs; [b] CTC occurrence was evaluated in CD45-depleted blood (CD45-DB) fractions through the absence or presence of epithelial and mesenchymal markers; [c] ER, PR was considered as positive in cases with ≥ 1% of positively responding cells; [d] HER2 positive cases were those that showed strong homogeneous and circumferential membrane expression in more than 10% of tumor cells (i.e., 3+ intensity) or those that showed a 2+ intensity and subsequent FISH analysis demonstrated amplification of the HER2 gene. HER2 negative cases were with a response intensity of 0 or 1+, or cases with a response intensity of 2+ without proven amplification; [e] Low and high Ki-67 expression according to the number of stained cancer cell with a cut-off 15%; [f] High E-cadherin expression was classified as homogenous 3+ and heterogeneous 3+ and 2+ staining; low E-cadherin expression were defined in samples with heterogeneous staining covering 1+ and no expression regardless of portion of cells with 3+, 2+, 1+ and no E-cadherin expression.

4.2. CD45 Depletion of Peripheral Blood and CTC Detection

Preparation of CD45-negative blood fractions was performed by RosetteSep Human CD45 Depletion Cocktail (StemCell Technologies, Vancouver, BC, Canada) based on depletion of CD45+ peripheral blood cells. Quantitative real-time polymerase chain reaction (qRT-PCR) was used for CTCs detection in CD45-DB samples as has been previously described [73,74]. RNA extraction from CD45-DB fractions was exposed to detection of EMT-inducing transcription factors gene transcripts (*TWIST1*, *SNAIL1*, *SLUG* and *ZEB1*) and epithelial antigen (*CK19*) by TaqMan assays (LifeTechnologies, Carlsbad, CA, USA). The higher expression levels of either epithelial and/or mesenchymal gene transcripts than those of healthy donors were considered as CTCs positive.

4.3. miRNA and mRNA Isolation and Real-Time PCR

For gene expression analyses, miRNA and mRNA from CD45-DB fraction and FFPE breast tissues were used. miRNAs from CD45-DB fraction were isolated using the miRNeasy Mini Kit (Qiagen, Hilden, Germany) and miRNAs from FFPE breast tissues were isolated using the miRNeasy FFPE Kit (Qiagen, Hilden, Germany) according to the manufacturer's instructions.

mRNAs from CD45-DB fractions were isolated using the miRNeasy Mini Kit–RNeasy MinElute Cleanup Kit (Qiagen, Hilden, Germany) and mRNAs from FFPE samples were extracted using the PureLink FFPE Total RNA Isolation Kit following the provided protocol (Invitrogen Corporation, Carlsbad, CA, USA). miRNAs and mRNA samples were reversely transcribed into cDNA using the miScript II RT Kit (Qiagen, Hilden, Germany) and RevertAid First Strand cDNA Synthesis Kit (Thermo Fisher Scientific, Vilnius, Lithuania), respectively.

For real-time polymerase chain reaction (RT-PCR) Custom miScript miRNA PCR Array (CMIHS02741, Qiagen, Germany) was used. For expression analyses of mature forms of hsa-miR-9-5p, hsa-miR-124-3p, hsa-miR-203a-3p, hsa-miR-200c-3p, hsa-miR-205-5p, hsa-miR-221-3p, and hsa-miR-720, the miScript SYBR Green PCR Kit (Qiagen, Germantown, MD, USA) was used. Reactions were performed in AriaMx Real-Time PCR System (Agilent, Santa Clara, CA, USA) using the following conditions: pre-denaturation at 95 °C for 15 min, followed by 40 cycles at 94 °C 15 s, 55 °C for 30 s, and 70 °C for 30 s, followed by melt cycle at 95 °C for 30 s, 65 °C for 30 s, and 95 °C for 30 s. Among three reference controls (Snord61, Snord72, and Snord95), Snord95, with the most stable expression, was selected for normalization of Ct values.

qRT- PCR detection and expression of *CDH1*, *TWIST1*, *SNAI1*, *SNAI2*, *ZEB1*, *ZEB2* and *18S* were performed using TaqMan Gene Expression Assays—single tube assays (Thermo Fisher Scientific, Pleasanton, CA, USA): *CDH1*–Hs01013959_m1, *TWIST1*–Hs00361186_m1, *SNAI1*–Hs00195591_m1, *SNAI2*–Hs00161904_m1, *ZEB1*–Hs01566408_m1, *ZEB2*–Hs002007691_m1, *18S*–Hs_9999991_s1. qRT-PCR reactions were carried out in an AriaMx Real-Time PCR System (Agilent, Santa Clara, CA, USA) at following settings: uracil-N-glycosylase incubation 1 cycle at 50 °C for 2 min, enzyme activation 1 cycle at 95 °C for 20 s, 40 cycles at 95 °C for 30 s denaturation and 60 °C for 30 s annealing. For all fluorescence-based RT-PCR, fluorescence was detected between 10 and 40 cycles for the reference (18 S) and target genes. Fold change was calculated as normalized relative gene expression using formula $2^{-\Delta\Delta Ct}$.

4.4. Immunohistochemical Analyses of E-Cadherin

Immunohistochemistry for detection of E-cadherin was performed on paraffin sections with ready to use reagents using an automated immunostainer, Autostainer Link 48 (Dako; Agilent Technologies, Inc., Santa Clara, CA, USA). Primary E-cadherin antibody (FLEX Monoclonal Mouse, clone NCH-38, RTU, IR05961) was supplied by Dako; Agilent Technologies, Inc. (Santa Clara, CA, USA). Antigen retrieval was performed using EnVision TM FLEX Target Retrieval Solution High pH (pH 9.0) for 20 min. at 97–98°C in PT Link instrument (Dako; Agilent Technologies, Inc., Santa Clara, CA, USA). Endogenous peroxidase activity was blocked by incubation for 10 min. in 3% hydrogen peroxide, followed by antibody incubation for 20 min. at room temperature. EnVision TM FLEX/HRP, High pH kit (K8000, Dako; Agilent Technologies, Inc., Santa Clara, CA, USA) was used as a detection system according to the manufacturer's instructions. High E-cadherin expression was classified as homogenous 3+ and heterogeneous 3+ and 2+ staining; low E-cadherin expression was defined in samples with heterogeneous staining covering 1+ and no expression regardless of the portion of cells with 3+, 2+, 1+, and no E-cadherin expression.

4.5. Statistical Analysis

IBM SPSS statistics 23.0 software was used for statistical analysis. qPCR data were analyzed using REST 2009 Software (Technical University Munich and Qiagen, Germany). The normality of distribution was assessed by the Shapiro–Wilk test. Normally distributed variables were tested using Student's t-test. Non-normally distributed data were tested by nonparametric Mann–Whitney U test. Pearson's or Spearman's correlations were used to assess the correlations between miRNA and mRNA expression of tested genes. Binary logistic regression was used to evaluate the influence of selected gene and miRNA expression on hematogenous and lymphogenous dissemination of tumor cells and to control for confounders. This determination included enumeration of the risk estimate presented as estimated odds ratio (OR) and 95% confidence interval (CI) for the OR. p-value < 0.05 was defined as statistically significant.

Supplementary Materials: The following are available online at https://www.mdpi.com/article/10.3390/ijms23010103/s1.

Author Contributions: Conceptualization, I.F.; Data curation, I.F.; Formal Analysis, L.K. and B.S.; Funding acquisition, I.F.; Investigation, L.K., N.N., K.K., S.C., V.H.K. and H.K.; Methodology, N.N., L.K. and G.M.; Project administration, I.F.; Resources, V.B., K.K. and I.F.; Supervision, I.F.; Writing—original draft, I.F.; Writing—review & editing, L.K., N.N., K.K. and S.C. All authors have read and agreed to the published version of the manuscript.

Funding: This work was supported by the Scientific Grant Agency of the Ministry of Education, Science, Research and Sport of the Slovak Republic and the Slovak Academy of Sciences under the project VEGA 2/0036/19.

Institutional Review Board Statement: The study was conducted according to the guidelines of the Declaration of Helsinki, and approved by the St. Elizabeth Cancer Institute Review Board (3-2019/EK OUSA, 20 March 2019).

Informed Consent Statement: Written informed consent has been obtained from all individual participants included in the study.

Acknowledgments: The authors would like to thank Dana Jurkovicova for methodology consultation, Viola Stevurkova for excellent technical assistance, and Rebecca Doherty for reading the manuscript carefully and helping with language editing.

Conflicts of Interest: The authors declare no conflict of interest.

Abbreviations

BC	Breast cancer
C-blood	CD45-depleted blood fraction from healthy women
C-breast	Non-neoplastic breast tissue
CD45-DB	CD45-depleted blood
CDH1	Cadherin 1
CI	Confidence interval
CTC	Circulating tumor cells
EMT	Epithelial-to-mesenchymal transition
ER	Estrogen receptor
FC	Fold change
FFPE	Formalin-fixed paraffin-embedded tissue
HER2	Human epidermal growth factor receptor 2
LN	Lymph node
LNM	Lymph node metastasis
LVI	Lymphovascular invasion
mRNA	Messenger RNA
miRNA	microRNA
MTS	Distant metastasis
OR	Odds ratio
PR	Progesterone receptor
r	Correlation coefficient
RT-PCR	Real time- Polymerase chain reaction
SNAI1	Snail Family Transcriptional Repressor 1
SNAI2	Snail Family Transcriptional Repressor 2
TNBC	Triple-negative breast cancer
TNM	Tumor Node Metastasis staging
TU-C	Tumor centrum
TU-IF	Tumor invasive front
TWIST1	Twist Family BHLH Transcription Factor 1
ZEB1	Zinc Finger E-Box Binding Homeobox 1
ZEB2	Zinc Finger E-Box Binding Homeobox 2

References

1. Bray, F.; Ferlay, J.; Soerjomataram, I.; Siegel, R.L.; Torre, L.A.; Jemal, A. Global cancer statistics 2018: GLOBOCAN estimates of incidence and mortality worldwide for 36 cancers in 185 countries. *CA Cancer J. Clin.* **2018**, *68*, 394–424. [CrossRef] [PubMed]
2. Wu, Q.; Li, J.; Zhu, S.; Wu, J.; Chen, C.; Liu, Q.; Wei, W.; Zhang, Y.; Sun, S. Breast cancer subtypes predict the preferential site of distant metastases: A SEER based study. *Oncotarget* **2017**, *8*, 27990–27996. [CrossRef] [PubMed]
3. Cummings, M.C.; Simpson, P.T.; Reid, L.E.; Jayanthan, J.; Skerman, J.; Song, S.; McCart Reed, A.E.; Kutasovic, J.R.; Morey, A.L.; Marquart, L.; et al. Metastatic progression of breast cancer: Insights from 50 years of autopsies. *J. Pathol.* **2014**, *232*, 23–31. [CrossRef] [PubMed]
4. Barinoff, J.; Hils, R.; Bender, A.; Groß, J.; Kurz, C.; Tauchert, S.; Mann, E.; Schwidde, I.; Ipsen, B.; Sawitzki, K.; et al. Clinicopathological diferences between breast cancer in patients with primary metastatic disease and those without: A multicentre study. *Eur. J. Cancer* **2013**, *49*, 305–311. [CrossRef] [PubMed]
5. Eng, L.G.; Dawood, S.; Sopik, V.; Haaland, B.; Tan, P.S.; Bhoo-Pathy, N.; Warner, E.; Iqbal, J.; Narod, S.A.; Dent, R. Ten-year survival in women with primary stage IV breast cancer. *Breast Cancer Res. Treat.* **2016**, *160*, 145–152. [CrossRef] [PubMed]
6. Paduch, R. The role of lymphangiogenesis and angiogenesis in tumor metastasis. *Cell Oncol.* **2016**, *39*, 397–410. [CrossRef] [PubMed]
7. Sleeman, J.P.; Nazarenko, I.; Thiele, W. Do all roads lead to Rome? Routes to metastasis development. *Int. J. Cancer* **2011**, *128*, 2511–2526. [CrossRef]
8. Wong, S.Y.; Hynes, R.O. Lymphatic or hematogenous dissemination: How does a metastatic tumor cell decide? *Cell Cycle* **2006**, *5*, 812–817. [CrossRef] [PubMed]
9. Witte, M.H.; Dellinger, M.T.; McDonald, D.M.; Nathanson, S.D.; Boccardo, F.M.; Campisi, C.C.; Sleeman, J.P.; Gershenwald, J.E. Lymphangiogenesis and hemangiogenesis: Potential targets for therapy. *J. Surg. Oncol.* **2011**, *103*, 489–500. [CrossRef] [PubMed]
10. Nathanson, S.D.; Kwon, D.; Kapke, A.; Alford, S.H.; Chitale, D. The role of lymph node metastasis in the systemic dissemination of breast cancer. *Ann. Surg. Oncol.* **2009**, *16*, 3396–3405. [CrossRef]
11. Nathanson, S.D.; Krag, D.; Kuerer, H.M.; Newman, L.A.; Brown, M.; Kerjaschki, D.; Pereira, E.R.; Padera, T.P. Breast cancer metastasis through the lympho-vascular system. *Clin. Exp. Metastasis* **2018**, *35*, 443–454. [CrossRef] [PubMed]
12. Cristofanilli, M.; Budd, G.T.; Ellis, M.J.; Stopeck, A.; Matera, J.; Miller, M.C.; Reuben, J.M.; Doyle, G.V.; Allard, W.J.; Terstappen, L.W.M.M.; et al. Circulating tumor cells, disease progression, and survival in metastatic breast cancer. *N. Engl. J. Med.* **2004**, *351*, 781–791. [CrossRef] [PubMed]
13. Giuliano, M.; Giordano, A.; Jackson, S.; De Giorgi, U.; Mego, M.; Cohen, E.N.; Gao, H.; Anfossi, S.; Handy, B.C.; Ueno, N.T.; et al. Circulating tumor cells as early predictors of metastatic spread in breast cancer patients with limited metastatic dissemination. *Breast Cancer Res.* **2014**, *16*, 440. [CrossRef] [PubMed]
14. Bidard, F.-C.; Proudhon, C.; Pierga, J.-Y. Circulating tumor cells in breast cancer. *Mol. Oncol.* **2016**, *10*, 418–430. [CrossRef] [PubMed]
15. Balic, M.; Lin, H.; Williams, A.; Datar, R.H.; Cote, R.J. Progress in circulating tumor cell capture and analysis: Implications for cancer management. *Expert Rev. Mol. Diagn.* **2012**, *12*, 303–312. [CrossRef]
16. Krebs, M.G.; Metcalf, R.L.; Carter, L.; Brady, G.; Blackhall, F.H.; Dive, C. Molecular analysis of circulating tumour cells-biology and biomarkers. *Nat. Rev. Clin. Oncol.* **2014**, *11*, 129–144. [CrossRef] [PubMed]
17. Kallergi, G.; Papadaki, M.A.; Politaki, E.; Mavroudis, D.; Georgoulias, V.; Agelaki, S. Epithelial to mesenchymal transition markers expressed in circulating tumour cells of early and metastatic breast cancer patients. *Breast Cancer Res.* **2011**, *13*, R59. [CrossRef]
18. Mego, M.; Mani, S.A.; Lee, B.N.; Li, C.; Evans, K.W.; Cohen, E.N.; Gao, H.; Jackson, S.A.; Giordano, A.; Hortobagyi, G.N.; et al. Expression of epithelial-mesenchymal transition-inducing transcription factors in primary breast cancer: The effect of neoadjuvant therapy. *Int. J. Cancer* **2012**, *130*, 808–816. [CrossRef]
19. Lustberg, M.B.; Balasubramanian, P.; Miller, B.; Garcia-Villa, A.; Deighan, C.; Wu, Y.; Carothers, S.; Berger, M.; Ramaswamy, B.; Macrae, E.R.; et al. Heterogeneous atypical cell populations are present in blood of metastatic breast cancer patients. *Breast Cancer Res.* **2014**, *16*, R23. [CrossRef] [PubMed]
20. Bulfoni, M.; Gerratana, L.; Del Ben, F.; Marzinotto, S.; Sorrentino, M.; Turetta, M.; Scoles, G.; Toffoletto, B.; Isola, M.; Beltrami, C.A.; et al. In patients with metastatic breast cancer the identification of circulating tumor cells in epithelial-to-mesenchymal transition is associated with a poor prognosis. *Breast Cancer Res.* **2016**, *18*, 30. [CrossRef] [PubMed]
21. Kalluri, R.; Weinberg, R.A. The basics of epithelial-mesenchymal transition. *J. Clin. Investig.* **2009**, *119*, 1420–1428. [CrossRef] [PubMed]
22. Pang, M.F.; Georgoudaki, A.M.; Lambut, L.; Johansson, J.; Tabor, V.; Hagikura, K.; Jin, Y.; Jansson, M.; Alexander, J.S.; Nelson, C.M.; et al. TGF-1-induced EMT promotes targeted migration of breast cancer cells through the lymphatic system by the activation of CCR7/CCL21-mediated chemotaxis. *Oncogene* **2016**, *35*, 748–760. [CrossRef]
23. Moyret-Lalle, C.; Ruiz, E.; Puisieux, A. Epithelial-mesenchymal transition transcription factors and miRNAs: "Plastic surgeons" of breast cancer. *World J. Clin. Oncol.* **2014**, *5*, 311–322. [CrossRef]
24. Nickel, A.; Stadler, S.C. Role of epigenetic mechanisms in epithelial-to-mesenchymal transition of breast cancer cells. *Transl. Res.* **2015**, *165*, 126–142. [CrossRef]
25. Berx, G.; Van Roy, F. The E-cadherin/catenin complex: An important gatekeeper in breast cancer tumorigenesis and malignant progression. *Breast Cancer Res.* **2001**, *3*, 289–293. [CrossRef]

26. Petridis, C.; Shinomiya, I.; Kohut, K.; Gorman, P.; Caneppele, M.; Shah, V.; Troy, M.; Pinder, S.E.; Hanby, A.; Tomlinson, I.; et al. Germline CDH1 mutations in bilateral lobular carcinoma in situ. *Br. J. Cancer* **2014**, *110*, 1053–1057. [CrossRef] [PubMed]
27. Caldeira, J.R.F.; Prando, E.C.; Quevedo, F.C.; Neto, F.A.M.; Rainho, C.A.; Rogatto, S.R. CDH1 promoter hypermethylation and E-cadherin protein expression in infiltrating breast cancer. *BMC Cancer* **2006**, *6*, 48. [CrossRef]
28. Sebova, K.; Zmetakova, I.; Bella, V.; Kajo, K.; Stankovicova, I.; Kajabova, V.; Krivulcik, T.; Lasabova, Z.; Tomka, M.; Galbavy, S.; et al. RASSF1A and CDH1 hypermethylation as potential epimarkers in breast cancer. *Cancer Biomark.* **2012**, *10*, 13–26. [CrossRef]
29. Fridrichova, I.; Zmetakova, I. MicroRNAs Contribute to Breast Cancer Invasiveness. *Cells* **2019**, *8*, 1361. [CrossRef] [PubMed]
30. Ma, F.; Li, W.; Liu, C.; Li, W.; Yu, H.; Lei, B.; Ren, Y.; Li, Z.; Pang, D.; Qian, C. MiR-23a promotes TGF-β-1-induced EMT and tumor metastasis in breast cancer cells by directly targeting CDH1 and activating Wnt/β-catenin signaling. *Oncotarget* **2017**, *8*, 69538–69550. [CrossRef]
31. Zhou, X.; Marian, C.; Makambi, K.H.; Kosti, O.; Kallakury, B.V.; Loffredo, C.A.; Zheng, Y.-L. MicroRNA-9 as potential biomarker for breast cancer local recurrence and tumor estrogen receptor status. *PLoS ONE* **2012**, *7*, e39011. [CrossRef]
32. Lambertini, E.; Lolli, A.; Vezzali, F.; Penolazzi, L.; Gambari, R.; Piva, R. Correlation between Slug transcription factor and miR-221 in MDA-MB-231 breast cancer cells. *BMC Cancer* **2012**, *12*, 445. [CrossRef]
33. Pan, Y.; Li, J.; Zhang, Y.; Wang, N.; Liang, H.; Liu, Y.; Zhang, C.Y.; Zen, K.; Gu, H. Slug-upregulated miR-221 promotes breast cancer progression through suppressing E-cadherin expression. *Sci. Rep.* **2016**, *6*, 25798. [CrossRef] [PubMed]
34. Niu, X.-Y.; Zhang, Z.-Q.; Ma, P.-L. MiRNA-221-5p promotes breast cancer progression by regulating E-cadherin expression. *Eur. Rev. Med. Pharm. Sci.* **2019**, *23*, 6983–6990. [CrossRef]
35. Stinson, S.; Lackner, M.R.; Adai, A.T.; Yu, N.; Kim, H.J.; O'Brien, C.; Spoerke, J.; Jhunjhunwala, S.; Boyd, Z.; Januario, T.; et al. TRPS1 targeting by miR-221/222 promotes the epithelial-to-mesenchymal transition in breast cancer. *Sci. Signal.* **2011**, *4*, ra41. [CrossRef]
36. Castilla, M.Á.; Díaz-Martín, J.; Sarrió, D.; Romero-Pérez, L.; López-García, M.Á.; Vieites, B.; Biscuola, M.; Ramiro-Fuentes, S.; Isacke, C.M.; Palacios, J. MicroRNA-200 family modulation in distinct breast cancer phenotypes. *PLoS ONE* **2012**, *7*, e47709. [CrossRef] [PubMed]
37. Hurteau, G.J.; Carlson, J.A.; Spivack, S.D.; Brock, G.J. Overexpression of the microRNA hsa-miR-200c leads to reduced expression of transcription factor 8 and increased expression of E-cadherin. *Cancer Res.* **2007**, *67*, 7972–7976. [CrossRef]
38. Sundararajan, V.; Gengenbacher, N.; Stemmler, M.P.; Kleemann, J.A.; Brabletz, T.; Brabletz, S. The ZEB1/miR-200c feedback loop regulates invasion via actin interacting proteins MYLK and TKS5. *Oncotarget* **2015**, *6*, 27083–27096. [CrossRef]
39. Chen, H.; Li, Z.; Zhang, L.; Zhang, L.; Zhang, Y.; Wang, Y.; Xu, M.; Zhong, Q. MicroRNA-200c inhibits the metastasis of triple-negative breast cancer by targeting ZEB2, an epithelial-mesenchymal transition regulator. *Ann. Clin. Lab. Sci.* **2020**, *50*, 519–527. [PubMed]
40. Lee, J.-Y.; Park, M.K.; Park, J.-H.; Lee, H.J.; Shin, D.H.; Kang, Y.; Lee, C.H.; Kong, G. Loss of the polycomb protein Mel-18 enhances the epithelial-mesenchymal transition by ZEB1 and ZEB2 expression through the downregulation of miR-205 in breast cancer. *Oncogene* **2014**, *33*, 1325–1335. [CrossRef] [PubMed]
41. Sun, E.-H.; Zhou, Q.; Liu, K.-S.; Wei, W.; Wang, C.-M.; Liu, X.-F.; Lu, C.; Ma, D.-Y. Screening miRNAs related to different subtypes of breast cancer with miRNAs microarray. *Eur. Rev. Med. Pharm. Sci.* **2014**, *18*, 2783–2788.
42. Moes, M.; Le Béchec, A.; Crespo, I.; Laurini, C.; Halavatyi, A.; Vetter, G.; Del Sol, A.; Friederich, E. A novel network integrating a miRNA-203/SNAI1 feedback loop which regulates epithelial to mesenchymal transition. *PLoS ONE* **2012**, *7*, e35440. [CrossRef]
43. Zhang, Z.; Zhang, B.; Li, W.; Fu, L.; Fu, L.; Zhu, Z.; Dong, J.-T. Epigenetic silencing of miR-203 upregulates SNAI2 and contributes to the invasiveness of malignant breast cancer cells. *Genes Cancer* **2011**, *2*, 782–791. [CrossRef]
44. Ji, H.; Sang, M.; Liu, F.; Ai, N.; Geng, C. miR-124 regulates EMT based on ZEB2 target to inhibit invasion and metastasis in triple-negative breast cancer. *Pathol. Res. Pr.* **2019**, *215*, 697–704. [CrossRef] [PubMed]
45. Liang, Y.-J.; Wang, Q.-Y.; Zhou, C.-X.; Yin, Q.-Q.; He, M.; Yu, X.-T.; Cao, D.-X.; Chen, G.-Q.; He, J.-R.; Zhao, Q. MiR-124 targets Slug to regulate epithelial-mesenchymal transition and metastasis of breast cancer. *Carcinogenesis* **2013**, *34*, 713–722. [CrossRef]
46. Li, L.-Z.; Zhang, C.Z.; Liu, L.-L.; Yi, C.; Lu, S.-X.; Zhou, X.; Zhang, Z.-J.; Peng, Y.-H.; Yang, Y.-Z.; Yun, J.-P. miR-720 inhibits tumor invasion and migration in breast cancer by targeting TWIST1. *Carcinogenesis* **2014**, *35*, 469–478. [CrossRef] [PubMed]
47. Jeschke, U.; Mylonas, I.; Kuhn, C.; Shabani, N.; Kunert-Keil, C.; Schindlbeck, C.; Gerber, B.; Friese, K. Expression of E-cadherin in human ductal breast cancer carcinoma in situ, invasive carcinomas, their lymph node metastases, their distant metastases, carcinomas with recurrence and in recurrence. *Anticancer Res.* **2007**, *27*, 1969–19674. [PubMed]
48. Borcherding, N.; Cole, K.; Kluz, P.; Jorgensen, M.; Kolb, R.; Bellizzi, A.; Zhang, W. Re-evaluating E-cadherin and β-catenin: A pan-cancer proteomic approach with an emphasis on breast cancer. *Am. J. Pathol.* **2018**, *188*, 1910–1920. [CrossRef]
49. Padmanaban, V.; Krol, I.; Suhail, Y.; Szczerba, B.M.; Aceto, N.; Bader, J.S.; Ewald, A.J. E-cadherin is required for metastasis in multiple models of breast cancer. *Nature* **2019**, *573*, 439–444. [CrossRef] [PubMed]
50. Prasad, C.P.; Mirza, S.; Sharma, G.; Prashad, R.; DattaGupta, S.; Rath, G.; Ralhan, R. Epigenetic alterations of CDH1 and APC genes: Relationship with activation of Wnt/beta-catenin pathway in invasive ductal carcinoma of breast. *Life Sci.* **2008**, *83*, 318–325. [CrossRef]
51. Cai, K.-T.; Feng, C.-X.; Zhao, J.-C.; He, R.-Q.; Ma, J.; Zhong, J.-C. Upregulated miR-203a-3p and its potential molecular mechanism in breast cancer: A study based on bioinformatics analyses and a comprehensive meta-analysis. *Mol. Med. Rep.* **2018**, *18*, 4994–5008. [CrossRef] [PubMed]

52. Gomes, B.C.; Martins, M.; Lopes, P.; Morujão, I.; Oliveira, M.; Araújo, A.; Rueff, J.; Rodrigues, A.S. Prognostic value of microRNA-203a expression in breast cancer. *Oncol. Rep.* **2016**, *36*, 1748–1756. [CrossRef] [PubMed]
53. Wu, H.-T.; Zhong, H.-T.; Li, G.-W.; Shen, J.-X.; Ye, Q.-Q.; Zhang, M.-L.; Liu, J. Oncogenic functions of the EMT-related transcription factor ZEB1 in breast cancer. *J. Transl. Med.* **2020**, *18*, 51. [CrossRef]
54. Lehmann, W.; Mossmann, D.; Kleemann, J.; Mock, K.; Meisinger, C.; Brummer, T.; Herr, R.; Brabletz, S.; Stemmler, M.P.; Brabletz, T. ZEB1 turns into a transcriptional activator by interacting with YAP1 in aggressive cancer types. *Nat. Commun.* **2016**, *7*, 10498. [CrossRef] [PubMed]
55. Zhang, Y.; Xu, L.; Li, A.; Han, X. The roles of ZEB1 in tumorigenic progression and epigenetic modifications. *Biomed. Pharm.* **2019**, *110*, 400–408. [CrossRef] [PubMed]
56. Scherbakov, A.M.; Andreeva, O.E.; Shatskaya, V.A.; Krasil'nikov, M.A. The relationships between snail1 and estrogen receptor signaling in breast cancer cells. *J. Cell Biochem.* **2012**, *113*, 2147–2155. [CrossRef]
57. Fu, J.; Zhang, L.; He, T.; Xiao, X.; Liu, X.; Wang, L.; Yang, L.; Yang, M.; Zhang, T.; Chen, R.; et al. TWIST represses estrogen receptor-alpha expression by recruiting the NuRD protein complex in breast cancer cells. *Int. J. Biol. Sci.* **2012**, *8*, 522–532. [CrossRef] [PubMed]
58. Cochrane, D.R.; Cittelly, D.M.; Howe, E.N.; Spoelstra, N.S.; McKinsey, E.L.; LaPara, K.; Elias, A.; Yee, D.; Richer, J.K. MicroRNAs link estrogen receptor alpha status and Dicer levels in breast cancer. *Horm. Cancer* **2010**, *1*, 306–319. [CrossRef] [PubMed]
59. Sakurai, M.; Masuda, M.; Miki, Y.; Hirakawa, H.; Suzuki, T.; Sasano, H. Correlation of miRNA expression profiling in surgical pathology materials, with Ki-67, HER2, ER and PR in breast cancer patients. *Int. J. Biol. Markers* **2015**, *30*, e190–e199. [CrossRef]
60. van Nes, J.G.H.; de Kruijf, E.M.; Putter, H.; Faratian, D.; Munro, A.; Campbell, F.; Smit, V.T.H.B.M.; Liefers, G.-J.; Kuppen, P.J.K.; van de Velde, C.J.H.; et al. Co-expression of SNAIL and TWIST determines prognosis in estrogen receptor-positive early breast cancer patients. *Breast Cancer Res. Treat.* **2012**, *133*, 49–59. [CrossRef] [PubMed]
61. Lv, X.-B.; Jiao, Y.; Qing, Y.; Hu, H.; Cui, X.; Lin, T.; Song, E.; Yu, F. miR-124 suppresses multiple steps of breast cancer metastasis by targeting a cohort of pro-metastatic genes in vitro. *Chin. J. Cancer* **2011**, *30*, 821–830. [CrossRef] [PubMed]
62. Cai, W.-L.; Huang, W.-D.; Li, B.; Chen, T.-R.; Li, Z.-X.; Zhao, C.-L.; Li, H.-Y.; Wu, Y.-M.; Yan, W.-J.; Xiao, J.-R. microRNA-124 inhibits bone metastasis of breast cancer by repressing Interleukin-11. *Mol. Cancer* **2018**, *17*, 9. [CrossRef]
63. Morel, A.P.; Ginestier, C.; Pommier, R.M.; Cabaud, O.; Ruiz, E.; Wicinski, J.; Devouassoux-Shisheboran, M.; Combaret, V.; Finetti, P.; Chassot, C.; et al. A stemness-related ZEB1-MSRB3 axis governs cellular pliancy and breast cancer genome stability. *Nat. Med.* **2017**, *23*, 568–578. [CrossRef]
64. Plantamura, I.; Cataldo, A.; Cosentino, G.; Iorio, M.V. miR-205 in breast cancer: State of the art. *Int. J. Mol. Sci.* **2020**, *22*, 27. [CrossRef] [PubMed]
65. Xiao, Y.; Humphries, B.; Yang, C.; Wang, Z. MiR-205 dysregulations in breast cancer: The complexity and opportunities. *Noncoding RNA* **2019**, *5*, 53. [CrossRef] [PubMed]
66. Xiao, Y.; Li, Y.; Tao, H.; Humphries, B.; Li, A.; Jiang, Y.; Yang, C.; Luo, R.; Wang, Z. Integrin α5 down-regulation by miR-205 suppresses triple negative breast cancer stemness and metastasis by inhibiting the Src/Vav2/Rac1 pathway. *Cancer Lett.* **2018**, *433*, 199–290. [CrossRef] [PubMed]
67. Chao, C.-H.; Chang, C.-C.; Wu, M.-J.; Ko, H.-W.; Wang, D.; Hung, M.-C.; Yang, J.-Y.; Chang, C.-J. MicroRNA-205 signaling regulates mammary stem cell fate and tumorigenesis. *J. Clin. Investig.* **2014**, *124*, 3093–3106. [CrossRef] [PubMed]
68. Hu, Y.; Qiu, Y.; Yague, E.; Ji, W.; Liu, J.; Zhang, J. miRNA-205 targets VEGFA and FGF2 and regulates resistance to chemotherapeutics in breast cancer. *Cell Death Dis.* **2016**, *7*, e2291. [CrossRef]
69. Smirnov, D.A.; Zweitzig, D.R.; Foulk, B.W.; Miller, M.C.; Doyle, G.V.; Pienta, K.J.; Meropol, N.J.; Weiner, L.M.; Cohen, S.J.; Moreno, J.G.; et al. Global gene expression profiling of circulating tumor cells. *Cancer Res.* **2005**, *65*, 4993–4997. [CrossRef] [PubMed]
70. Lang, J.E.; Scott, J.H.; Wolf, D.M.; Novak, P.; Punj, V.; Magbanua, M.J.; Zhu, W.; Mineyev, N.; Haqq, C.M.; Crothers, J.R.; et al. Expression profiling of circulating tumor cells in metastatic breast cancer. *Breast Cancer Res. Treat.* **2015**, *149*, 121–131. [CrossRef] [PubMed]
71. Onstenk, W.; Sieuwerts, A.M.; Weekhout, M.; Mostert, B.; Reijm, E.A.; van Deurzen, C.H.M.; Bolt-de Vries, J.B.; Peeters, D.J.; Hamberg, P.; Seynaeve, C.; et al. Gene expression profiles of circulating tumor cells versus primary tumors in metastatic breast cancer. *Cancer Lett.* **2015**, *362*, 36–44. [CrossRef] [PubMed]
72. Pereira-Veiga, T.; Martínez-Fernández, M.; Abuin, C.; Piñeiro, R.; Cebey, V.; Cueva, J.; Palacios, P.; Blanco, C.; Muinelo-Romay, L.; Abalo, A.; et al. CTCs expression profiling for advanced breast cancer monitoring. *Cancers* **2019**, *11*, 1941. [CrossRef] [PubMed]
73. Cierna, Z.; Mego, M.; Janega, P.; Karaba, M.; Minarik, G.; Benca, J.; Sedláčková, T.; Cingelova, S.; Gronesova, P.; Manasova, D.; et al. Matrix metalloproteinase 1 and circulating tumor cells in early breast cancer. *BMC Cancer* **2014**, *14*, 472. [CrossRef] [PubMed]
74. Kalinkova, L.; Zmetakova, I.; Smolkova, B.; Minarik, G.; Sedlackova, T.; Horvathova Kajabova, V.; Cierna, Z.; Mego, M.; Fridrichova, I. Decreased methylation in the SNAI2 and ADAM23 genes associated with de-differentiation and haematogenous dissemination in breast cancers. *BMC Cancer* **2018**, *18*, 875. [CrossRef] [PubMed]

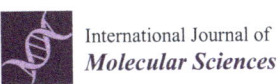

International Journal of Molecular Sciences

Article

Gene Expression Profile in Primary Tumor Is Associated with Brain-Tropism of Metastasis from Lung Adenocarcinoma

Yen-Yu Lin [1,2,†], Yu-Chao Wang [3,†], Da-Wei Yeh [3], Chen-Yu Hung [3], Yi-Chen Yeh [1,3], Hsiang-Ling Ho [1,4], Hsiang-Chen Mon [1], Mei-Yu Chen [5], Yu-Chung Wu [6] and Teh-Ying Chou [1,2,4,7,*]

1. Department of Pathology and Laboratory Medicine, Taipei Veterans General Hospital, Taipei 112201, Taiwan; b91401116@ntu.edu.tw (Y.-Y.L.); ycyeh2@vghtpe.gov.tw (Y.-C.Y.); hlho5@vghtpe.gov.tw (H.-L.H.); jennifer620jennifer620@gmail.com (H.-C.M.)
2. Cancer Progression Research Center, National Yang Ming Chiao Tung University, Taipei 112304, Taiwan
3. Institute of Biomedical Informatics, National Yang Ming Chiao Tung University, Taipei 112304, Taiwan; yuchao@ym.edu.tw (Y.-C.W.); dustin3141@gmail.com (D.-W.Y.); candy1234234@gmail.com (C.-Y.H.)
4. Department of Biotechnology and Laboratory Science in Medicine, National Yang Ming Chiao Tung University, Taipei 112304, Taiwan
5. Institute of Biochemistry and Molecular Biology, National Yang Ming Chiao Tung University, Taipei 112304, Taiwan; meychen@ym.edu.tw
6. Department of Thoracic Surgery, Taipei Medical University Hospital, Taipei 110301, Taiwan; yuchungwu@tmu.edu.tw
7. Institute of Clinical Medicine, National Yang Ming Chiao Tung University, Taipei 112304, Taiwan
* Correspondence: tychou@vghtpe.gov.tw
† These authors contributed equally to this work.

Abstract: Lung adenocarcinoma has a strong propensity to metastasize to the brain. The brain metastases are difficult to treat and can cause significant morbidity and mortality. Identifying patients with increased risk of developing brain metastasis can assist medical decision-making, facilitating a closer surveillance or justifying a preventive treatment. We analyzed 27 lung adenocarcinoma patients who received a primary lung tumor resection and developed metastases within 5 years after the surgery. Among these patients, 16 developed brain metastases and 11 developed non-brain metastases only. We performed targeted DNA sequencing, RNA sequencing and immunohistochemistry to characterize the difference between the primary tumors. We also compared our findings to the published data of brain-tropic and non-brain-tropic lung adenocarcinoma cell lines. The results demonstrated that the targeted tumor DNA sequencing did not reveal a significant difference between the groups, but the RNA sequencing identified 390 differentially expressed genes. A gene expression signature including CDKN2A could identify 100% of brain-metastasizing tumors with a 91% specificity. However, when compared to the differentially expressed genes between brain-tropic and non-brain-tropic lung cancer cell lines, a different set of genes was shared between the patient data and the cell line data, which include many genes implicated in the cancer-glia/neuron interaction. Our findings indicate that it is possible to identify lung adenocarcinoma patients at the highest risk for brain metastasis by analyzing the primary tumor. Further investigation is required to elucidate the mechanism behind these associations and to identify potential treatment targets.

Keywords: lung adenocarcinoma; brain metastasis; omics data analysis; CDKN2A; p16

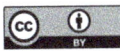

1. Introduction

Lung cancer is the world-leading cause of cancer-related death [1], and lung adenocarcinoma has recently surpassed squamous cell carcinoma as the most common histology type [2]. Despite efforts in prevention, screening and treatment, many lung cancer patients still die of the disease, mostly because of distant metastasis. Among the metastatic sites, metastasis to the central nervous system, mainly the brain, is a major problem in patient care. Lung cancer, especially lung adenocarcinoma, has a strong propensity to metastasize to the brain. About 15% of patients already have brain metastasis at the time of the initial diagnosis [3]; more than 20% of all lung adenocarcinoma patients develop brain metastasis along their disease courses [4]. Of all cancer metastases to the brain, lung adenocarcinoma is the most common primary tumor, constituting 37% of all the cases [3]. The brain metastases can cause neurological deficits and increased intracranial pressure, resulting in significant morbidity and mortality. However, the current clinical practice has limited tools for the early detection and treatment of brain metastasis [5]. Because of the cost and radiation exposure related to brain imaging modalities, lung adenocarcinoma patients often do not receive regular brain imaging examinations until they develop symptoms and signs suspicious of brain metastasis. By this time point, multiple brain metastasis foci may have already developed, sometimes to a significant size, and surgical resection or stereotactic radiosurgery may not be feasible. Whole-brain irradiation and systemic therapy may be the patient's only choices, but the irradiation may cause a significant cognitive function decline, and the chemotherapeutic agents and targeted therapies for driver mutations (such as tyrosine kinase inhibitors) invariably encounter the problem of tumor resistance. These treatments can control the brain metastasis temporarily at best, and most patients eventually die of disease progression.

One possible way to improve the management of lung adenocarcinoma-derived brain metastasis is to identify patients who are at the highest risk of developing brain metastasis. If such patients can be identified, implementing a regular brain imaging schedule may be justified, and the metastatic disease may be detected at an earlier time point to allow for a more effective treatment. A preventive treatment, either with irradiation or pharmaceutical agents, may also be considered for this selected group. To achieve this goal, several possible approaches may be taken. Many studies attempted to investigate the mechanism of lung adenocarcinoma brain metastasis by comparing the same patient's primary lung tumor and a tumor from the brain metastatic site [6–9]. The rationale behind such an approach is that the "brain-tropic" clone of cells may be a minor clone in the primary tumor, which should be enriched in the brain site, and this phenomenon may allow us to identify genes and pathways important for this process. Indeed, studies by this method showed that *MYC*, *YAP1*, *MMP13* and other genes may contribute to the development of brain metastasis, and these may be potential treatment targets [6]. However, the information gained from this approach may not be useful for a risk stratification of patients before brain metastasis occurs, since detecting the minor clone in the primary tumor may be difficult. Another possibility is that some lung adenocarcinomas may have an inherently higher likelihood of metastasizing to the brain, either because of specific driver oncogenes or because of the tumor–host interaction. In this situation, the genotype or phenotype associated with the brain tropism should be present in both the entire primary tumor and the metastatic site, and a prediction of the brain metastasis by analyzing the primary tumor may be more feasible in this kind of situation. Indeed, studies have found genes that are altered in this manner [6], indicating that at least some brain metastases develop in this fashion. It is this group of patients that is the focus of our current study. We further hypothesized that, instead of comparing patients with brain metastasis to lung adenocarcinoma patients in general, comparing patients with brain metastasis to patients with non-brain metastasis may help us identify features specifically related to brain-tropism. Since both groups of patients have metastatic diseases, any difference remaining may be more likely related to the brain-metastasizing mechanisms.

In order to address the unmet clinical need and to test our hypothesis, we retrospectively analyzed lung adenocarcinoma patients who received a surgical primary tumor resection and later developed brain or non-brain metastasis within 5 years in a single medical center. We first performed a targeted next-generation sequencing of the tumors to investigate their genetic composition. We also performed a comprehensive transcriptome analysis of the primary tumor tissue by RNA sequencing (RNA-seq) to identify differentially expressed genes (DE genes) between the two groups. Based on the difference between the groups, we proposed algorithms to segregate lung adenocarcinoma patients into the high risk/low risk categories for brain metastasis. We further compared our patient study results with the difference found in the study of brain-tropic and non-brain-tropic lung adenocarcinoma cell lines in animal models to look for common mechanisms between the two systems.

2. Results

2.1. Basic Clinical and Pathological Characteristics

The basic characteristics of the patients are summarized in Table 1. A total of 16 patients who developed brain metastasis within 5 years after a surgical resection of the primary lung adenocarcinoma were identified, while 11 patients developed only non-brain metastasis in the same time window. These two groups of patients had similar age, size of primary tumor and experience of adjuvant chemotherapy. Of notice, a larger proportion of patients with brain metastasis were female (male to female ratio = 6:10), while more patients with non-brain metastasis were male than female (male to female ratio = 8:3). On the contrary, fewer patients with brain metastasis had a smoking history compared to those with non-brain metastasis (43.8 % vs. 63.6%).

Table 1. Basic clinical and pathological information of patients.

Attribute		Brain Metastasizing	Non-Brain Metastasizing	p Value
n		16	11	
Mean age (range)		62 (45–78)	67 (46–77)	0.19
Male sex (%)		6 (37.5)	8 (72.7)	0.12
Smoking history (%)		7 (43.8)	7 (63.6)	0.44
Mean tumor size (S.D.)		2.9 (1.1)	3.4 (1.9)	0.40
Received adjuvant chemotherapy (%)		11 (68.8)	8 (72.7)	1
Predominant growth pattern in primary tumor	Acinar (%)	7 (43.7)	5 (45.4)	0.55
	Papillary (%)	1 (6.3)	1 (9.1)	
	Micropapillary (%)	5 (31.3)	1 (9.1)	
	Solid (%)	3 (18.7)	4 (36.4)	
T stage (%)	T1a	1 (6.3)	1 (9.1)	0.28
	T1b	3 (18.7)	3 (27.3)	
	T2a	11 (68.7)	4 (36.3)	
	T2b	1 (6.3)	1 (9.1)	
	T3	0 (0)	2 (18.2)	
N stage (%)	N0	8 (50.0)	5 (45.5)	1
	N1	3 (18.7)	3 (27.3)	
	N2	5 (31.3)	3 (27.3)	

S.D.: standard deviation. T stage was reported according to AJCC 7th Ed.

About the pathological features of their diseases, the predominant growth pattern in the primary tumors was mostly acinar in both groups. Regarding the growth patterns traditionally considered of high risk for metastasis (micropapillary and solid), 50% of the brain-metastasizing tumors contained predominantly either one of these two patterns, compared to 45.5% of the non-brain metastasizing tumors, although micropapillary-predominance was more common in the brain-metastasizing group. The distribution of the T stage and the N stage at the time of surgery was similar between the two groups, except that the brain-metastasizing group had more N2 cases (31.3% vs. 27.3%). Overall, some difference was observed in sex ratio, smoking history, frequency of histological micropapillary predominance and N2 stage, but none of these differences was of sufficient magnitude to allow for its use as clinical guidance for brain metastasis risk stratification, and the differences were all statistically non-significant ($p > 0.05$). The actual timeline of the brain/non-brain-metastasis occurrence and the follow-up length for each individual case are shown in Figure S1.

2.2. No significant Genomic Difference Was Identified between Brain-Metastasizing and Non-Brain-Metastasizing Lung Adenocarcinomas by Targeted Next-Generation Sequencing

We compared the genomic composition of the primary lung tumors of the two groups of patients with the FoundationOne CDx targeted DNA sequencing panel (Foundation Medicine, Cambridge, MA, USA) (Figure 1). In our patient population, we found that a *EGFR* gene alteration was present in 68.75% of the patients with brain metastasis and 54.55% of those with non-brain metastasis. Among those with the *EGFR* alteration, the two most common alterations were equally found in both groups (five cases each for L858R mutation and exon 19 deletion in the brain metastasis group; two cases each in the non-brain metastasis group). The other, less common *EGFR* alterations were observed in single patients. In summary, there is no significant correlation between the *EGFR* gene alteration and brain metastasis (Fisher's exact test, $p = 0.49$). Chromosome rearrangements involving *ALK* and *ROS1* were found in only one patient in the brain metastasis group (*ALK-EML4*) and one in the non-brain metastasis group (*CD74-ROS1*). Variants of *K-RAS* and *BRAF* mutations also occurred in single patients in each group. We did not find any other single genomic alteration that was significantly different between the two groups; other than the *EGFR* alterations mentioned above, no other genetic alteration was found in more than three cases (Table S1). None of the sequenced cases showed microsatellite instability (MSI). As for the tumor mutation burden, the average mutations per megabase were 4.59 in the brain-metastasizing group and 5.30 in the non-brain-metastasizing group; the difference was not significant using the Wilcoxon rank sum test ($p = 0.7221$).

a

Attribute		Brain metastasizing	Non-brain metastasizing
n		16	11
EGFR mutation status (%)	Wild type	5 (31.25)	5 (45.45)
	L858R	5 (31.25)	2 (18.18)
	Exon 19 deletion	5 (31.25)	2 (18.18)
	G719A	1 (6.25)	0 (0)
	L861Q	0 (0)	1 (9.09)
	Exon 20 insertion	0 (0)	1 (9.09)
K-RAS mutation	G12C	1 (6.25)	1 (9.09)
	G12R	1 (6.25)	0 (0)
	Q61H	0 (0)	1 (9.09)
BRAF mutation	Y472C	1 (6.25)	0 (0)
ALK-EML4 fusion		1 (6.25)	0 (0)
ROS1-CD74 fusion		0 (0)	1 (9.09)

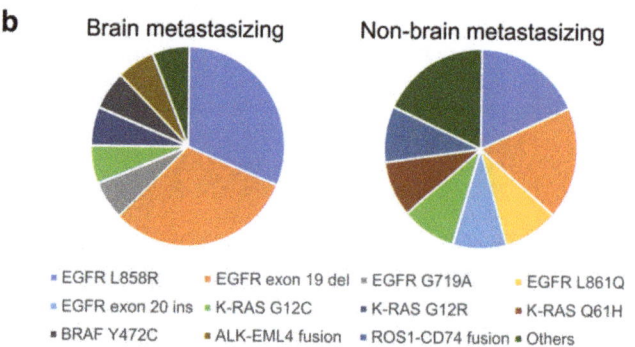

Figure 1. Presence of common lung adenocarcinoma driver mutations and gene fusions in the patient cohort. Panel (**a**) lists the number and percentage of patient tumors carrying each common driver mutations and gene fusions. Panel (**b**) shows the distribution of the above-mentioned genetic alterations in pie chart format.

2.3. The mRNA Expression Profile, including CDKN2A, Is Significantly Different between Brain-Metastasizing and Non-Brain-Metastasizing Lung Adenocarcinomas

We next compared the transcriptome of the two groups of primary tumors via a RNA-seq of fresh-frozen tumor tissue (Figure 2). A volcano plot (Figure 2a) showed the differentially expressed genes (DE genes) with an at least two-fold expression difference and a p value less than 0.05, as determined by the DESeq2 program. A total of 390 DE genes were identified. A Gene Ontology (GO) enrichment analysis (Figure 2b, Table S2) showed multiple biological processes varying between the two groups of tumors, notably including an "extracellular matrix organization", which may be related to their metastasis behavior. Interestingly, biological processes related to the nervous system, such as synaptic transmission and assembly, are also highlighted by the analysis, while a Kyoto Encyclopedia of Genes and Genomes (KEGG) enrichment analysis also showed that neuroactive ligand-receptor interaction-related genes are differentially expressed between the groups (Figure 2c). The Gene Set Enrichment Analysis (GSEA) based on GO (Figure 2d, Table S2) and KEGG (Figure 2e, Table S2) also pointed out that genes related to cell adhesion and the extracellular matrix were differentially expressed. When Receiver Operating Characteristic (ROC) curves were used to analyze the ability of individual genes to correctly segregate cases into brain-metastasizing and non-brain-metastasizing, the gene with top performance was *CDKN2A*, with an area under curve (AUC) of 0.86. Using the expression of this single gene in the primary tumor could correctly segregate cases into brain-metastasizing and non-brain metastasizing with a sensitivity of 93.8%, a specificity of 81.8%, a positive predictive value (PPV) of 88.2% and a negative predictive value (NPV) of 90% (Table S3). A dot plot (Figure 2f) showed that the brain metastasizing tumors demonstrated a range of *CDKN2A* expression, while most of the non-brain-metastasizing tumors showed a low *CDKN2A* expression. The difference was statistically significant ($p = 0.002$). Based on the gene list ranked with AUC, a stepwise method was used to build a 17-gene brain-metastasizing signature (Figure 2g, Table S3). With the optimal threshold -1.89 determined by the ROC curve (Figure 2h), the brain-metastasizing signature was shown to identify 100% of brain-metastasizing tumors with a 91% specificity (Figure 2i). A leave-one-out cross validation was further applied, demonstrating that the signature had a 60% precision and a 75% recall. In addition, the expression of *ARL9* was significantly lower in brain-metastasizing tumors than in non-brain-metastasizing tumors. (Figure 2j). The significance of this gene will be explained later in the article.

To assess the RNA expression difference at the protein level, we performed immunohistochemistry (IHC) for p16, the protein product of the *CDKN2A* gene, on a tissue microarray constructed from the patients' archived formalin-fixed, paraffin-embedded (FFPE) lung tumor tissue. (Figure 3a,b). We specifically chose this target because among the protein products of the genes in our list of high AUC candidates, p16 immunohistochemistry is the most widely performed in pathology laboratories. However, the correlation between the tumor *CDKN2A* mRNA expression level, p16-positive cell percentage and p16 immunohistochemistry H-score was only moderate (Figure 3c,d). The Pearson correlation coefficient between the p16-positive cell percentage and the *CDKN2A* expression was 0.47 ($p = 0.014$), while the correlation coefficient between the p16 immunohistochemistry H-score and the *CDKN2A* expression was 0.32 ($p = 0.099$). We noticed a few cases with very diffuse (100%) and strong p16 immunostaining but low mRNA expression (CPM < 12 in RNA-seq). These include two cases in the brain-metastasizing group and two cases in the non-brain-metastasizing group. Other than these cases, we found that the rest of brain-metastasizing tumors are more frequently positive for p16 staining with variable positive percentages and intensity, while the non-brain-metastasizing tumors show limited or no p16 staining. Nevertheless, the overall p16 staining was not significantly different between the two groups, either looking at the p16-positive cell percentage or the H-score ($p = 0.21$ and 0.26, respectively) (Figure 3e,f).

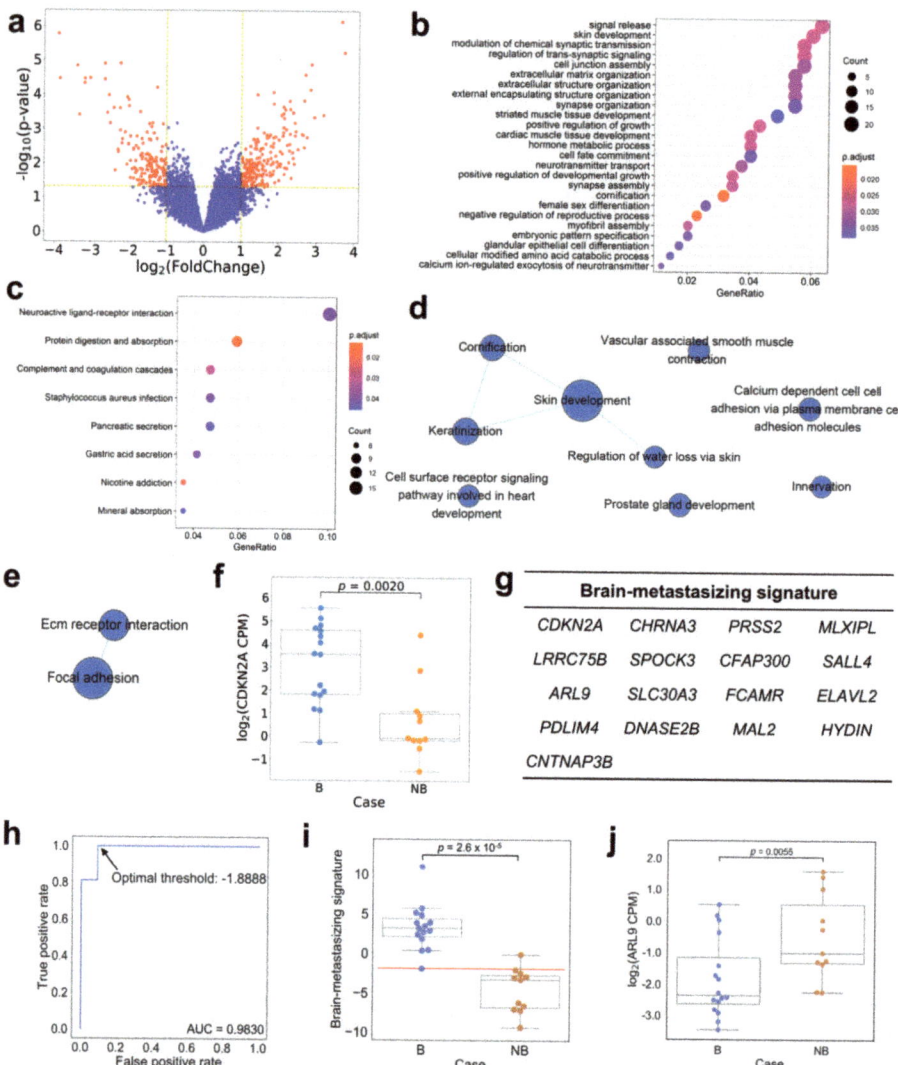

Figure 2. Comparing the gene expression profile of brain-metastasizing and non-brain-metastasizing lung adenocarcinomas using RNA-seq. The Volcano plot (panel (**a**)) showed differentially expressed genes (DE genes) with at least two-fold expression difference and $p < 0.05$ between the two groups by DESeq2. A total of 390 genes were identified. The GO enrichment analysis (panel (**b**)) and the KEGG pathway enrichment analysis (panel (**c**)) of the DE genes highlighted multiple groups of genes and pathways, notably the cellular interaction with extracellular matrix. The visualization of enriched GO terms or KEGG pathways were presented with clusterProfiler [10], and only the top 10 enriched GO terms were shown. The GSEA with GO (panel (**d**)) and KEGG (panel (**e**)) also found an enrichment of several similar gene sets, which were visualized by EnrichmentMap [11]. However, when the ability of the individual DE gene to segregate the two groups of tumors was analyzed, the top gene with the greatest AUC value in the ROC analysis was *CDKN2A*. The dot plot (panel (**f**)) of *CDKN2A* expression showed that while brain-metastasizing tumors have a range of expression levels, most non-brain-metastasizing tumors express very little of this gene ($p = 0.0020$, Mann–Whitney U test). A 17-gene brain-metastasizing signature (panel (**g**)) was identified for classification. The optimal threshold was determined as -1.89, as indicated in the ROC curve (panel (**h**)). The dot plot (panel (**i**)) showed that the brain-metastasizing signature was

significantly higher in the brain-metastasizing group ($p = 2.6 \times 10^{-5}$, Mann–Whitney U test). The red line indicated the optimal threshold for classification. The dot plot (panel (**j**)) of *ARL9* expression showed that the expression was significantly lower in brain-metastasizing tumors ($p = 0.0055$, Mann–Whitney U test). B: brain-metastasizing, NB: non-brain-metastasizing.

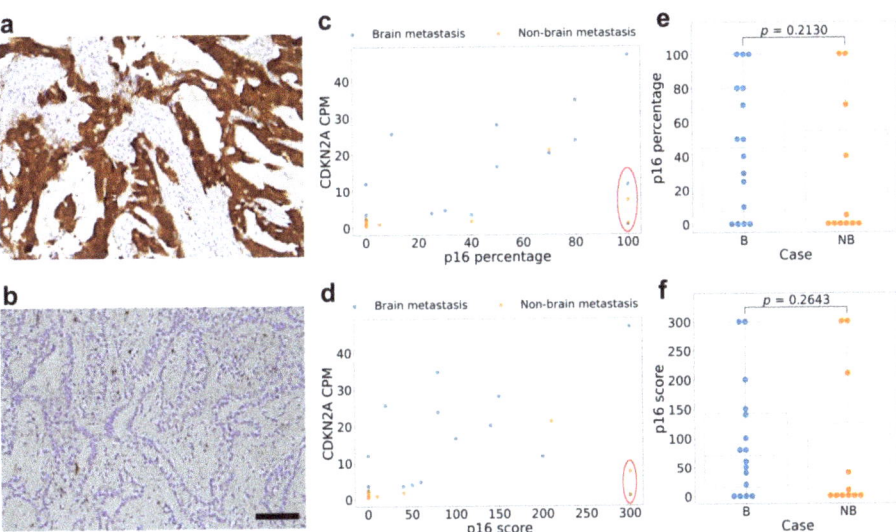

Figure 3. The p16 immunohistochemical staining of lung adenocarcinoma tissue shows a moderate correlation with the *CDKN2A* RNA expression. Representative photographs show one tumor with 100% strong-intensity (3+) p16 staining (panel (**a**)) compared to another tumor with 0% (negative, 0 intensity) staining (panel (**b**)). The percentage of tumor cells positive for p16 shows a moderate correlation with the *CDKN2A* RNA expression level (panel (**c**)), but the correlation is not significant for the p16 staining H-score (panel (**d**)). Note that 4 cases deviating from the correlation form a group and share the feature of low *CDKN2A* RNA expression and high p16 positive percentage and score (red circle). Of these cases, 2 belong to the brain metastasizing group and 2 belong to the non-brain-metastasizing group. Box plots of p16-positive percentage (panel (**e**)) and p16 H-score (panel (**f**)) show that the brain-metastasizing cases tend to have a variable staining of p16, some reaching high levels, while non-brain-metastasizing cases tend to have low p16 staining. However, the difference was not clear-cut nor statistically significant ($p = 0.21$ for the percentage and 0.26 for the H-score, Mann–Whitney U test). Scale bar: 100 micrometer. B: brain-metastasizing, NB: non-brain-metastasizing.

2.4. Comparing the Gene Expression Pattern between Brain-Metastasizing Patient Tumors and Brain-Tropic Lung Adenocarcinoma Cell Lines Showed a Small Set of Shared Differentially Expressed Genes

We hypothesized that lung adenocarcinoma cell lines with a higher propensity to metastasize to the brain may share common gene expression features with the lung adenocarcinoma patients' lung tumors that produced brain metastases. We examined the recently published MetMap [12] database to look for lung adenocarcinoma cell lines with a different metastasis tropism. In this database, various cell lines were genetically barcoded and intracardiac-injected into immunodeficient mice, then traced in different organs using single-cell sequencing technology. Among the tested cell lines, there were 11 derived from primary lung adenocarcinoma tumors with metastasis potential, and five of them were determined to have higher brain metastasis potential (Figure 4a). We retrieved the gene expression profile of these 11 cell lines from the Cancer Cell Line Encyclopedia (CCLE) database [13] and compared those with higher brain metastasis potential to those with lower potential. We found 1079 genes differentially expressed between the two groups (Figure 4b). The GO enrichment and KEGG pathway enrichment analysis results are shown in Figure 4c,d. Interestingly, we found that multiple biological processes highlighted the overlap with those found in our patient cohort analysis. In the GO enrichment analysis, "signal release", "modulation of chemical synaptic transmission", "regulation of trans-synaptic signaling", "extracellular matrix organization", "extracellular structure organization" and "extracellular encapsulating structure organization" were also enriched in our patient cohort analysis and appear to be related to the nervous system or cell adhesion. The overlapping results in the KEGG pathway analysis include "complement and coagulation cascades" and "Staphylococcus aureus infection", which may also contribute to brain metastasis (see Discussion below). We further compared individual genes on the cell line DE gene list with the DE gene list derived from our patient cohort. We found 28 genes that were differentially expressed both between the brain-tropic/non-brain-tropic cell lines and between the brain-metastasizing/non-brain-metastasizing patient tumors, and with the difference in the same direction (e.g., higher in the brain-tropic cell lines and higher in the brain-metastasizing patient tumors) (Figure 4e). Noticeably, only one gene in the patient cohort-derived brain-metastasizing signature, *ARL9*, was included in this 28-gene set (Figure 2j). In fact, the expression of classical immune-related genes, such as CD3 (hallmark of T lymphocytes) and CD20 (hallmark of B lymphocytes), are detected in our patient cohort (average CPM: CD20 14.99, CD3D 35.59, CD3E 30.58, CD3G 15.40) but not detected in the cell line experiment (average CPM: CD20 0.16, CD3D 0.04, CD3E 0.07, CD3G 0.01), highlighting the absence of the role of the immune system in the cell line experiment. This reflects the fundamental difference between patient tumors and cancer cell line behavior in animal models, yet those 28 differentially expressed genes shared between these two very different systems may warrant further study because they may be related to fundamental principles of lung cancer brain metastasis.

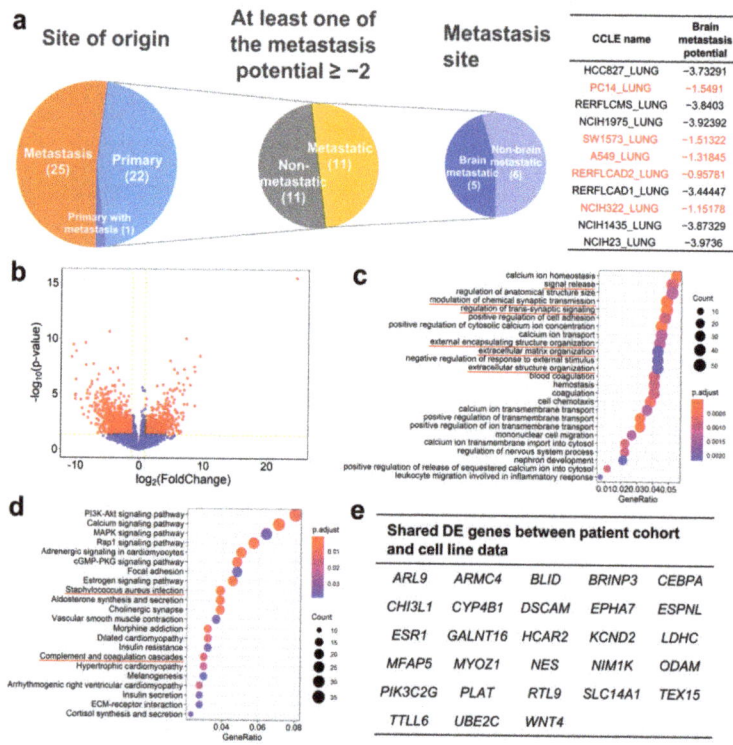

Figure 4. Analysis of brain-tropic and non-brain-tropic lung adenocarcinoma cell lines identified by the MetMap project showed differentially altered pathways and genes in common with lung cancer

patient data. (**a**) Among the 48 lung adenocarcinoma cell lines analyzed by the MetMap project, 22 were from primary tumors, and among them 11 were found to have substantial metastatic potential. Five of these 11 were found to have a higher brain metastasis potential, while 6 were considered to have a low brain metastasis potential. (**b**) Analysis of cell line RNA-seq data from the CCLE database showed that the brain-tropic and non-brain-tropic cell lines have 1079 differentially expressed genes with an at least 2-fold expression difference and a p value lower than 0.05. The GO enrichment analysis (**c**) and the KEGG pathway enrichment analysis (**d**) showed multiple differences between the two groups of cell lines; the representative GO terms or KEGG pathways that were also identified in our patient cohort analysis were highlighted with red color. (**e**) Twenty-eight genes were found to be differentially expressed in the same direction in both the cell line analysis and the patient cohort analysis.

3. Discussion

We proposed an algorithm to stratify lung adenocarcinoma patients into those with high risk for brain metastasis development and those with low risk, potentially useful for guiding the clinical management of patients receiving curative primary lung tumor resection. If the algorithm can be verified in a larger, statistically powered cohort in a prospective study, at the detection of the first metastasis, if not in the brain, the patient's primary tumor may be analyzed according to our algorithm, and the patient's brain metastasis risk assessed. If the risk is high, then the patient may begin to receive regular brain imaging even without neurological signs and symptoms, for the purpose of early detection. Preventive treatment may also be considered, although the risk and benefit of such treatments may require further studies to confirm. For neurologically asymptomatic patients who received brain imaging either during re-staging, because of a non-brain metastasis, or for surveillance only, sometimes small, equivocal lesions will be detected. Our algorithm may also provide the clinician and patient with more risk-stratification information in terms of how to manage such image findings. In a broader sense, any lung adenocarcinoma patient with distant metastasis may be analyzed for their risk of brain metastasis. However, whether our findings still hold true in this population may require further confirmation, and it is of interest to know if needle biopsies of the primary tumor or even a non-brain metastatic site can be used for this purpose.

Among the genes included in our prediction model, CDKN2A is most well-known for its role in tumor development. However, unlike the previous report that showed CDKN2A mutation was associated with brain metastasis [6], we found its over-expression is. Although many previous studies have characterized the phenomenon of CDKN2A/p16 loss in lung adenocarcinoma and its relationship with a poor prognosis [14–16], many studies also reported that CDKN2A/p16 expression is not related to the prognosis [17–19], or even that an over-expression is related to a poor prognosis [20]. Indeed, the role of CDKN2A/p16 in the formation of brain metastasis by lung adenocarcinoma has rarely been specifically studied. One report showed that the metastatic adenocarcinoma cells from the brain site express more p16 than the primary lung tumor [21]. To our knowledge, our study is the first to demonstrate a relationship between CDKN2A expression and the brain tropism of metastasis. The difference between our findings and the previous report [6] may be attributed to the different patient population studied; in our cohort, a high proportion (63%) of patients have EGFR gene alterations, which is common in east Asian lung adenocarcinoma patients in general but uncommon in Western countries. As for the mechanism whereby CDKN2A expression contributes to brain metastasis, it is conspicuous that traditional genes and pathways related to the CDKN2A function, i.e., cell-cycle-related genes and pathways, are not significantly differentially expressed between brain-metastasizing and non-brain-metastasizing tumors in this study. A possible explanation is that the CDKN2A expression difference may indicate a compensatory mechanism to various cell cycle dysregulations (e.g., responding to RB loss or CDK4/CDK6 gene amplification), and its function in brain metastasis lies in non-cell-cycle regulatory roles.

One study on head and neck squamous cell carcinoma showed that p16 expression can stimulate lymphangiogenesis but inhibit angiogenesis, which may correlate with the strong tendency of p16-positive head and neck squamous cell carcinoma to spread through the lymphatic system [22]. However, such a mechanism cannot explain the brain metastasis behavior of lung adenocarcinoma, which most likely occurs via the hematogenous route. In a mouse non-small-cell lung-cancer model, the inhibition of CDK4/6, the downstream target of p16, resulted in increased CD4 and CD8 T cell infiltration in the tumor [23]. It is now known that adaptive immune cells influence tumor angiogenesis and metastasis behavior [24]. Inflammation-associated angiogenesis may contribute to the establishment of metastasis specifically in the brain's microenvironment, which is reported to be the most inefficient and therefore crucial step in brain metastasis establishment [25]. Further studies are required to elucidate the mechanism behind the association we discovered.

The regulation of *CDKN2A*/p16 expression in cancer cells is complex [26]. Its loss is often ascribed to the deletion of the gene or the methylation of its promoter, but its over-expression is less understood. The cellular response to stress or other oncogenic environmental factors may drive its expression, and its normal function of inhibiting cell proliferation is negated by other mechanisms. In lung cancer, smoking has been linked to p16 over-expression [27]. Some studies reported the detection of human papilloma virus, a known cause of p16 over-expression, in lung cancer [28–30], while others did not [31,32]. In addition, we also noted in our study a group of patients with a low *CDKN2A* RNA level but high p16 immunohistochemistry staining. The post-translational regulation of p16 is not very well understood. The protein is generally considered short-lived and rapidly degraded by the proteasome in minutes to hours [26]. The interaction between p16 and proteasome activator REGγ has been shown to be required for its degradation [33]. Whether such interactions were disrupted in our cases with discrepant *CDKN2A* RNA-p16 protein levels requires further investigation. Another pathway of p16 degradation is through autophagy [34]. We found that in three of the four cases with low *CDKN2A* mRNA expression but strong p16 protein staining, the tumor harbors either *PIK3CA* mutation, *PIK3CB* amplification or loss of *PTEN* gene (Table S2, case B6, NB7, NB8). These genomic alterations can potentially increase the activity of the PI3K signal transduction pathway, which is known to be able to suppress autophagy [35]. *PIK3CA*, *PIK3CB* or *PTEN* alteration was not observed in cases without the *CDKN2A*/p16 discrepancy. The correlation between the PI3K pathway, autophagy and p16 requires further study to clarify.

The analysis of brain-tropic vs. non-brain-tropic lung adenocarcinoma cell lines based on their behavior in immunodeficient mice demonstrated a different gene expression pattern between the two groups, yet not many of these differentially expressed genes were found in our analysis of patient tumors. We think this is because the patient tumors and the cell line/mouse model systems have many important differences, notably the absence of immune surveillance in the cell line/mouse model. A significant limitation of our study is the relatively small number of patients studied, and a lack of testing cohort to verify the brain metastasis-related gene expression signature we identified, a role that the comparison with the cancer cell line data can only partially fill. However, despite these differences, we still identified 28 genes that were differentially expressed in the same manner in both systems, many of which were related to neurological processes. The GO enrichment analysis also found that genes related to synaptic transmission and signaling were enriched among the differentially expressed genes in both the patient cohort data and the cell line data. It is known that cancer cells can interact with cells in the central nervous system, such as neurons and glia cells, to facilitate the establishment of brain metastasis [29]. One gene, *DSCAM*, is more highly expressed in both the brain-metastasizing patient tumors and brain-tropic cell lines in our analyses. This gene encodes a cell adhesion molecule involved in glutamate synapse formation [36]. It has been reported in breast cancer that cancer cells can mimic the reciprocal relationship between astrocytes and neurons, metabolize glutamate to GABA and promote tumor cell proliferation [37]. On the contrary, our analysis found that both the brain-metastasizing patient tumors and brain-tropic cell lines express less mRNA of *PLAT* than their non-brain-metastasizing/tropic counterparts. *PLAT* encodes a tissue type plasminogen activator, and it has been shown that its activation target, plasmin, can inhibit brain metastasis by releasing FasL from astrocytes to promote cancer cell death, as well as inactivating the adhesion molecule L1CAM important for cancer spreading [38]. These findings demonstrate that cancer-glia/neuron interaction may play a fundamental role in lung cancer brain metastasis development, which transcends different species such as mouse and man.

In summary, it is possible to identify lung adenocarcinoma patients with a high risk of brain metastasis by analyzing the primary tumor. Our current study is limited by its relatively small sample size and its retrospective nature. Our RNA analysis was performed with fresh frozen tissue obtained during primary tumor surgery. Whether archived tissue can generate similar results is not known. A prospective study with larger patient numbers using FFPE tissue is required to validate these findings and to prove their clinical utility. An animal experiment comparing brain-tropic and non-brain-tropic metastatic lung adenocarcinoma in an immune-competent environment using genetically engineered models [39] is also required to validate our findings and further dissect the biological mechanisms. Therapies targeting the p16/CDK/Rb pathway may be evaluated for its role in the prevention or treatment of brain metastasis.

4. Materials and Methods

4.1. Patient Selection

We retrospectively enrolled patients who were at least 20 years old and received surgery for lung adenocarcinoma at Taipei Veterans General Hospital from 2007 to 2012. The inclusion and exclusion criteria are: (1) The patient received a primary lung tumor resection during this period, either by lobectomy or wedge resection. During surgery, the tumor was judged by the surgeon to be of sufficient size to allow the direct freezing of a portion of tumor specimen in liquid nitrogen. (2) The pathological diagnosis of the primary lung tumor was a pure adenocarcinoma of lung origin, with no squamous component, small cell component, mucinous phenotype or other special histology types. (3) The patient did not have another malignancy diagnosed from 5 years before to 5 years after the lung tumor resection date. (4) The patient did not receive neoadjuvant therapy before surgery (adjuvant therapy was allowed). (5) The patient had clinically or pathologically documented distant metastasis detected within 5 years after the surgery. Patients with only lung-to-lung metastasis were excluded because of the possible confounding factor of multiple primary lung carcinoma. Similarly, patients with multiple lung tumors at the time of surgery, in whom the primary tumor cannot be clearly determined by a clinical or pathological examination, were also excluded. Patients with only pleural metastasis were also excluded, considering the possible route difference (direct seeding versus hematogenous spreading) between pleural metastasis and other distal organ metastasis. (6) Follow up period: patients who developed brain metastasis within 5 years were all included, regardless of whether they had metastasis to another organ. Those who developed only non-brain metastasis were included only if the patients had at least 2.5 years of clinical follow-up after the surgery, or if the patient died within 5 years. This study was approved by the Institutional Review Board (IRB) of Taipei Veterans General Hospital (ID No. 2016-09-031AC) in accordance with the Declaration of Helsinki. The informed consent requirement was waived.

4.2. Targeted DNA Next-Generation Sequencing to Detect Genomic Alterations

Formalin-fixed, paraffin-embedded primary lung tumor sections from the patients were sent to Foundation Medicine (MA, USA) for targeted DNA sequencing using the FoundationOne CDx panel, which includes 324 known cancer-related genes for substitution, insertion/deletion, copy number variations and rearrangements. Microsatellite stability and tumor mutation burden were also assessed. The sample preparation and analysis process were performed according to the Foundation Medicine protocol.

4.3. Transcriptome Analysis and Identification of Differentially Expressed Genes

Total RNA was extracted from the lung tumor tissue fragments (approximately $0.5 \times 0.5 \times 0.5$ cm) preserved in liquid nitrogen at the time of the surgery. The extraction was performed using a QIAGEN RNeasy Mini Kit (QIAGEN, Germantown, MD, USA). The cDNA library was built from the RNA with Illumina TruSeq RNA Exome Kit (Illumina, San Diego, CA, USA). 150bp paired-end sequencing, 50 million reads per sample, was performed on the Illumina HiSeq 4000 platform.

The raw sequencing data were aligned to the reference human genome (GRch38) using the STAR software (version 2.7.2a) [40]. The reads mapped to each gene were enumerated using HTSeq (version 0.11.1) [41]. After low-count filtering by edgeR [42], the read counts of protein-coding genes were fed into DESeq2 [43] to determine the differentially expressed genes between brain-metastasizing and non-brain-metastasizing tumors. Meanwhile, the CPM (counts per million) or log_2CPM value was calculated for each DE gene. The list of DE genes was subjected to a GO (Gene Ontology) enrichment analysis a and KEGG (Kyoto Encyclopedia of Genes and Genomes) pathway enrichment analysis by clusterProfiler [10]. A Gene Set Enrichment Analysis (GSEA) [44] was also applied to investigate the enriched function/pathways. The receiver operating characteristic (ROC) curve of each individual DE gene for its ability to segregate cases into brain-metastasizing and non-brain-metastasizing was plotted, and DE genes with top area under curve (AUC) values were identified. Additionally, a stepwise selection method based on a principal component analysis (PCA) was proposed to identify the optimal gene set for classifying brain-metastasizing samples. Specifically, according to the gene list with a ranked AUC value, one gene with a top AUC value was added into the gene set in each round. Then, PCA was applied using the expression profiles of the gene set. Consequently, the value of the first principal component for each sample was used for classification and the corresponding AUC was calculated for the specific gene set. This gene-adding process continued until the AUC could not be increased in the next five rounds. In this way, the gene set with the highest AUC was defined as the brain-metastasizing signature for classification. A leave-one-out cross validation was further employed to test the classification performance.

4.4. Immunohistochemistry

We examined the differentially expressed genes and identified genes of particular interest, i.e., genes with a top AUC value in the ROC plots, and for which there are antibodies commercially available against their protein products. We chose *CDKN2A* (p16, clone E6H4, Ventana Medical Systems, Oro Valley, AZ, USA) as our target. Immunohistochemistry was performed to corroborate the RNA expression differences on tissue microarrays.

Tissue microarrays were constructed from archived formalin-fixed, paraffin-embedded (FFPE) lung tumor tissue from the patients. All specimens were fixed for 6–72 h before embedding in paraffin. Two cores, each with a diameter of 2 mm, were taken from representative tumor areas of each patient. Four micrometer-thick sections were cut from the arrays and attached onto slides. One section was stained with hematoxylin and eosin for morphology evaluation. The other section was stained with the primary antibody on the Leica Bond-Max (Leica Biosystems, Mount Waverley, VIC, Australia) automated staining platform. The slides were stained with a primary antibody at room temperature for 15 min and then treated with the Bond Polymer Refine Detection Kit (Leica Microsystems, Milton Keynes, UK). The sections were counter-stained with hematoxylin. The percentage of tumor cells positive for p16 was recorded, and the immunohistochemistry H-score was calculated.

4.5. Comparison of Gene Expression Profile between Brain-Tropic Lung Adenocarcinoma Cell Lines and Patients with Brain-Metastasizing Lung Adenocarcinoma

A recently published database (MetMap) [12] described the metastasis organ tropism of various human cancer cell lines in an immunodeficient mouse model based on single-cell sequencing technology. In this database, 11 human lung adenocarcinoma cell lines derived from primary tumors with metastatic potential were identified. These cell lines were separated into brain-tropic versus non-brain-tropic based on their brain metastasis potential determined by the MetMap project. A potential greater than -2 (on a $\log_{10}$ scale) is considered brain-tropic, and a value less than -2 is considered non-brain tropic. The RNA-seq-based gene expression profile of these cell lines was retrieved from the Cancer Cell Line Encyclopedia (CCLE) database [13]. Differentially expressed genes between the brain-tropic and non-brain-tropic cell lines were determined with DEseq2, similarly to the analysis performed on our lung cancer patient specimen RNA-seq data. A GO enrichment analysis and a KEGG pathway enrichment analysis were also performed for the identified DE genes. We compared the DE genes from the MetMap/CCLE cell line data to our patient tumor data and identified the overlapping DE genes with the same direction of difference (e.g., higher in both the brain-tropic cell line and the brain-metastasizing patient tumor).

4.6. Statistical Analysis

In general, a Student's t test was performed for the continuous variables, and a Chi-squared test or Fisher's exact test was performed for the categorical variables to determine whether there was a significant difference between the brain-metastasizing and non-brain-metastasizing groups. A Mann–Whitney U test was performed to compare the *CDKN2A* RNA expression level and p16 immunohistochemistry staining between the two groups. A Pearson correlation coefficient was calculated to demonstrate the correlation between the *CDKN2A* mRNA expression and p16 immunohistochemistry results. A Wilcoxon rank sum test was performed to compare the tumor mutation burden between the two groups. A *p* value less than 0.05 was considered significant.

Supplementary Materials: The following are available online at https://www.mdpi.com/article/10.3390/ijms222413374/s1.

Author Contributions: Conceptualization, Y.-Y.L., Y.-C.W. (Yu-Chao Wang), Y.-C.Y., T.-Y.C.; methodology, Y.-Y.L., Y.-C.W. (Yu-Chao Wang), D.-W.Y.; software, D.-W.Y., C.-Y.H.; validation, Y.-Y.L.; formal analysis, Y.-Y.L., Y.-C.W. (Yu-Chao Wang), D.-W.Y., C.-Y.H.; investigation, Y.-Y.L., Y.-C.W. (Yu-Chao Wang), Y.-C.Y.; resources, Y.-C.W. (Yu-Chung Wu), T.-Y.C.; data curation, Y.-Y.L., H.-C.M.; writing—original draft preparation, Y.-Y.L., Y.-C.W. (Yu-Chao Wang); writing—review and editing, T.-Y.C.; visualization, D.-W.Y., C.-Y.H.; supervision, T.-Y.C.; project administration, H.-L.H., M.-Y.C., T.-Y.C.; funding acquisition, T.-Y.C. All authors have read and agreed to the published version of the manuscript.

Funding: This work was supported by the "Cancer Progression Research Center, National Yang-Ming University", from The Featured Areas Research Center Program within the framework of the Higher Education Sprout Project by the Ministry of Education (MOE); Ministry of Health and Welfare, Taiwan [MOHW108-TDU-B-211-124019, MOHW109-TDU-B-211-134019]; Ministry of Science and Technology, Taiwan [MOST 107-2221-E-010-019-MY3, MOST 109-2221-E-010-013-MY3]; Taipei Veterans General Hospital, Taiwan [V109C-002, V108E-008-2 and VTA108-V1-4-3]; and the cost of the Foundation Medicine's FoundationOne CDx test was covered by F. Hoffmann-La Roche Ltd., Basel, Switzerland.

Institutional Review Board Statement: The study was conducted according to the guidelines of the Declaration of Helsinki and approved by the Institutional Review Board of Taipei Veterans General Hospital (ID No. 2016-09-031AC).

Informed Consent Statement: Patient consent was waived.

Data Availability Statement: The RNA-seq data obtained in the current study were deposited in the NCBI Sequence Read Archive (SRA) under the accession number PRJNA649988. The FoundationOne CDx panel DNA sequencing data that support the findings of this study are available from Foundation Medicine (MA, USA), but restrictions apply to the availability of these data, which were used under license for the current study, and so are not publicly available. However, the data are available from the authors upon reasonable request and with the permission of Foundation Medicine.

Acknowledgments: The authors appreciate the excellent technical assistance from Yu-Chi Su and thank Lee H. Chen, from the Department of Pathology, Duke University, USA, for critically reviewing the manuscript and providing valuable suggestions.

Conflicts of Interest: The authors declare no conflict of interest.

References

1. Global Burden of Disease Cancer Collaboration; Fitzmaurice, C.; Abate, D.; Abbasi, N.; Abbastabar, H.; Abd-Allah, F.; Abdel-Rahman, O.; Abdelalim, A.; Abdoli, A.; Abdollahpour, I.; et al. Global, Regional, and National Cancer Incidence, Mortality, Years of Life Lost, Years Lived with Disability, and Disability-Adjusted Life-Years for 29 Cancer Groups, 1990 to 2017: A Systematic Analysis for the Global Burden of Disease Study. *JAMA Oncol.* **2019**, *5*, 1749–1768. [CrossRef]
2. Dela Cruz, C.S.; Tanoue, L.T.; Matthay, R.A. Lung cancer: Epidemiology, etiology, and prevention. *Clin. Chest Med.* **2011**, *32*, 605–644. [CrossRef]
3. Cagney, D.N.; Martin, A.M.; Catalano, P.J.; Redig, A.J.; Lin, N.U.; Lee, E.Q.; Wen, P.Y.; Dunn, I.F.; Bi, W.L.; Weiss, S.E.; et al. Incidence and prognosis of patients with brain metastases at diagnosis of systemic malignancy: A population-based study. *Neuro-Oncol.* **2017**, *19*, 1511–1521. [CrossRef] [PubMed]
4. Barnholtz-Sloan, J.S.; Sloan, A.E.; Davis, F.G.; Vigneau, F.D.; Lai, P.; Sawaya, R.E. Incidence proportions of brain metastases in patients diagnosed (1973 to 2001) in the Metropolitan Detroit Cancer Surveillance System. *J. Clin. Oncol.* **2004**, *22*, 2865–2872. [CrossRef] [PubMed]
5. Owen, S.; Souhami, L. The management of brain metastases in non-small cell lung cancer. *Front. Oncol.* **2014**, *4*, 248. [CrossRef] [PubMed]
6. Shih, D.J.H.; Nayyar, N.; Bihun, I.; Dagogo-Jack, I.; Gill, C.M.; Aquilanti, E.; Bertalan, M.; Kaplan, A.; D'Andrea, M.R.; Chukwueke, U.; et al. Genomic characterization of human brain metastases identifies drivers of metastatic lung adenocarcinoma. *Nat. Genet.* **2020**, *52*, 371–377. [CrossRef]
7. Wang, H.; Ou, Q.; Li, D.; Qin, T.; Bao, H.; Hou, X.; Wang, K.; Wang, F.; Deng, Q.; Liang, J.; et al. Genes associated with increased brain metastasis risk in non-small cell lung cancer: Comprehensive genomic profiling of 61 resected brain metastases versus primary non-small cell lung cancer (Guangdong Association Study of Thoracic Oncology 1036). *Cancer* **2019**, *125*, 3535–3544. [CrossRef] [PubMed]
8. Sun, G.; Ding, X.; Bi, N.; Wang, Z.; Wu, L.; Zhou, W.; Zhao, Z.; Wang, J.; Zhang, W.; Fan, J.; et al. Molecular predictors of brain metastasis-related microRNAs in lung adenocarcinoma. *PLoS Genet.* **2019**, *15*, e1007888. [CrossRef]
9. Su, H.; Lin, Z.; Peng, W.; Hu, Z. Identification of potential biomarkers of lung adenocarcinoma brain metastases via microarray analysis of cDNA expression profiles. *Oncol. Lett.* **2019**, *17*, 2228–2236. [CrossRef]
10. Yu, G.; Wang, L.G.; Han, Y.; He, Q.Y. clusterProfiler: An R package for comparing biological themes among gene clusters. *OMICS* **2012**, *16*, 284–287. [CrossRef] [PubMed]
11. Merico, D.; Isserlin, R.; Stueker, O.; Emili, A.; Bader, G.D. Enrichment map: A network-based method for gene-set enrichment visualization and interpretation. *PLoS ONE* **2010**, *5*, e13984. [CrossRef]
12. Jin, X.; Demere, Z.; Nair, K.; Ali, A.; Ferraro, G.B.; Natoli, T.; Deik, A.; Petronio, L.; Tang, A.A.; Zhu, C.; et al. A metastasis map of human cancer cell lines. *Nature* **2020**, *588*, 331–336. [CrossRef] [PubMed]
13. Ghandi, M.; Huang, F.W.; Jane-Valbuena, J.; Kryukov, G.V.; Lo, C.C.; McDonald, E.R., 3rd; Barretina, J.; Gelfand, E.T.; Bielski, C.M.; Li, H.; et al. Next-generation characterization of the Cancer Cell Line Encyclopedia. *Nature* **2019**, *569*, 503–508. [CrossRef] [PubMed]
14. Rotolo, F.; Zhu, C.Q.; Brambilla, E.; Graziano, S.L.; Olaussen, K.; Le-Chevalier, T.; Pignon, J.P.; Kratzke, R.; Soria, J.C.; Shepherd, F.A.; et al. Genome-wide copy number analyses of samples from LACE-Bio project identify novel prognostic and predictive markers in early stage non-small cell lung cancer. *Transl. Lung Cancer Res.* **2018**, *7*, 416–427. [CrossRef]
15. Bradly, D.P.; Gattuso, P.; Pool, M.; Basu, S.; Liptay, M.; Bonomi, P.; Buckingham, L. CDKN2A (p16) promoter hypermethylation influences the outcome in young lung cancer patients. *Diagn Mol. Pathol.* **2012**, *21*, 207–213. [CrossRef] [PubMed]
16. Bian, C.; Li, Z.; Xu, Y.; Wang, J.; Xu, L.; Shen, H. Clinical outcome and expression of mutant P53, P16, and Smad4 in lung adenocarcinoma: A prospective study. *World J. Surg. Oncol.* **2015**, *13*, 128. [CrossRef]
17. Drilon, A.; Sugita, H.; Sima, C.S.; Zauderer, M.; Rudin, C.M.; Kris, M.G.; Rusch, V.W.; Azzoli, C.G. A prospective study of tumor suppressor gene methylation as a prognostic biomarker in surgically resected stage I to IIIA non-small-cell lung cancers. *J. Thorac. Oncol.* **2014**, *9*, 1272–1277. [CrossRef]
18. Tong, J.; Sun, X.; Cheng, H.; Zhao, D.; Ma, J.; Zhen, Q.; Cao, Y.; Zhu, H.; Bai, J. Expression of p16 in non-small cell lung cancer and its prognostic significance: A meta-analysis of published literatures. *Lung Cancer* **2011**, *74*, 155–163. [CrossRef] [PubMed]
19. Okamoto, T.; Kohno, M.; Ito, K.; Takada, K.; Katsura, M.; Morodomi, Y.; Toyokawa, G.; Shoji, F.; Maehara, Y. Clinical Significance of DNA Damage Response Factors and Chromosomal Instability in Primary Lung Adenocarcinoma. *Anticancer Res.* **2017**, *37*, 1729–1735. [CrossRef]
20. Hsu, Y.L.; Hung, J.Y.; Lee, Y.L.; Chen, F.W.; Chang, K.F.; Chang, W.A.; Tsai, Y.M.; Chong, I.W.; Kuo, P.L. Identification of novel gene expression signature in lung adenocarcinoma by using next-generation sequencing data and bioinformatics analysis. *Oncotarget* **2017**, *8*, 104831–104854. [CrossRef]
21. Fabian, K.; Nemeth, Z.; Furak, J.; Tiszlavicz, L.; Papay, J.; Krenacs, T.; Timar, J.; Moldvay, J. Protein expression differences between lung adenocarcinoma and squamous cell carcinoma with brain metastasis. *Anticancer Res.* **2014**, *34*, 5593–5597.
22. Dok, R.; Glorieux, M.; Holacka, K.; Bamps, M.; Nuyts, S. Dual role for p16 in the metastasis process of HPV positive head and neck cancers. *Mol. Cancer* **2017**, *16*, 113. [CrossRef] [PubMed]

23. Deng, J.; Wang, E.S.; Jenkins, R.W.; Li, S.; Dries, R.; Yates, K.; Chhabra, S.; Huang, W.; Liu, H.; Aref, A.R.; et al. CDK4/6 Inhibition Augments Antitumor Immunity by Enhancing T-cell Activation. *Cancer Discov.* **2018**, *8*, 216–233. [CrossRef]
24. Solimando, A.G.; Summa, S.; Vacca, A.; Ribatti, D. Cancer-Associated Angiogenesis: The Endothelial Cell as a Checkpoint for Immunological Patrolling. *Cancers* **2020**, *12*, 3380. [CrossRef]
25. Kienast, Y.; von Baumgarten, L.; Fuhrmann, M.; Klinkert, W.E.; Goldbrunner, R.; Herms, J.; Winkler, F. Real-time imaging reveals the single steps of brain metastasis formation. *Nat. Med.* **2010**, *16*, 116–122. [CrossRef]
26. Li, J.; Poi, M.J.; Tsai, M.D. Regulatory mechanisms of tumor suppressor P16(INK4A) and their relevance to cancer. *Biochemistry* **2011**, *50*, 5566–5582. [CrossRef]
27. Ko, E.; Kim, Y.; Lee, B.B.; Han, J.; Song, S.Y.; Shim, Y.M.; Park, J.; Kim, D.H. Relationship of phospho-pRb (Ser-807/811) level to exposure to tobacco smoke in primary non-small cell lung cancer. *Cancer Lett.* **2009**, *274*, 225–232. [CrossRef] [PubMed]
28. Robinson, L.A.; Jaing, C.J.; Pierce Campbell, C.; Magliocco, A.; Xiong, Y.; Magliocco, G.; Thissen, J.B.; Antonia, S. Molecular evidence of viral DNA in non-small cell lung cancer and non-neoplastic lung. *Br. J. Cancer* **2016**, *115*, 497–504. [CrossRef]
29. Baba, M.; Castillo, A.; Koriyama, C.; Yanagi, M.; Matsumoto, H.; Natsugoe, S.; Shuyama, K.Y.; Khan, N.; Higashi, M.; Itoh, T.; et al. Human papillomavirus is frequently detected in gefitinib-responsive lung adenocarcinomas. *Oncol. Rep.* **2010**, *23*, 1085–1092. [CrossRef] [PubMed]
30. Wu, M.F.; Cheng, Y.W.; Lai, J.C.; Hsu, M.C.; Chen, J.T.; Liu, W.S.; Chiou, M.C.; Chen, C.Y.; Lee, H. Frequent p16INK4a promoter hypermethylation in human papillomavirus-infected female lung cancer in Taiwan. *Int. J. Cancer* **2005**, *113*, 440–445. [CrossRef] [PubMed]
31. Chang, S.Y.; Keeney, M.; Law, M.; Donovan, J.; Aubry, M.C.; Garcia, J. Detection of human papillomavirus in non-small cell carcinoma of the lung. *Hum. Pathol.* **2015**, *46*, 1592–1597. [CrossRef]
32. van Boerdonk, R.A.; Daniels, J.M.; Bloemena, E.; Krijgsman, O.; Steenbergen, R.D.; Brakenhoff, R.H.; Grunberg, K.; Ylstra, B.; Meijer, C.J.; Smit, E.F.; et al. High-risk human papillomavirus-positive lung cancer: Molecular evidence for a pattern of pulmonary metastasis. *J. Thorac. Oncol.* **2013**, *8*, 711–718. [CrossRef] [PubMed]
33. Chen, X.; Barton, L.F.; Chi, Y.; Clurman, B.E.; Roberts, J.M. Ubiquitin-independent degradation of cell-cycle inhibitors by the REGgamma proteasome. *Mol. Cell* **2007**, *26*, 843–852. [CrossRef]
34. Coryell, P.R.; Goraya, S.K.; Griffin, K.A.; Redick, M.A.; Sisk, S.R.; Purvis, J.E. Autophagy regulates the localization and degradation of p16(INK4a). *Aging Cell* **2020**, *19*, e13171. [CrossRef] [PubMed]
35. Kwon, Y.; Kim, M.; Jung, H.S.; Kim, Y.; Jeoung, D. Targeting Autophagy for Overcoming Resistance to Anti-EGFR Treatments. *Cancers* **2019**, *11*, 1374. [CrossRef]
36. Stachowicz, K. The role of DSCAM in the regulation of synaptic plasticity: Possible involvement in neuropsychiatric disorders. *Acta Neurobiol. Exp.* **2018**, *78*, 210–219. [CrossRef]
37. Neman, J.; Termini, J.; Wilczynski, S.; Vaidehi, N.; Choy, C.; Kowolik, C.M.; Li, H.; Hambrecht, A.C.; Roberts, E.; Jandial, R. Human breast cancer metastases to the brain display GABAergic properties in the neural niche. *Proc. Natl. Acad. Sci. USA* **2014**, *111*, 984–989. [CrossRef]
38. Valiente, M.; Obenauf, A.C.; Jin, X.; Chen, Q.; Zhang, X.H.; Lee, D.J.; Chaft, J.E.; Kris, M.G.; Huse, J.T.; Brogi, E.; et al. Serpins promote cancer cell survival and vascular co-option in brain metastasis. *Cell* **2014**, *156*, 1002–1016. [CrossRef] [PubMed]
39. Zheng, S.; El-Naggar, A.K.; Kim, E.S.; Kurie, J.M.; Lozano, G. A genetic mouse model for metastatic lung cancer with gender differences in survival. *Oncogene* **2007**, *26*, 6896–6904. [CrossRef]
40. Dobin, A.; Davis, C.A.; Schlesinger, F.; Drenkow, J.; Zaleski, C.; Jha, S.; Batut, P.; Chaisson, M.; Gingeras, T.R. STAR: Ultrafast universal RNA-seq aligner. *Bioinformatics* **2013**, *29*, 15–21. [CrossRef] [PubMed]
41. Anders, S.; Pyl, P.T.; Huber, W. HTSeq—A Python framework to work with high-throughput sequencing data. *Bioinformatics* **2015**, *31*, 166–169. [CrossRef]
42. Robinson, M.D.; McCarthy, D.J.; Smyth, G.K. edgeR: A Bioconductor package for differential expression analysis of digital gene expression data. *Bioinformatics* **2010**, *26*, 139–140. [CrossRef] [PubMed]
43. Love, M.I.; Huber, W.; Anders, S. Moderated estimation of fold change and dispersion for RNA-seq data with DESeq2. *Genome Biol.* **2014**, *15*, 550. [CrossRef] [PubMed]
44. Subramanian, A.; Tamayo, P.; Mootha, V.K.; Mukherjee, S.; Ebert, B.L.; Gillette, M.A.; Paulovich, A.; Pomeroy, S.L.; Golub, T.R.; Lander, E.S.; et al. Gene set enrichment analysis: A knowledge-based approach for interpreting genome-wide expression profiles. *Proc. Natl. Acad. Sci. USA* **2005**, *102*, 15545–15550. [CrossRef] [PubMed]

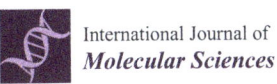

Article

Reduced *Zeb1* Expression in Prostate Cancer Cells Leads to an Aggressive Partial-EMT Phenotype Associated with Altered Global Methylation Patterns

Jenna Kitz [1], Cory Lefebvre [1], Joselia Carlos [2], Lori E. Lowes [3] and Alison L. Allan [1,4,5,*]

1. London Regional Cancer Program, London Health Sciences Centre, Department of Anatomy & Cell Biology, Western University, London, ON N6A 5W9, Canada; jkitz@uwo.ca (J.K.); clefebvre2019@meds.uwo.ca (C.L.)
2. Department of Medical Biophysics, Western University, London, ON N6A 5C1, Canada; jcarlos6@uwo.ca
3. Flow Cytometry, London Health Sciences Centre, London, ON N6A 5W9, Canada; lori.lowes@lhsc.on.ca
4. Department of Oncology, Western University, London, ON N6A 5W9, Canada
5. Cancer Research Laboratory Program, Lawson Health Research Institute, London, ON N6C 2R5, Canada
* Correspondence: alison.allan@lhsc.on.ca; Tel.: +1-519-685-8600 (ext. 55134)

Abstract: Prostate cancer is the most common cancer in American men and the second leading cause of cancer-related death. Most of these deaths are associated with metastasis, a process involving the epithelial-to-mesenchymal (EMT) transition. Furthermore, growing evidence suggests that partial-EMT (p-EMT) may lead to more aggressive disease than complete EMT. In this study, the EMT-inducing transcription factor *Zeb1* was knocked down in mesenchymal PC-3 prostate cancer cells (Zeb1^{KD}) and resulting changes in cellular phenotype were assessed using protein and RNA analysis, invasion and migration assays, cell morphology assays, and DNA methylation chip analysis. Inducible knockdown of *Zeb1* resulted in a p-EMT phenotype including co-expression of epithelial and mesenchymal markers, a mixed epithelial/mesenchymal morphology, increased invasion and migration, and enhanced expression of p-EMT markers relative to PC-3 mesenchymal controls ($p \leq 0.05$). Treatment of Zeb1^{KD} cells with the global de-methylating drug 5-azacytidine (5-aza) mitigated the observed aggressive p-EMT phenotype ($p \leq 0.05$). DNA methylation chip analysis revealed 10 potential targets for identifying and/or targeting aggressive p-EMT prostate cancer in the future. These findings provide a framework to enhance prognostic and/or therapeutic options for aggressive prostate cancer in the future by identifying new p-EMT biomarkers to classify patients with aggressive disease who may benefit from 5-aza treatment.

Keywords: prostate cancer; metastasis; epithelial-to-mesenchymal transition (EMT); partial-EMT (p-EMT); *Zeb1*; DNA methylation; 5-azacytidine

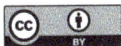

1. Introduction

Prostate cancer is the second leading cause of cancer related deaths in American men [1]. Most of these deaths are caused by metastasis, which allows cancer to spread beyond the prostate to other parts of the body [2]. Metastasis is associated with an epithelial-to mesenchymal transition (EMT), where epithelial cells lose their epithelial characteristics and gain a mesenchymal phenotype, which aids in the process of metastasis [2–8].

Transcription factors bind to specific promoter sequences within the DNA to influence the expression of target genes [9]. Master EMT-inducing transcription factors upregulate mesenchymal genes and/or inhibit epithelial genes, which can cause the cell to undergo EMT [10]. An example of this is zinc finger E-box-binding homeobox 1 (Zeb1), which binds to the E-box promoter sequence, regulates neuronal differentiation, and has important roles in promoting EMT to allow for cell movement during gestation [11,12]. In cancer progression, Zeb1 promotes metastasis and a loss of cell polarity by repressing the epithelial proteins E-Cadherin and EpCAM and promotes tumorigenicity by repressing stemness-inhibiting microRNAs [10,13].

It is well-established that EMT is a dynamic state, utilizing both EMT and a reverse mesenchymal-to-epithelial (MET) transition to switch between epithelial and mesenchymal states during the process of metastasis [2–8]. In addition to EMT and MET, recent studies have demonstrated that there is an intermediate state called partial EMT (p-EMT), a phenotype that may result in the most aggressive cancer cells [14]. Partial EMT is associated with increased cell-cell interactions and cell proliferation in migrating circulating tumor cells (CTC). Growing evidence suggests that migrating cell clusters and CTC clusters in the blood are more aggressive and have higher metastatic potential than migrating single cells or single CTCs, and that these clusters often exhibit a p-EMT phenotype rather than complete EMT [15]. It has also been suggested that epigenetic modifications such as DNA methylation of the promoter region of essential genes may be responsible for this increased cell aggressiveness, and that treatment with a global de-methylating agent may aid in treatment of aggressive prostate cancers [16].

In the current study, we tested the hypothesis that knockdown of the EMT-inducing transcription factor *Zeb1* in mesenchymal PC-3 cells would produce an MET leading to a more epithelial, less aggressive phenotype compared to control cells. Unexpectedly, we observed that inducible knockdown of *Zeb1* in PC-3 cells (Zeb1^{KD} cells) resulted in a p-EMT phenotype including co-expression of epithelial and mesenchymal markers, a mixed epithelial/mesenchymal morphology, increased invasion and migration, and enhanced expression of p-EMT markers relative to PC-3 mesenchymal controls (ctrl cells). Treatment of Zeb1^{KD} cells with the global de-methylating drug 5-azacytidine (5-aza) [17] mitigated the observed aggressive p-EMT phenotype. DNA methylation chip analysis revealed 10 potential targets for identifying and/or targeting aggressive p-EMT prostate cancer in the future. These novel findings provide a framework to enhance prognostic and/or therapeutic options for aggressive prostate cancer in the future by identifying new p-EMT biomarkers to classify patients who may benefit from combination treatment with the clinically relevant inhibitor 5-azacitadine.

2. Results

2.1. Inducible Knockdown of Zeb1 in PC-3 Human Prostate Cancer Cells Results in Enhanced Expression of Epithelial Proteins

Mesenchymal human PC-3 prostate cancer cells were engineered with an inducible lentiviral shRNA system to knockdown expression of the master EMT regulator *Zeb1*. The following cell lines were created: PC-3 ctrl cells with a non-targeting control sequence of scrambled shRNA, and Zeb1^{KD} cells with shRNA targeting the 3′UTR of *Zeb1*. This was achieved using the SMARTvector inducible lentiviral shRNA (Dharmacon), which features Tet-on® induction of the target shRNA in the presence of doxycycline (Dox) and validation by concurrent induction of TurboGFP (green fluorescent protein). Following Dox induction (72 h), we observed that Zeb1 protein (Figure 1A,B) and RNA (Supplementary Figure S1A) expression were significantly decreased compared to all ctrl cells ($p \leq 0.05$), down to a level equivalent to that of human LNCaP cells, an epithelial prostate cancer cell line. Immunofluorescence confirmed successful knockdown of Zeb1 via TurboGFP expression following Dox induction (Supplementary Figure S1B). Immunoblotting (Figure 1C,D) and qRT-PCR (Supplementary Figure S1C) was used to assess EMT phenotypic marker expression following Dox induction of Zeb1^{KD} cells. Zeb1^{KD} cells had significantly higher expression of epithelial (EpCAM, E-Cadherin) proteins relative to ctrl cells ($p \leq 0.05$), with no change in expression of mesenchymal proteins (Vimentin, N-Cadherin) (Figure 1C,D).

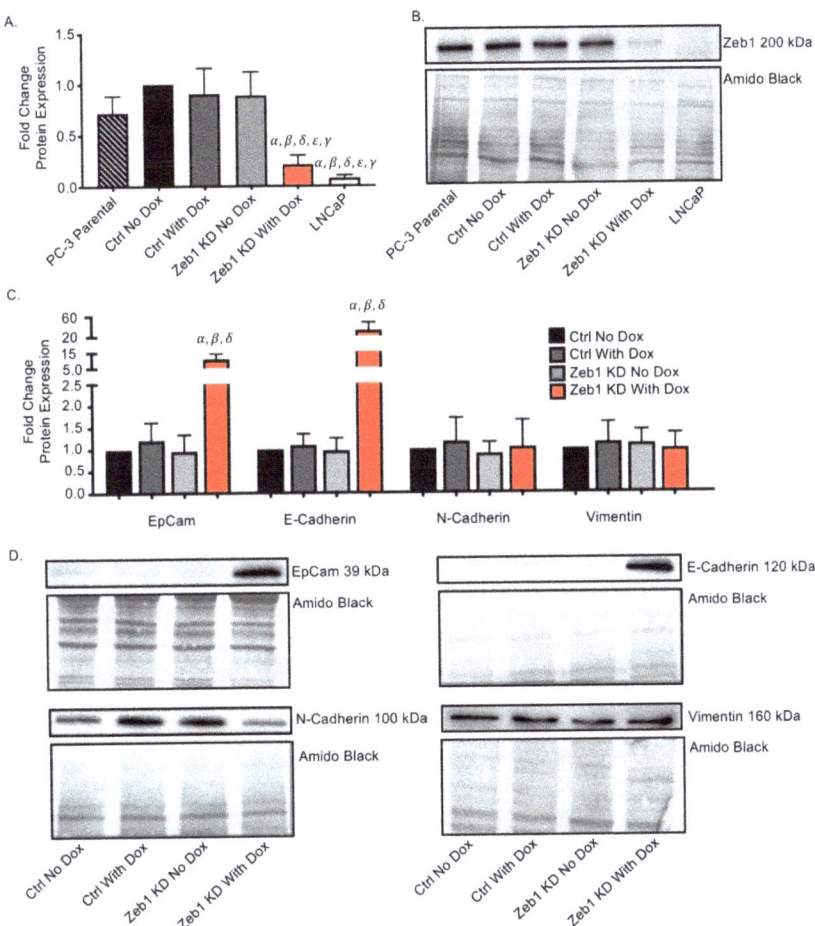

Figure 1. Inducible knockdown of *Zeb1* in PC-3 human prostate cancer cells results in enhanced expression of epithelial proteins. Mesenchymal human PC-3 prostate cancer cells were engineered to knockdown expression of the master epithelial-to-mesenchymal (EMT) regulator *Zeb1* using the SMARTvector inducible lentiviral shRNA system (Dharmacon), which features Tet-on® induction of the target shRNA in the presence of doxycycline (Dox). (**A**,**B**) Immunoblot analysis of Zeb1 protein expression in the presence or absence of Dox (72 h) in Zeb1^{KD} (*Zeb1* knockdown), control (ctrl) PC-3 cells, or LNCaP cells. (**C**,**D**) Immunoblot analysis of E-Cadherin, EpCAM, Vimentin and N-cadherin in Zeb1^{KD} or ctrl cells 72 h after Dox induction. Representative immunoblots are shown and amido black staining of total protein was used as a loading control. Quantitative data is presented as mean ± standard error of the mean (SEM) fold-change in expression relative to ctrl cells ($n = 3$). α = significantly different than ctrl no Dox. β = significantly different than ctrl with Dox. δ = significantly different than Zeb1^{KD} no Dox. γ = significantly different than PC-3 parental ε = significantly different than LNCaP ($p \leq 0.05$).

2.2. Knockdown of Zeb1 in PC-3 Prostate Cancer Cells Increases Migration and Invasion but Does Not Alter Proliferation

Next, we assessed the effect of *Zeb1* knockdown on migration and invasion of PC-3 prostate cancer cells using transwell migration (gelatin) and physical barrier wound healing assays. Unexpectedly, we observed that Zeb1^{KD} cells with Dox exhibit significantly increased migration compared to ctrl cells in both transwell (Figure 2A,B) and wound healing assays (Figure 2C,D) ($p \leq 0.05$). When Zeb1^{KD} cells were assessed for changes in cell invasion using transwell invasion and spheroid invasion (Matrigel) assays, we similarly observed that Zeb1^{KD} cells with Dox demonstrate significantly enhanced invasion into Matrigel in both the transwell (Figure 3A,B) and spheroid invasion assays (Figure 3C,D) ($p \leq 0.05$). BrdU proliferation assays were used to assess differences in cell proliferation between Zeb1^{KD} and ctrl cells, however no significant differences in proliferation were observed (Supplementary Figure S2A).

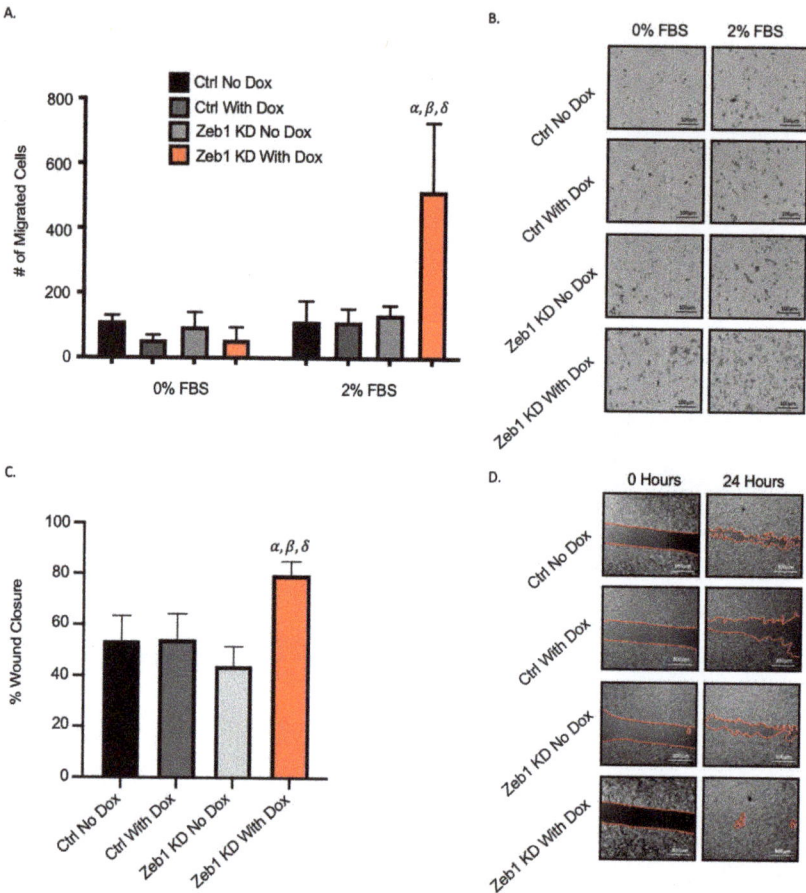

Figure 2. Knockdown of *Zeb1* in PC-3 prostate cancer cells increases cell migration. (**A,B**) Transwells were coated with 6 µg/well of gelatin. Cells (5×10^4/well) were added to wells and either control media (0% fetal bovine serum [FBS]) or chemoattractant media (2% FBS) was added and cells were allowed to migrate for 18 h. Cells were fixed with 1% glutaraldehyde and mounted with DAPI-containing mounting media. (**C,D**) For physical barrier wound healing assays, cells were seeded and grown to 90–100% confluency. The physical barrier was removed and cells were allowed to migrate into the wound for 36 h. Representative images are shown for each assay; with migration calculated based on 5 high-powered fields of view (HP-FOV) per well. Black scale bars = 100µm, white scale bars = 300µm. Data is presented as the mean ± standard error of the mean (SEM) ($n = 3$). α = significantly different than control (ctrl) no doxycycline (Dox). β = significantly different than ctrl with Dox. δ = significantly different than Zeb1^{KD} (*Zeb1* knockdown) no Dox ($p \leq 0.05$).

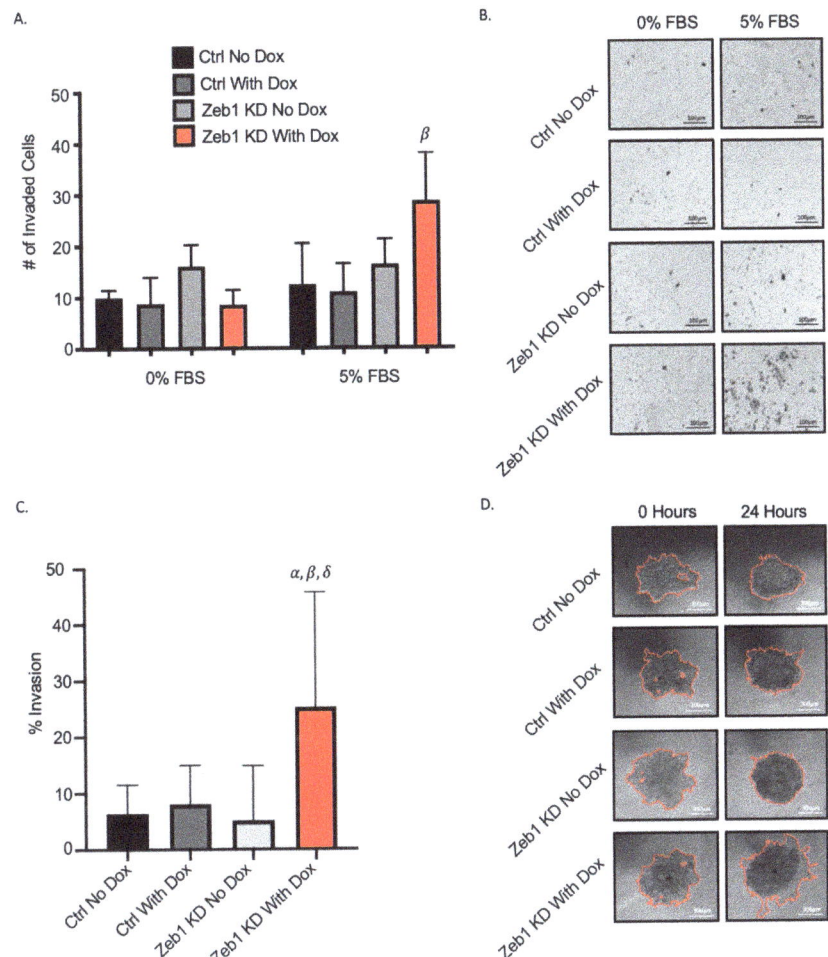

Figure 3. Knockdown of *Zeb1* in PC-3 prostate cancer cells increases cell invasion. (**A,B**) Transwells were coated with 4 µg/well of Matrigel. Cells (5 × 10^4/well) were added to wells and either control media (0% fetal bovine serum [FBS]) or chemoattractant media (5% FBS) was added and cells were allowed to invade for 24 h. Cells were fixed with 1% glutaraldehyde and mounted with DAPI-containing mounting media. (**C,D**) For spheroid invasion assays, cells were seeded onto ultra-low attachment plates and allowed to grow for 96 h to create spheroids. Matrigel was then added and invasion was quantified after 48 h. Representative images are shown for each assay; with invasion calculated based on 5 high-powered fields of view (HP-FOV) per well. Black scale bars = 100 µm, white scale bars = 300 µm. Data is presented as the mean ± standard error of the mean (SEM) (n = 3). α = significantly different than PC-3 control (ctrl) no doxycycline (Dox). β = significantly different than ctrl with Dox. δ = significantly different than Zeb1^{KD} (*Zeb1* knockdown) no Dox ($p \leq 0.05$).

2.3. Knockdown of Zeb1 in PC-3 Prostate Cancer Cells Leads to a Partial EMT Phenotype at the Cellular and Molecular Level

We had originally expected that knockdown of *Zeb1* in mesenchymal PC-3 prostate cancer cells would lead to a mesenchymal-to-epithelial (MET) transition and reduced metastatic cell behaviors such as migration and invasion. Our observation that knockdown of *Zeb1* instead actually led to more aggressive cell behavior led us to investigate the potential for a partial EMT (p-EMT) phenotype [14]. Zeb1^{KD} cells with Dox were assessed for changes in cell morphology as described in the Materials & Methods section and in Supplementary Figure S3. We observed that Zeb1^{KD} cells with Dox demonstrate a mixed cell morphology, with a significantly higher percentage of epithelial cells and significantly lower percentage of mesenchymal cells compared to ctrl cells ($p \leq 0.05$) (Figure 4A,B). We next assessed changes in expression of the p-EMT markers P-Cadherin (P-Cad) and integrin β4 (ITGβ4) [18,19]. We observed that both P-Cad and ITGβ4 protein expression was significantly enhanced in Zeb1^{KD} cells with Dox compared to ctrl cells ($p \leq 0.05$) (Figure 4C), while *P-Cad* RNA expression was also significantly increased in Zeb1^{KD} cells with Dox compared to ctrl cells ($p \leq 0.05$) (Figure 4D).

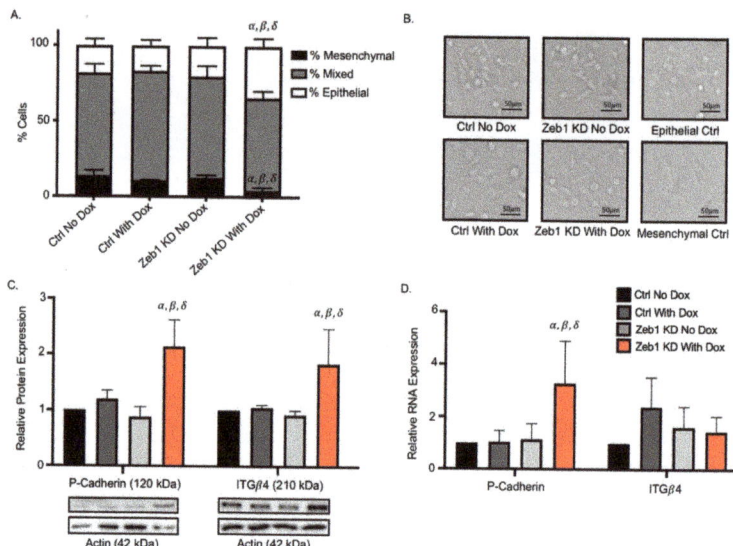

Figure 4. Knockdown of *Zeb1* in PC-3 prostate cancer cells leads to a partial-EMT phenotype at the cellular and molecular level. (**A,B**) Cultured PC-3 Zeb1^{KD} (Zeb1 knockdown) and control (ctrl) cells were assessed for cell morphology characteristics as described in the Materials & Methods and in Supplementary Figure S3 (N = 3; n = 250/cells per group). Representative images of each cell group and epithelial (MDA-MB-468) and mesenchymal (primary lung fibroblasts) controls are shown. (**C**) Immunoblot analysis of P-Cadherin and ITGβ4 in Zeb1^{KD} or ctrl cells. Actin was used as a loading control and representative immunoblots are shown. (**D**) qRT-PCR analysis of p-EMT marker expression in the presence of absence of Dox in Zeb1^{KD} or ctrl cells. Data is presented as the mean ± standard error of the mean (SEM) (n = 3) relative to ctrl no Dox. Scale bars = 50 μm. α = significantly different than PC-3 ctrl no Dox. β = significantly different than ctrl with Dox. δ = significantly different than Zeb1^{KD} no Dox ($p \leq 0.05$).

2.4. Treatment of PC-3 Zeb1^{KD} Prostate Cancer Cells with the Global Demethylating Agent 5-Azacitadine Results in Decreased DNA Methylation, Migration, and Invasion

It has been suggested that epigenetic modifications such as DNA methylation of the promoter region of essential genes may be responsible for increased cell aggressiveness in cancer [16]. The global demethylating agent 5-aza is currently used to treat myelodysplastic syndrome [20] and is in many phase III clinical trials for cancer (ClinicalTrials.gov (accessed on 7 September 2021). To begin investigating whether DNA methylation is involved in the p-EMT phenotype observed in our Zeb1^{KD} cells, we treated cells with 5-aza ± Dox to assess the effects on cell phenotype. We observed that DNA methylation was decreased (based on decreased expression of 5-mC) in Zeb1^{KD} with Dox and ctrl cells treated with 5-aza compared to DMSO ($p \leq 0.05$) (Figure 5A,B). We next assessed the effects of demethylation on cell aggressiveness, and observed that treatment with 5-aza significantly mitigated both migration (Figure 5C,D) and invasion (Figure 5E,F) compared to treatment with DMSO ($p \leq 0.05$), although there was no change in proliferation (Supplemental Figure S2B).

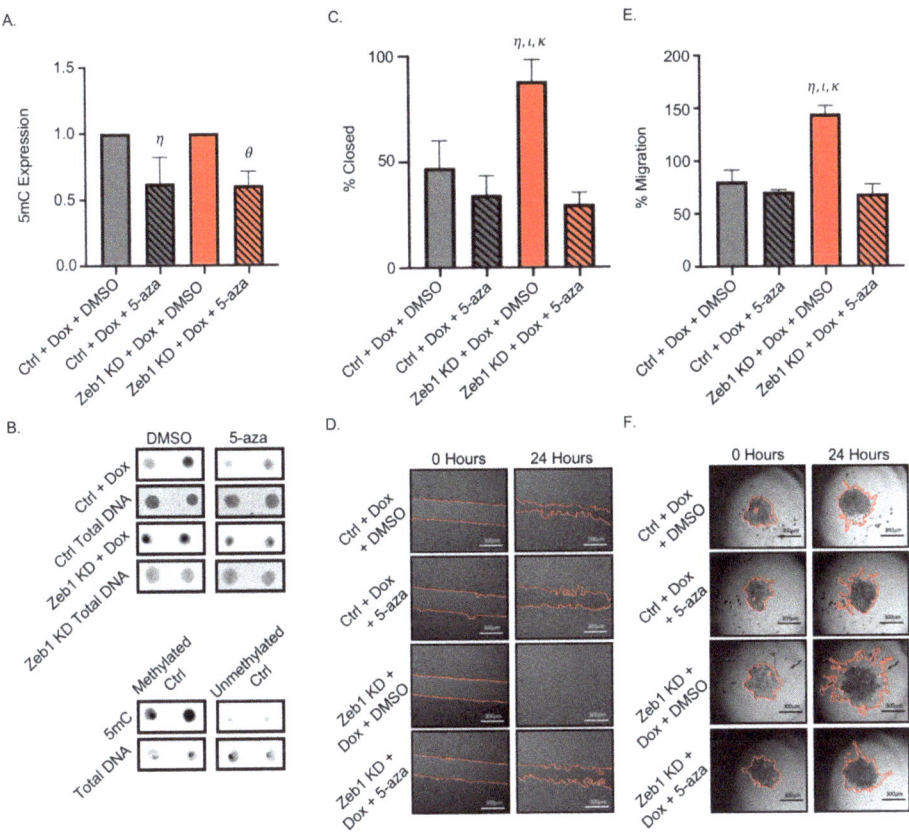

Figure 5. Treatment of PC-3 Zeb1^{KD} prostate cancer cells with the global demethylating agent 5-azacitadine (5-aza) results in decreased DNA methylation, migration and invasion. (**A,B**) PC-3 Zeb1^{KD} (Zeb1 knockdown) with doxycycline (Dox) or control (ctrl) cells were treated with either dimethyl sulfoxide (DMSO) or 5-aza (5 µM) for 24 h and DNA was extracted to assess for global DNA methylation via dot blot assays. Representative dot blots are shown. Methylated and unmethylated DNA controls were used to validate 5-methylcytosine (5mC) expression. (**C,D**) Cells were seeded onto physical barrier cell culture dishes and grown to 90–100% confluency. Treatments (5 µM 5-aza or DMSO) were added to cells, the physical barrier was removed, and cells were allowed to migrate into the wound. (**E,F**) Cells were seeded onto ultra-low attachment plates and allowed to grow for 96 h to create spheroids. After 96 h of growth, Matrigel and 5 µM 5-aza or DMSO were added. Representative images are shown for each assay; with migration or invasion calculated based on 5 high-powered fields of view (HP-FOV) per well. Scale bars = 300 µm. Data is presented as the mean ± standard error of the mean (SEM) (n = 3). η = significantly different than ctrl with Dox and treated with DMSO. θ = significantly different than Zeb1^{KD} with Dox and treated with DMSO. ι = significantly different than ctrl with Dox treated with 5 µM 5-aza. κ = significantly different than Zeb1^{KD} with Dox treated with 5 µM 5-aza ($p \leq 0.05$).

2.5. Methylation Chip Analysis of Zeb1^{KD} PC-3 Prostate Cancer Cells Identified 10 Genes Associated with a p-EMT Phenotype

To explore specific molecular characteristics in Zeb1^{KD} cells that are being affected by demethylation, DNA was extracted from Dox-induced Zeb1^{KD} cells treated with DMSO

(Z0) or 5 µM of 5-aza (Z5), and from Dox-induced ctrl cells treated with DMSO (C0) or 5-aza (C5) and assessed for global changes in DNA methylation using an Infinium MethylationEPIC chip. We observed over 100,000 differentially methylated sites between ctrl + DMSO cells (C0) and Zeb1^{KD} + DMSO cells (Z0) (false discovery rate (FDR) cutoff value = 0.05) (Figure 6A). We then further assessed only those sites which had an increase in DNA methylation between C0 and Z0 that also demonstrated rescued demethylation in Zeb1^{KD} cells + 5-aza (Z5); resulting in 51 potential sites of importance (FDR cutoff value = 0.05) (Figure 6B). Of these, 10 sites (*LRPPRC, CLDN11, MTOR, EPB41, DAPK1, PPZR2B, ZDHHC2, HSD17B13, MYOM2* and *MAN1A1*) were linked to decreased expression and increased aggressiveness/p-EMT, which may be of clinical importance for identifying an aggressive p-EMT phenotype in prostate cancer patients in the future (Figure 6C, Table 1).

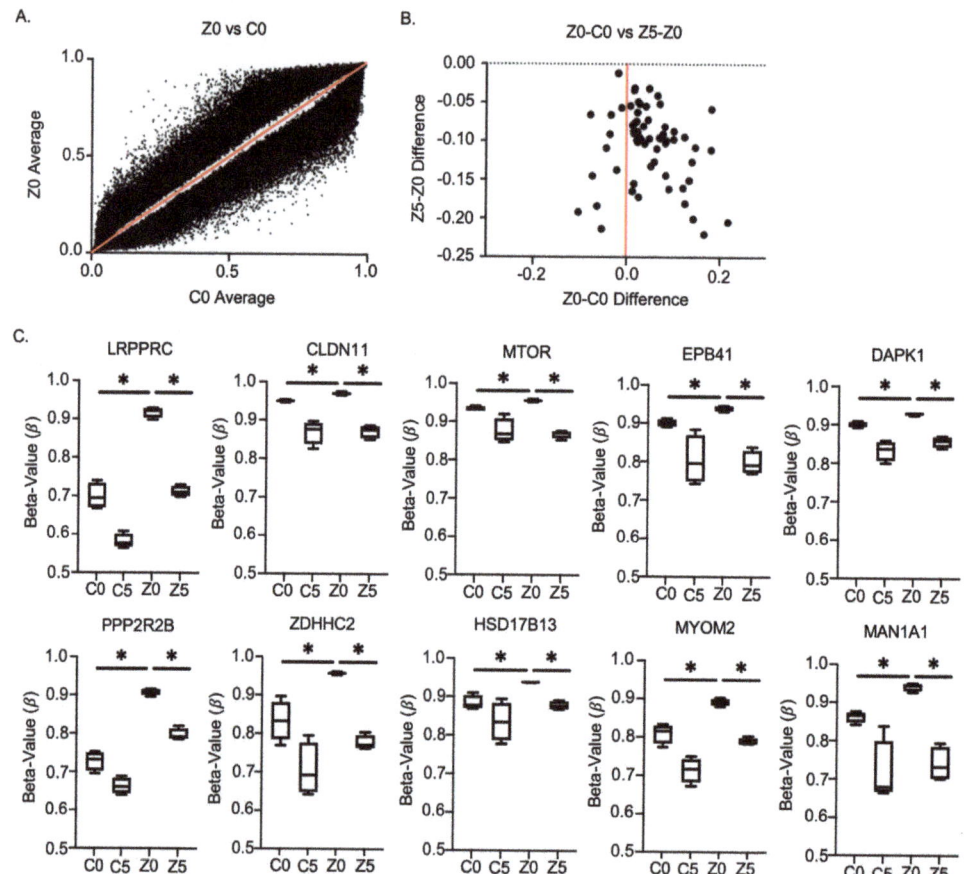

Figure 6. DNA methylation chip analysis of Zeb1^{KD} PC-3 prostate cancer cells identified 10 genes associated with a p-EMT phenotype. DNA was extracted from PC-3 Zeb1^{KD} (Zeb1 knockdown) cells with doxycycline (Dox) treated with dimethyl sulfoxide (DMSO) (Z0) or 5-azacitadine (5-aza; Z5; 5µM), and from Dox-induced control (ctrl) cells treated with DMSO (C0) or 5-aza (C5; 5 µM) and was assessed for global changes in DNA methylation using an Infinium Methylation EPIC chip. (**A**) A two-tailed, unpaired, equal variance *t*-test was completed with FDR cut-off value = 0.05 (Benjamini-Hochberg FDR)

between C0 and Z0. This was filtered for significant Z0-C0 differences, and 107,971 cg sites were observed. (**B**) A two-tailed, unpaired, equal variance *t*-test was completed with FDR cut-off value = 0.05 (Benjamini-Hochberg FDR) between Z0 vs. Z5. This was filtered for significant Z0-Z5 differences, and 62 cg sites were observed. Among the C0-Z0 and Z0-Z5 significant differences, we wanted to identify rescue changes, so we filtered the dataset for cg sites where Z0-C0 = -(Z5-Z0) and identified 51 cg sites (right side of graph (**B**)). (**C**) Genes identified in DNA methylation chip analysis (increased DNA methylation from C0 versus Z0 with a corresponding demethylation in Z5). β-value represents the estimate of DNA methylation level at a given locus. Data is presented as the mean ± standard error of the mean (SEM) (n = 4). * = significant difference between conditions.

Table 1. Functional relevance of genes identified in DNA methylation chip analysis.

Gene	Function Relative to Cancer Aggressiveness
LRPPRC	Dysregulation is related to various diseases ranging from tumors to viral infections [21].
Claudin-11	Plays an important role in cellular proliferation and migration [22].
mTOR	Regulates cell growth, proliferation, motility, survival, protein synthesis, autophagy, and transcription [23].
EPB41	Expression is significantly decreased in HCC tissue specimens, especially in portal vein metastasis or intrahepatic metastasis, compared to normal tissues [24].
DAPK1	Downregulation promotes the stemness of cancer stem cells and EMT process by activating ZEB1 in colorectal cancer [25].
PPP2RR2B	Negative control of cell growth and division [26].
ZDHHC2	Tumor suppressor in metastasis and recurrence of HCC [27].
HSD17B13	Downregulated in hepatocellular carcinoma [28].
MYOM2	Downregulation was observed in a clinical assessment of breast cancer patients [29].
MAN1A1	Reduced expression leads to impaired survival in breast cancer [30].

2.6. MAN1A1, EPB41, HSD17B13 and MYOM2 Are Altered in Prostate Cancer Patients

Finally, we were interested in determining the potential clinical relevance of the identified DNA methylation targets in prostate cancer patients. We analyzed the 10 identified target p-EMT genes using available Ualcan (http://ualcan.path.uab.edu (accessed on 10 September 2021) and cBioportal (https://www.cbioportal.org (accessed on 10 September 2021) online clinical databases. We observed significant hypermethylation in 4 of the 10 target genes (*MAN1A1*, *EPB41*, *HSD17B13*, and *MYOM2*) in primary prostate cancer patient tumors (n = 503) compared to normal prostatic samples (n = 50) ($p < 0.05$) (Figure 7A). Expression of *MAN1A1* was also observed to be significantly decreased in metastatic prostate cancer patients (n = 42) relative to non-metastatic prostate cancer patients (n = 44) ($p \leq 0.05$) (Figure 7B). Lastly, we observed that decreased expression of *MYOM2* correlates with decreased overall survival in prostate cancer patients (Figure 7C). Taken together, these observations in prostate cancer patients support our pre-clinical findings in aggressive Zeb1[KD] cells and suggest that these genes merit future investigation as potential biomarkers for combination treatment of prostate cancer patients with 5-aza.

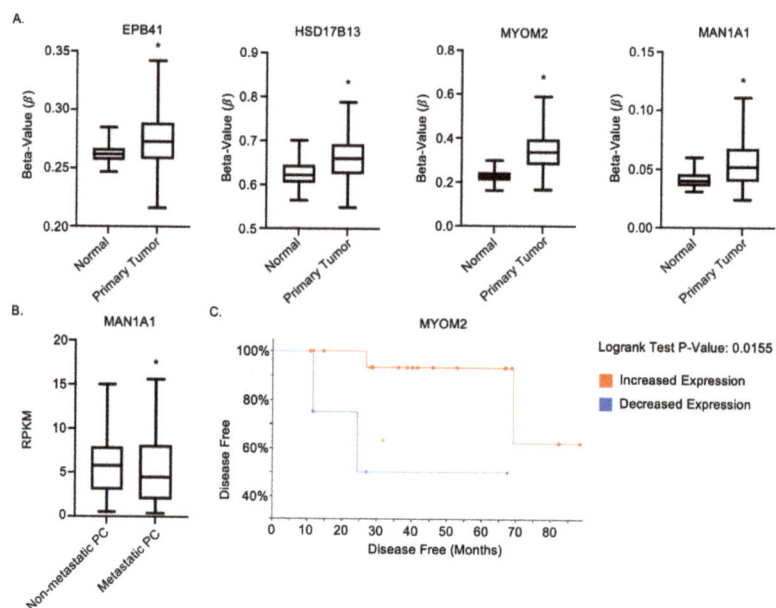

Figure 7. *MAN1A1, EPB41, HSD17B13* and *MYOM2* are altered in prostate cancer patients. (**A,B**) Ualcan analysis in prostate adenocarcinoma identified (**A**) 4 target genes (*MAN1A1, EPB41, HSD17B13* and *MYOM2*) with increased promoter methylation in primary prostate cancer tumors (n = 502) compared to normal prostatic samples (n = 50) and (**B**) *MAN1A1* RNA expression in metastatic prostate cancer (PC) (n = 42) vs. non-metastatic prostate cancer (n = 44). (**C**) cBioportal analysis of relationship between *MYOM2* expression and progression free survival. * = significantly different between conditions.

3. Discussion

Prostate cancer is the most common cancer in American men and the second leading cause of cancer-related death. The majority of these deaths are associated with metastasis, a process involving the epithelial-to-mesenchymal (EMT) transition. Furthermore, growing evidence suggests that a partial-EMT (p-EMT) phenotype, whereby cells are able to simultaneously maintain both epithelial and mesenchymal characteristics, may lead to more aggressive disease than complete EMT [14]. Gaining a greater understanding of p-EMT may thus provide insights into the mechanisms of metastatic disease progression, which currently has no cure. In the current study, we observed that inducible knockdown of *Zeb1* in mesenchymal PC-3 cells resulted in a p-EMT phenotype including co-expression of epithelial and mesenchymal markers, a mixed epithelial/mesenchymal morphology, increased invasion and migration, and enhanced expression of p-EMT markers.

In addition to changes in gene and protein expression, the p-EMT phenotype is commonly associated with aberrant hypermethylation [31,32]. The global de-methylating agent 5-azacytidine (5-aza) is FDA-approved for treating myelodysplastic syndrome and is currently in 42 phase III clinical trials for treating cancer patients (ClinincalTrials.gov (accessed on 7 September 2021), as well as 4 phase II clinical trials specifically for prostate cancer patients (ClinicalTrials.gov (accessed on 7 September 2021). When we treated our p-EMT prostate cancer cells with 5-aza, we observed a significant decrease in aggressive phenotype. Furthermore, our DNA methylation chip analysis revealed 10 potential markers for further investigation in association with p-EMT.

Our observations included increased DNA methylation of *EPB41* and *HSD17B13*. *EPB41* has been identified as a tumor suppressor in the molecular pathogenesis of meningiomas [24]. *HSD17B13* expression has also been shown to inhibit the progression and recurrence of hepatocellular carcinomas [28]. Additionally, Ualcan online database analysis showed increased promoter methylation of both *EPB41* and *HSD17B13* in prostate cancer patients compared to healthy controls. Silencing of these genes due to increased DNA methylation could result in tumor progression and poor patient survival [24,28].

We also observed increased DNA methylation of *MAN1A1*, which correlated with decreased gene expression. Reduced *MAN1A1* expression has previously been associated with reduced survival in breast cancer patients [30]. In our study, Ualcan online database analysis showed increased promoter methylation of *MAN1A1* in prostate cancer patients compared to healthy controls and in metastatic prostate cancer patients compared to non-metastatic prostate cancer patients. This suggests that decreased expression of *MAN1A1* may be associated with increased prostate cancer aggressiveness and could be a novel marker for identifying a p-EMT phenotype in patient tumors.

Lastly, we demonstrated increased DNA methylation of *MYOM2*. *MYOM2* has been previously been observed to be downregulated in breast cancer patients, as determined by multiplex RT-PCR [29]. Our assessment using the cBioportal online database revealed that decreased *MYOM2* expression is associated with significantly worse progression free survival in prostate cancer patients compared to those with high *MYOM2* expression, suggesting that *MYOM2* may be another potential marker for identifying aggressive prostate cancer.

In summary, in this study we developed a stable, inducible p-EMT prostate cancer model that provides the opportunity to investigate the aggressive p-EMT phenotype, a cell state that often occurs transiently in vivo. In addition, we have identified 4 potential biomarkers related to p-EMT for which decreased expression may be an indicator of metastatic disease and may warrant consideration for use in identifying patients who would benefit from 5-aza treatment to target hypermethylation. Currently, there is no cure for metastatic prostate cancer, however, early detection and targeted treatment with agents that target hypermethylation may slow down the progression towards metastasis and improved patient outcomes.

4. Materials and Methods

4.1. Cell Culture

Human mesenchymal PC-3 prostate cancer cells (parental PC-3 cells [#CRL-1435]; ATCC, Manassas, VA, USA) were cultured in F12K media + 10% fetal bovine serum (FBS). Human epithelial LNCaP prostate cancer cells (#CRL-1740, ATCC) were cultured in RPMI-1640 media + 10% FBS. Human epithelial MDA-MB-468 breast cancer cells (#HTB-132, ATCC) were cultured in alpha minimum essential media (αMEM) + 10% FBS. Cell lines were authenticated via third party testing (IDEXX BioAnalytics, Columbia, MO, USA). Primary lung fibroblasts (Lonza, Basel, Switzerland) were cultured in RPMI-1640 media + 5% FBS, 1% 4-(2-hydroxyethyl)-1-piperazineethanesulfonic acid (HEPES), 0.1% bovine serum albumin (BSA) (10%), 0.5% insulin, and 0.05% hydrocortisone. Media and reagents are from Life Technologies (Carlsbad, CA, USA), and FBS is from Sigma (St. Louis, MO, USA).

4.2. Cell Transductions

To create PC-3 Zeb1^{KD} and ctrl cells, 1×10^6 PC-3 cells/mL were seeded into each well of a 6-well dish 24 h prior to transduction. Twenty-five µL of SMARTvector Lentiviral *Zeb1* shRNA stock (target region; 3' untranslated region, target sequence 5'-TCTAAACCCAGGCTTCCCT-3') or scrambled control (non-targeting control sequence) (Dharmacon, Lafayette, CO, USA) was added to each well and growth media was exchanged for transduction media containing 0.01% polybrene. After 24 h, transduction media was exchanged for growth media. One day later, growth media was exchanged for selection media containing 0.025% puromycin. Cells were then cultured as usual, supplementing growth media with 0.025% puromycin to continue selective pressure. Resulting changes in inducible Zeb1 expression (± Dox) were analyzed using immunoblotting and qRT-PCR as described below.

4.3. Immunoblotting

Cells were harvested by cell scraping, collected in lysis buffer, and quantified using a Lowry Assay. Protein (10 µg) was subjected to sodium dodecyl sulfate polyacrylamide gel electrophoresis (SDS-PAGE) and transferred onto polyvinylidene difluoride membranes (PVDF; Millipore, Billerica, MA, USA). Membranes were blocked using 5% bovine serum albumin (BSA) in Tris-buffered saline + 0.1% Tween-20 (TBS-T). Anti-human primary antibodies were diluted in 5% BSA in TBS-T prior to use as detailed in Supplementary Table S1. Goat anti-mouse IgG and goat anti-rabbit IgG secondary antibodies (Calbiochem, Billerica, MA, USA) conjugated to horseradish peroxidase and diluted in 5% BSA/TBS-T were used at concentrations of 1:2000 and 1:5000. Protein expression was visualized using Amersham ECL Prime Detection Reagent (GE Healthcase, Wauwatosa, WI, USA), and normalized to total protein based on amido black (Sigma) staining of membranes or actin immunoblotting.

4.4. Quantitative Real-Time PCR

Total RNA was isolated using TRIzol (Life Technologies), and reverse transcribed using SuperScript™ IV VILO Master Mix (Invitrogen, Waltham, MA, USA; 11766050). Samples were then subjected to subsequent RNA analysis using Advanced qPCR Master Mix with Supergreen LO-ROX (Wisent Bioproducts, Saint-Jean-Baptiste, QC, Canada) on a QuantStudio™ 3 Real-Time PCR system (Applied Biosystems, Waltham, WA, USA) with primers detailed in Supplementary Table S2. *GAPDH* was used as a control.

4.5. Transwell Migration and Invasion Assays

Changes in cell migration and invasion were assessed using transwell migration and invasion assays. Transwell plates were coated with either gelatin (4 µg/well, migration) or Matrigel (6 µg/well, invasion). Media in the bottom well included normal media supplemented with puromycin and 2% FBS (migration) or 5% FBS (invasion) with or without 1 µg/mL Dox treatment as required. Human PC-3 prostate cancer cells (parental, ctrl or Zeb1^{KD}; 5×10^4 cells/mL) were seeded onto the top portion of each transwell chamber and incubated for 18 h at 37 °C, 5% CO_2 prior to staining and assessment of differences in migration and invasion. Five high powered fields of view (HP-FOVs) were captured for each well, and the mean number of migrated or invaded cells/HP-FOV was calculated using ImageJ software (National Health Institute, Bethesda, MD, USA).

4.6. Physical Barrier Wound Healing Assay

Changes in migratory capacity were also assessed using physical barrier wound healing assays. Cells (3×10^5/mL) were plated in F12K media supplemented with puromycin and doxycycline, DMSO, and/or 5-aza, onto 24 well plates. Cells were incubated at 37 °C, 5% CO_2. After 24 h the physical barrier was removed from each well. Images were captured at 0, 12, 24, and 36 h time points using 5 HP-FOVs for each well. Cell migration, calculated by percent wound closure, was analyzed using ImageJ. software.

4.7. Spheroid Invasion Assay

Changes in invasion were also assessed using spheroid invasion assays. Cells (5×10^3) were plated onto 96-well ultra-low attachment plates spheroid microplates (Corning, Kennebunk, ME, USA) using growth media supplemented with puromycin, doxycycline, DMSO, and/or 5-aza and allowed to grow into spheroids for 96 h. Matrigel was added to the spheroids and images were captured at 0, 24, and 48 h time points using 5 HP-FOVs for each well. ImageJ software was used to calculate the area of invasion from spheroids into surrounding Matrigel.

4.8. BrdU Proliferation Assay

Cell proliferation was assessed using a bromodeoxyuridine (BrdU) incorporation assay. Cells were plated on 8-well chamber slides, allowed to adhere, and serum-starved for 72 h. Media was then replaced with F12K supplemented with puromycin and 10% FBS ± Dox, 5-aza, and/or DMSO for 24 h. Following incubation, Cell Proliferation Labelling Reagent (BrdU) (GE Healthcare, Chicago, IL, USA) was added for 30 min, cells were formalin fixed and stained with a 100 µL/well anti-BrdU primary antibody (BD-347580) and a 1:400 concentration of a PE-conjugated goat anti-mouse IgG secondary antibody was used for immunofluorescent visualization. Images were captured using 5 HP-FOVs for each well, and nuclei were counted using ImageJ, with results expressed as a percentage of BrdU positive cells to total nuclei (DAPI$^+$).

4.9. Cell Morphology Assay

Changes in cell morphology were determined by analyzing the roundness versus spindle-like shape of each cell. High powered FOVs were used to capture cell images, and 250 cells per HP-FOV (n = 3) were analyzed for cell shape. The actual area (AA) of each cell was calculating by outlining and measuring the entire cell in ImageJ, which was also used to trace the diameter between the longest two points of each cell and the expected area (EA) was calculating using the equation πr^2. The AA was then divided by EA to assign each cell with a number from 0 to 1. If AA was equal to the expected area then the number is 1, and the cell is more round in shape. If the AA is less than the expected area then the number is closer to 0, and the cell is more spindle shaped. To determine the limits of what number represented a round or spindle-shaped cell control, epithelial MDA-MB-468 breast cancer cells and mesenchymal primary lung fibroblasts were used as controls for cell shape (250 cells/FOV, n = 3). The average of the epithelial/mesenchymal control cells was attained, and the standard deviation was either added or subtracted from the average respectively in order to create a cutoff point for an epithelial cell, a mesenchymal cell, and a cell of "mixed" morphology (i.e., neither epithelial nor mesenchymal) (Supplementary Figure S3).

4.10. DNA Extraction and Dot-Blot DNA Analysis

DNA was extracted using a Blood & Cell Culture DNA Mini Kit (Qiagen, Hilden, Germany) and the manufacturer's protocol. For the dot-blot analysis, 180 ng of DNA was added to 3 M NaOH and incubated at 42 °C for 12 min to denature the DNA. Samples were immediately transferred to positively charged nylon membranes (Roche, Mannheim, Germany) in the dot-blot apparatus. Membranes were then baked at 120 °C for 30 min to allow DNA-membrane crosslinking. The membrane was then blocked in 1× TBS + 0.05% Tween-20 and 5% powdered milk for 1 h prior to incubation with the anti-5mC primary antibody (ab179898; 1:500 in blocking solution) and agitated for 1.5 h. Membranes were washed 3× with TBS-T for 10 min, and then incubated with a goat anti-mouse IgG secondary antibody (Calbiochem, Billerica, MA, USA; 1:1000) for 1 h. Expression of 5 mC was visualized using Amersham ECL Prime Detection Reagent (GE Healthcare) on a ChemiDoc™ MP Imaging System, and normalized to total DNA based on methylene blue staining of membranes.

4.11. DNA Methylation Chip Analysis

Changes in global DNA methylation profile were analyzed using the Illumina Methylation EPIC BeadChip (Illumina, San Diego, CA, USA) and 1000 ng of DNA input (n = 4 per cell group) using the manufacturer's protocol [33]. In total, 3 different QC methods were carried out. First, raw methylation betas were generated using the Minfi package in R [34] and no QC was performed in order to retain flexibility for analysis. Secondly, quality control was performed with the Chip Analysis Methylation Pipeline (ChAMP) [35]. This method filtered probes with a detection p-value above 0.01 (removing 3337 probes), bead count <3 in at least 5% of samples (removing 26,519 probes), only keeping CpG methylation measurements (removing 2931 probes), filtering probes with SNPs (removing

95,596 probes), probes that align to multiple locations (removing 11 probes), filtering XY chromosome probes (removing 16,109 probes). The last method of QC still used ChAMP, but only removed probes failing detection p-value, bead count and non-cpg sites (as explained above). After probe filtering with ChAMP, no samples were removed due to QC issues, and values for each sample were normalized with BMIQ normalization [36].

4.12. Patient Sample Analysis

Follow-up analysis was completed using Ualcan and cBioportal online clinical patient databases. Using the gene analysis Ulcan database (accessed on 10 September 2021), each aberrantly methylated gene identified was analyzed. Utilizing the TCGA dataset, genes were assessed for promoter methylation in prostate adenocarcinoma compared to normal tissue as well as for expression in metastatic prostate cancer (MET500 dataset) compared to non-metastatic prostate cancer. Additionally, cBioportal (accessed on 10 September 2021) was used to assess for association with survival using mRNA expression level comparisons of aberrantly methylated genes in prostate adenocarcinoma. First, the sample set was identified using Onco Query Language on cBioportal (accessed on 10 September 2021). Patients were stratified based on expression of each identified gene, an mRNA profile was added to the query, and "example gene: EXP > 2 EXP < −2" was written in the gene set box. After running the query, the "samples affected" list was downloaded. Next the list of sample IDs was pasted into the homepage into the "user-defined case list" in the "select patient/case set": dropdown. This query only looks at samples with high or low expression. To stratify into high versus low survival analysis, "example gene: EXP > 2" was entered in the gene set box and the same (prostate adenocarcinoma) mRNA profile was selected. The query was run, and the survival tab was selected for results.

4.13. Statistical Analysis

Statistical analysis was performed using GraphPad Prism 9 (GraphPad, San Diego, CA, USA) and Microsoft Excel 16.5.2 (Microsoft, Redmond, WA, USA). Unless otherwise stated, data is presented as the mean ± standard error of the mean (SEM), with $p \leq 0.05$ considered to be statistically significant. For normally distributed comparisons of 2 groups, t-tests were performed and for comparisons of more than 2 groups a one-way ANOVA with follow up t-tests for multiple comparisons was performed. Non-matched, non-parametric data of more than two groups was assessed with a one-way Krustral-Wallis ANOVA with follow up Mann-Whitney tests for multiple comparisons, with a false discovery rate cutoff = 0.05 considered to be statistically significant.

5. Conclusions

In the current manuscript we created and characterized a stable inducible p-EMT cell line model by decreasing *Zeb1* expression in mesenchymal PC-3 prostate cancer cells. This resulted in an increased aggressive phenotype compared to mesenchymal controls. We identified 10 potential p-EMT markers which had aberrant DNA methylation in these p-EMT cells which may be used as a screening panel for p-EMT patients in the future to allow for earlier detection of aggressive prostate cancer and/or potentially serve to identify patients who might benefit from 5-aza therapy.

Supplementary Materials: The following are available online at https://www.mdpi.com/article/10.3390/ijms222312840/s1.

Author Contributions: Conceptualization, A.L.A., J.K. and L.E.L.; methodology, A.L.A., J.K. and L.E.L.; validation, J.K.; formal analysis, C.L. and J.K.; investigation, J.K.; data curation, J.K. and J.C.; writing—original draft preparation, J.K. and A.L.A.; writing—review and editing, A.L.A., J.K., C.L., J.C. and L.E.L.; visualization, J.K.; supervision, A.L.A.; funding acquisition, A.L.A. All authors have read and agreed to the published version of the manuscript.

Funding: This research was funded by a Movember Discovery Grant from Prostate Cancer Canada (grant # D2017-1974) and by a Catalyst Grant from the London Regional Cancer Program. J.K. has been the recipient of scholarship from the Lawson Health Research Institute (IRF Award) and the Province of Ontario (Ontario Graduate Scholarship). C.L. has been the recipient of a Vanier Canada Graduate Scholarship from the Canadian Institutes of Health Research.

Data Availability Statement: Infinium Methylation EPIC chip dataset can be found archived in the GEO repository, series number GSE186782, "Treatment of p-EMT prostate cancer cell with the demethylating drug 5-azacytidine reduces cell aggressiveness and changes methylation profile".

Acknowledgments: We thank Reina Ditta and Nathan Cawte from the Clinical Research Laboratory and Biobank (CRLB) and the Genetic and Molecular Epidemiology Laboratory (GMEL) at McMaster University (Hamilton, ON, Canada) for their assistance in generating and analyzing the methylation chip data and their advice with archiving the resulting datasets. We also thank Vasudeva Bhat, Bart Kolendowski, and Michael Levy at the London Health Sciences Centre for their advice with study design and data analysis.

Conflicts of Interest: The authors declare no conflict of interest.

References

1. Siegel, R.L.; Miller, K.D.; Jemal, A. Cancer statistics, 2020. *CA Cancer J. Clin.* **2020**, *70*, 7–30. [CrossRef]
2. Pantel, K.; Brakenhoff, R.H.; Brandt, B. Detection, clinical relevance and specific biological properties of disseminating tumour cells. *Nat. Rev. Cancer* **2008**, *8*, 329–340. [CrossRef] [PubMed]
3. Fidler, I.J. The pathogenesis of cancer metastasis: The "seed and soil" hypothesis revisited. *Nat. Rev. Cancer* **2003**, *3*, 453–458. [CrossRef] [PubMed]
4. Kalluri, R.; Weinberg, R.A. The basics of epithelial-mesenchymal transition. *J. Clin. Investig.* **2009**, *119*, 1420–1428. [CrossRef] [PubMed]
5. Kano, A. Tumor cell secretion of soluble factor(s) for specific immunosuppression. *Sci. Rep.* **2015**, *5*, srep08913. [CrossRef]
6. Weidner, N.; Semple, J.P.; Welch, W.R.; Folkman, J. Tumor angiogenesis and metastasis–Correlation in invasive breast carcinoma. *N. Engl. J. Med.* **1991**, *324*, 1–8. [CrossRef]
7. Scott, J.; Kuhn, P.; Anderson, A.R.A. Unifying metastasis-integrating intravasation, circulation and end-organ colonization. *Nat. Rev. Cancer* **2012**, *12*, 445–446. [CrossRef] [PubMed]
8. Hou, J.M.; Krebs, M.; Ward, T.; Sloane, R.; Priest, L.; Hughes, A.; Clack, G.; Ranson, M.; Blackhall, F.; Dive, C. Circulating tumor cells as a window on metastasis biology in lung cancer. *Am. J. Pathol.* **2011**, *178*, 989–996. [CrossRef] [PubMed]
9. Palstra, R.J.; Grosveld, F. Transcription factor binding at enhancers: Shaping a genomic regulatory landscape in flux. *Front. Genet.* **2012**, *3*, 195. [CrossRef] [PubMed]
10. Takeyama, Y.; Sato, M.; Horio, M.; Hase, T.; Yoshida, K.; Yokoyama, T.; Nakashima, H.; Hashimoto, N.; Sekido, Y.; Gazdar, A.F.; et al. Knockdown of ZEB1, a master epithelial-to-mesenchymal transition (EMT) gene, suppresses anchorage-independent cell growth of lung cancer cells. *Cancer Lett.* **2010**, *296*, 216–224. [CrossRef]
11. Graham, T.R.; Yacoub, R.; Taliaferro-Smith, L.; Osunkoya, A.O.; Odero-Marah, V.A.; Liu, T.; Kimbro, K.S.; Sharma, D.; O'Regan, R.M. Reciprocal regulation of ZEB1 and AR in triple negative breast cancer cells. *Breast Cancer Res. Treat.* **2010**, *123*, 139–147. [CrossRef] [PubMed]
12. Jiang, Y.; Yan, L.; Xia, L.; Lu, X.; Zhu, W.; Ding, D.; Du, M.; Zhang, D.; Wang, H.; Hu, B. Zinc finger E-box–binding homeobox 1 (ZEB1) is required for neural differentiation of human embryonic stem cells. *J. Biol. Chem.* **2018**, *293*, 19317–19329. [CrossRef] [PubMed]
13. Liao, T.T.; Yang, M.H. Revisiting epithelial-mesenchymal transition in cancer metastasis: The connection between epithelial plasticity and stemness. *Mol. Oncol.* **2017**, *11*, 792–804. [CrossRef]
14. Jolly, M.K.; Somarelli, J.A.; Sheth, M.; Biddle, A.; Tripathi, S.C.; Armstrong, A.J.; Hanash, S.M.; Bapat, S.A.; Rangarajan, A.; Levine, H. Hybrid epithelial/mesenchymal phenotypes promote metastasis and therapy resistance across carcinomas. *Pharmacol. Ther.* **2019**, *194*, 161–184. [CrossRef] [PubMed]
15. Yu, M.; Bardia, A.; Wittner, B.S.; Stott, S.L.; Smas, M.E.; Ting, D.T.; Isakoff, S.J.; Ciciliano, J.C.; Wells, M.N.; Shah, A.M.; et al. Circulating breast tumor cells exhibit dynamic changes in epithelial and mesenchymal composition. *Science* **2013**, *339*, 580–584. [CrossRef] [PubMed]
16. DeAngelis, J.T.; Farrington, W.J.; Tollefsbol, T.O. An overview of epigenetic assays. *Mol. Biotechnol.* **2008**, *38*, 179–183. [CrossRef]
17. Kitagawa, Y.; Kyo, S.; Takakura, M.; Kanaya, T.; Koshida, K.; Namiki, M.; Inoue, M. Demethylating reagent 5-azacytidine inhibits telomerase activity in human prostate cancer cells through transcriptional repression of hTERT. *Clin. Cancer Res.* **2000**, *6*, 2868–2875.
18. Ribeiro, A.S.; Paredes, J. P-Cadherin Linking Breast Cancer Stem Cells and Invasion: A Promising Marker to Identify an "Intermediate/Metastable" EMT State. *Front. Oncol.* **2015**, *4*, 371. [CrossRef] [PubMed]

19. Bierie, B.; Pierce, S.E.; Kroeger, C.; Stover, D.G.; Pattabiraman, D.R.; Thiru, P.; Liu Donaher, J.; Reinhardt, F.; Chaffer, C.L.; Keckesova, Z.; et al. Integrin-β4 identifies cancer stem cell-enriched populations of partially mesenchymal carcinoma cells. *Proc. Natl. Acad. Sci. USA* **2017**, *114*, E2337–E2346. [CrossRef] [PubMed]
20. Czibere, A.; Bruns, I.; Kröger, N.; Platzbecker, U.; Lind, J.; Zohren, F.; Fenk, R.; Germing, U.; Schröder, T.; Gräf, T.; et al. 5-Azacytidine for the treatment of patients with acute myeloid leukemia or myelodysplastic syndrome who relapse after allo-SCT: A retrospective analysis. *Bone Marrow Transplant.* **2010**, *45*, 872–876. [CrossRef] [PubMed]
21. Cui, J.; Wang, L.; Ren, X.; Zhang, Y.; Zhang, H. LRPPRC: A multifunctional protein involved in energy metabolism and human disease. *Front. Physiol.* **2019**, *10*, 1–10. [CrossRef] [PubMed]
22. Agarwal, R.; Mori, Y.; Cheng, Y.; Jin, Z.; Olaru, A.V.; Hamilton, J.P.; David, S.; Selaru, F.M.; Yang, J.; Abraham, J.M.; et al. Silencing of claudin-11 is associated with increased invasiveness of gastric cancer cells. *PLoS ONE* **2009**, *4*, e8002. [CrossRef] [PubMed]
23. Kohn, E.C.; Liotta, L.A. Molecular insights into cancer invasion: Strategies for prevention and intervention. *Cancer Res.* **1995**, *55*, 1856–1862. [PubMed]
24. Liu, S.; Liu, J.; Yu, X.; Shen, T.; Fu, Q. Identification of a Two-Gene (PML-EPB41) Signature With Independent Prognostic Value in Osteosarcoma. *Front. Oncol.* **2020**, *9*, 1–11. [CrossRef]
25. Yuan, W.; Ji, J.; Shu, Y.; Chen, J.; Liu, S.; Wu, L.; Zhou, Z.; Liu, Z.; Tang, Q.; Zhang, X.; et al. Downregulation of DAPK1 promotes the stemness of cancer stem cells and EMT process by activating ZEB1 in colorectal cancer. *J. Mol. Med.* **2019**, *97*, 89–102. [CrossRef] [PubMed]
26. Vazquez, A.; Kulkarni, D.; Grochola, L.F.; Bond, G.L.; Barnard, N.; Toppmeyer, D.; Levine, A.J.; Hirshfield, K.M. A genetic variant in a PP2A regulatory subunit encoded by the PPP2R2B gene associates with altered breast cancer risk and recurrence. *Int. J. Cancer* **2011**, *128*, 2335–2343. [CrossRef]
27. Peng, C.; Zhang, Z.; Wu, J.; Lv, Z.; Tang, J.; Xie, H.; Zhou, L.; Zheng, S. A critical role for ZDHHC2 in metastasis and recurrence in human hepatocellular carcinoma. *BioMed Res. Int.* **2014**, *2014*, 832712. [CrossRef]
28. Chen, J.; Zhuo, J.Y.; Yang, F.; Liu, Z.K.; Zhou, L.; Xie, H.Y.; Xu, X.; Zheng, S. Sen 17-Beta-Hydroxysteroid Dehydrogenase 13 Inhibits the Progression and Recurrence of Hepatocellular Carcinoma. *Hepatobiliary Pancreat. Dis. Int.* **2018**, *17*, 220–226. [CrossRef] [PubMed]
29. Yamamoto, F.; Yamamoto, M. Identification of genes that exhibit changes in expression on the 8p chromosomal arm by the Systematic Multiplex RT-PCR (SM RT-PCR) and DNA microarray hybridization methods. *Gene Expr.* **2008**, *14*, 217–227. [CrossRef] [PubMed]
30. Legler, K.; Rosprim, R.; Karius, T.; Eylmann, K.; Rossberg, M.; Wirtz, R.M.; Müller, V.; Witzel, I.; Schmalfeldt, B.; Milde-Langosch, K.; et al. Reduced mannosidase MAN1A1 expression leads to aberrant N-glycosylation and impaired survival in breast cancer. *Br. J. Cancer* **2018**, *118*, 847–856. [CrossRef] [PubMed]
31. Tam, W.L.; Weinberg, R.A. The epigenetics of epithelial-mesenchymal plasticity in cancer. *Nat. Med.* **2013**, *19*, 1438–1449. [CrossRef] [PubMed]
32. Lu, W.; Kang, Y. Epithelial-Mesenchymal Plasticity in Cancer Progression and Metastasis. *Dev. Cell* **2019**, *49*, 361–374. [CrossRef] [PubMed]
33. Point, S.S. *Infinium HD Methylation Assay Manual Workflow Checklist Convert DNA Create the BCD Plate Infinium HD Methylation Assay Manual Workflow Checklist Incubate DNA Fragment DNA*; Illumina: San Diego, CA, USA, 2019; pp. 1–5.
34. Hansen, K.D.; Aryee, M.; Irizarry, R.A.; Jaffe, A.E.; Maksimovic, J.; Houseman, E.A.; Fortin, J.-P.; Triche, T.; Andrews, S.V.; Hickey, P.F. Available online: https://bioconductor.org/packages/release/bioc/html/minfi.html (accessed on 10 September 2021).
35. Tian, Y.; Morris, T.J.; Webster, A.P.; Yang, Z.; Beck, S.; Feber, A.; Teschendorff, A.E. The Chip Analysis Methylation Pipeline. Available online: https://www.bioconductor.org/packages/devel/bioc/vignettes/ChAMP/inst/doc/ChAMP.html (accessed on 10 September 2021).
36. Teschendorff, A.E.; Marabita, F.; Lechner, M.; Bartlett, T.; Tegner, J.; Gomez-Cabrero, D.; Beck, S. A beta-mixture quantile normalization method for correcting probe design bias in Illumina Infinium 450 k DNA methylation data. *Bioinformatics* **2013**, *29*, 189–196. [CrossRef] [PubMed]

MDPI
St. Alban-Anlage 66
4052 Basel
Switzerland
Tel. +41 61 683 77 34
Fax +41 61 302 89 18
www.mdpi.com

International Journal of Molecular Sciences Editorial Office
E-mail: ijms@mdpi.com
www.mdpi.com/journal/ijms

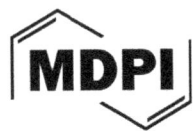

www.ingramcontent.com/pod-product-compliance
Lightning Source LLC
LaVergne TN
LVHW070733100526
838202LV00013B/1222